Environmentally Induced
Induced
DISORDERS
SOURCEBOOK

Health Reference Series

Volume Twenty-eight

Environmentally Induced
DISORDERS
SOURCEBOOK

*Basic Information about Diseases
and Syndromes Linked to
Exposure to Pollutants and Other
Substances in Outdoor and Indoor
Environments Such as Lead,
Asbestos, Formaldehyde, Mercury,
Emissions, Noise, and More*

Edited by
Allan R. Cook

Omnigraphics, Inc.

Penobscot Building / Detroit, MI 48226

BIBLIOGRAPHIC NOTE

This volume contains individual publications issued by the National Institutes of Health (NIH), its sister agencies, and sub-agencies. Numbered or dated publications are: NIH 87-861, 91-2241, 93-1209, NIH Technology Assessment Workshop April 1994, ON-0878, Office of Noise Abatement Control, K93008,(EPA) K94001, (EPA), 19945232, (EPA), ANR445, (EPA Indoor Air Facts No.3), ANR445W, (EPA Indoor Air Facts No.4), TS-793, (EPA). It also contains unnumbered and undated documents from EPA, NCI Cancerfax, Centers for Disease Control and Prevention, and the Consumer Product Safety Commission. Also used are selected non-copyrighted articles from the *FDA Consumer, Environmental Health Perspectives, Environmental Health Perspectives Supplements,* and RACHEL (Remote Access Chemical Hazards Electronic Library) and copyrighted articles from *American Academy of Environmental Medicine,* the American Academy of Otolaryngology, the American Lung Association, *Healthline,* the *Journal of Environmental Health* and *Research Horizons.* All copyrighted articles are reprinted with permission.

Edited by Allan R. Cook

Peter D. Dresser, Managing Editor, Health Reference Series
Karen Bellenir, Series Editor, Health Reference Series

Omnigraphics, Inc.

Matthew P. Barbour, Production Manager
Laurie Lanzen Harris, Vice President, Editorial
Peter E. Ruffner, Vice President, Administration
James A. Sellgren, Vice President, Operations and Finance
Jane J. Steele, Marketing Consultant

Frederick G. Ruffner, Jr., Publisher

Copyright © 1997, Omnigraphics, Inc.

∞
This book is printed on acid-free paper meeting the ANSI Z39.48 Standard. The infinity symbol that appears above indicates that the paper in this book meets that standard.

Printed in the United States of America

Table of Contents

Part III: Water Pollution

Part IV: Indoor Pollution

Part V: Occupational Risks

Part VI: Chemicals and Poisons

Part VII: Radiation and Noise Pollution

Part VIII: Environmental Pollutants and Food

Part IX: Environmental Risks to Children

Part X: Global Concerns

Preface

About This Book

As humanity has learned to harness its environment to produce more abundant foods and materials, it has also brought upon itself unforeseen threats to human life and health. In many cases, these harmful conditions can be termed pollution, and that is a key term for this volume. These health hazards can also be thought of as selective sensitivities. In some cases, the operation of these sensitivities is so poorly understood that they are often rejected by the mainstream medical profession. This book examines many of the probable sources of environmentally induced disorders and introduces some of the most common controversies that mark the newly emerging fields of environmental medicine and clinical ecology.

This book contains basic information for the layperson on a wide range of common complaints often associated with environmental triggers and some methods of treating, avoiding, and coping with environmentally induced illnesses. Patients, friends, family members, and the interested general public will find this volume a good place to begin to understand the complex and delicate web of dependency that is environmental health.

How to Use This Book

This book is divided into parts and chapters. Parts focus on broad areas of interest and chapters on specific topics within those areas.

Part I: *Medicine in the Environmental Balance* begins the discussion of the nature of Environmental Medicine by surveying the boundaries, uncertain as they are, of the field and presenting the debate between proponents and opponents.

Part II: *Outdoor Air Pollution* considers the air we breath and the ways science and government assess its degradation along with our ability to cope with pollutants.

Part III: *Water Pollution* looks at the water we drink, bathe with, and play in and highlights some particularly worrying concerns like lead, mercury, and biological contaminants as well as introducing the debate over fluoridation of our drinking water.

Part IV: *Indoor Air Pollution* examines the quality of air in homes and offices.

Part V: *Occupational Risks* focuses on contaminants and triggers of environmental illness found in the workplace.

Part VI: *Chemicals and Poisons* highlights some specific compounds that have been identified as potentially harmful. This section also includes information on multiple chemical sensitivity.

Part VII: *Radiation and Noise Pollution* considers two important and common elements of environmental health that often go overlooked: the effects of electromagnetic radiation and of environmental noise levels.

Part VIII: *Environmental Pollutants and Food* presents some concerns about keeping the food supply safe and nutritious.

Part IX: *Environmental Risks to Children* examines issues involving children and environmental pollutants.

Part X: *Global Concerns* considers how changes in the environment caused by such factors as global warming and ozone depletion could have effects on our health.

Index: gives page references and cross-references for key words and phrases used in the various articles.

Acknowledgements

The editor gratefully acknowledges the assistance of the many people who helped produce this volume and the private organizations that agreed to grant permission to reprint their articles: American Academy of Otolaryngology—Head and Neck Surgery, Inc., Healthline Publishing, American Academy of Environmental Medicine, the American Lung Association, the *Journal of Environmental Health*, and *Research Horizons*. Special thanks to Margaret Mary Missar for her patient search for the documents that make up this volume, Karen Bellenir for her technical assistance and advice, Bruce the Scanman and special assistant Mike for their digitally correct representations and Valerie Cook for her sharp-eyed text verification.

Note from the Editor

This book is part of Omnigraphics' *Health Reference Series*. The series provides basic information about a broad range of medical concerns. It is not intended to serve as a tool for diagnosing illness, in prescribing treatments, or as a substitute for the physician/patient relationship. All persons concerned about medical symptoms or the possibility of disease are encouraged to seek professional care from an appropriate health care provider.

Part One

Medicine in the Environmental Balance

Chapter 1

Issues and Challenges in Environmental Health

"Man is embedded in nature. The biologic science of recent years has been making this a more urgent fact of life. The new, hard problem will be to cope with the dawning, intensifying realization of just how interlocked we are."

Lewis Thomas, M.D. "The Lives of a Cell"

Human beings have always had a close, interdependent relationship with the soil, water, atmosphere, and food chains that make up their environment. Imbalances in rainfall that have affected crops, lightning-sparked forest fires, and volcanic eruptions have always exerted powerful influences on the lives of humans and the other creatures that inhabit the earth. So have diseases caused by harmful bacteria and viruses that also make up the human environment.

But in recent decades, as sophisticated technology has given people increasing awareness of the complex webs of dependency with the environment, scientists and policy makers have come to see "environmental health" in broader perspective. The environment in which we live includes not only air, water, and soil, but just about every other external factor that can affect our health and quality of life. Thus today the word "environment" includes a person's place and type of occupation; personal habits; diet; use of alcohol, tobacco, and drugs; exposure to toxic wastes; exposure to natural and medical chemicals and radiation; climate; and geologic phenomena such as volcanoes and earthquakes.

NIH Publication No. 87-861.

3

Implicit in the term "environmental health" is the growing awareness that the very technology that has given us some ability to affect our environment with climate-adjusted homes, disease-resistant agricultural crops, and more effective medicines may also pose potential hazards for our health.

Even as better sanitation and the development of life-saving antibiotics and vaccines have contributed to increased longevity by decreasing disability from communicable diseases, new and different potential threats to human health have been identified: toxic wastes, cigarette smoke, acid rain, smog, and drugs such as thalidomide that can cause birth defects. These are examples of some of the products of a highly developed technology which may obviously harm, as well as enhance, our well being.

For two decades the National Institute of Environmental Health Sciences (NIEHS)—the lead agency supporting basic and applied research for characterizing environmentally provoked illnesses—has recognized the need for effective planning of long-term research and prevention strategies in environmental health. In the spring of 1968, a task force of leaders in environmental health was established to advise the Institute on future directions for research. The work of the first Task Force led to the publication of a major report, "Man's Health and the Environment: Some Research Needs," in 1970. The Task Force recommended research on a broad array of environmental areas (including air pollution, food, water, consumer products) and of disease mechanisms.

In 1975, mindful of rapidly expanding knowledge and the growing impact of environmental factors on health, a congressional committee requested an updated version of the Institute's 1970 Task Force report on research planning. Thus a second Task Force of leaders in the field of environmental health was appointed by the Institute to study the issues and to produce a second Task Force report on research strategies in the environmental health sciences. This second report— "Human Health and the Environment: Some Research Needs"— stressed the central focus of toxicology in all environmental health issues and addressed the areas of occupational health and safety, selected health problems of special environments from hospitals to homes, waste disposal, disease mechanisms, and, among other subjects, methods for estimating disease risk in humans.

In 1983, Congress again called for a Task Force study on research planning in environmental health sciences, but this time the charge was more exact: to identify specific research opportunities in areas

4

where increased knowledge would improve the ability of scientists to deal with environmental issues most likely to affect human health through the end of the century. Thus the third Task Force was not to be as broadly based as the first two in examining potential environmental health problems; rather, the intended focus was on areas of particular research promise, building on the work of the two previous Task Forces and on the expanding base of new knowledge.

In following its congressional mandate, the Third Task Force focused its energies on five topical areas:

1. biological mechanisms through which physical and chemical agents give rise to disease,

2. methods for assessing the health significance of exposure to toxic agents,

3. research strategies for preventing environmentally provoked disease,

4. organization and structure of environmental health research in the United States, and

5. information exchange in the environmental health sciences.

The main thrust of the Task Force report was to recommend research efforts that are likely to provide the greatest benefit to human health through prevention of environmentally induced diseases. In humans, the range of diseases that can be partially or completely initiated or caused by environmental factors is broad. The range includes, among other diseases:

- Cardiovascular diseases;
- Cancers;
- Birth defects, malformations, and reproductive disorders;
- Respiratory illnesses;
- Deficiencies in the immune system, the built-in defense against substances or organisms the body perceives as foreign;
- Allergies and hypersensitivity disorders;
- Nervous system abnormalities; and
- Diseases of other organs, especially all the excretory organs including the kidney, liver, and intestine.

While it is not practical to determine exactly how much disability, medical expense, salary loss, and other costs environmentally associated diseases cause, the health impact is enormous. For example, experimental studies have shown that kidney failure can be produced in laboratory animals following exposure to some common chemicals, such as toxic metals, chlorinated hydrocarbons, and certain drugs. Although about 30 to 40 percent of renal disease in humans is thought to be linked to high blood pressure or diabetes mellitus, the causes of the other 60 to 70 percent are poorly known and may involve environmental influences. Some cases of high blood pressure may likewise have an environmental component. For example, elevated blood lead levels have been shown to correlate with hypertension.

Through research, specific environmental factors may be identified which contribute to disorders such as end-stage renal disease. A primary reason for supporting environmental health research is to learn how to prevent or ameliorate such disease. This, in turn, could lead to substantial savings. For example, the costs of the end-stage renal disease program—a major Social Security Administration program enabling patients with kidney failure to receive blood-cleansing treatments with dialysis machines that act as artificial kidneys—are rising at a rapid rate. In 1974 the cost to taxpayers for the end-stage renal disease program was nearly $300 million, while in 1984 the cost was estimated to be more than $2 billion—approximately a four-fold increase in terms of 1974 dollars.

Because every potentially harmful environmental substance has not been and cannot be studied extensively, the sources of harmful exposure that have been identified may represent only a fraction of those with the potential to harm human health. It is important for environmental scientists to make informed judgments as to which substances are most likely to pose the greatest hazard to human health, and then to concentrate their research efforts on those that have the highest priority because of potential adverse health impacts.

It has been estimated that a high proportion of cancer is linked to factors in the environment, defined broadly to include all nonhereditary influences such as air, diet, water, use of tobacco, other personal habits and lifestyle, occupation, etc. But while cancer is the most feared of all diseases, it represents only a fraction of the large variety of serious and costly environmentally linked diseases that plague mankind. Allergic reactions and hypersensitivity diseases, for instance, are among the most common and costly of U.S. health problems, afflicting at least 35 million Americans at an annual medical cost of $1 billion. Indirect costs, such as wages lost because of illness, are estimated at $800 million per year for asthma alone, with more than 35 million sick days lost each year. A partial list of occupationally related substances causing hypersensitivity reactions includes: platinum salts, cotton dust, copper-ammonia solutions, toluene diisocyanate, organic gold compounds, formaldehyde, beryllium, nickel sulfate, and turpentine.

Some reproductive problems are increasing in incidence and are of growing concern to scientists, physicians, and the public; a special worry is the fact that the interwoven and complex processes involved in human reproduction can be adversely affected by a toxic agent at virtually any point in the lifetime of a prospective parent or at any point during gestation. Such an interruption can result in, for instance, an inability to conceive, as well as the loss or malformation of a fetus.

Because the environmental health sciences encompass such a broad research area, environmental scientists face special challenges when attempting to evaluate a potential hazard to human health. The complexities arise in part from new technological processes and products, hence the task facing these scientists is more difficult today than a decade ago. Dealing with a growing array of new chemicals, additives, and industrial compounds, environmental scientists may try to predict with as much certainty as possible which substances in the environment—synthetic as well as natural—pose the greatest risks to human health. Unless they are in public policy positions, research scientists rarely make regulatory decisions about environmental substances; but they must attempt to determine what degree of hazard is posed by a given activity or exposure situation in order that society may judge whether the risk is acceptable or unacceptable.

There are many difficult challenges in this task. Consider the problem in assessing a sample of air. A sample taken from one city block may be quite different from one taken from the next block. Furthermore, the factors relating to air quality are constantly changing and the air is breathed by people who differ in susceptibility because of differences in age, sex, personal lifestyle, genetic makeup, and health status.

The task of assessing health risk from a particular environmental source or pathway (food, air, water, etc.) is also made difficult by the complexity of human exposures. Human beings are often exposed continually to many different potentially harmful substances, not just one. Substances may interact with one another synergistically (for example asbestos and cigarette smoke), thus increasing the combined toxic effects disproportionately.

Assessing environmental risks is made difficult also because it is often not possible to predict whether a given substance will cause a particular effect in a single individual or group of people who are known to have been exposed. Nevertheless, postponement of preventive action until a cause-effect relation can be demonstrated unequivocally may not be justified, because it may take decades to do so. In the case of most cancers, for example, a period of 20 to 40 years usually elapses following exposure to a cancer-causing substance before the resulting cancer becomes detectable. Hence the postponement of preventive steps to limit exposure to a suspected carcinogen or to a possible mutagen or teratogen may significantly increase the incidence of adverse health outcomes which could otherwise have been avoided in an entire generation.

Today, environmental scientists have increasingly useful laboratory techniques for evaluating potentially harmful substances. Although laboratory experiments usually do not provide a full or certain answer of how a substance will behave in people, most substances that have been shown to cause harm to human health are also proved harmful when studied in experimental animals. Consequently it is possible to take the results of carefully designed studies in experimental animals (usually specially bred rat and mouse species) and extrapolate the results to forecast whether a chemical may be harmful to human beings. All mammals share certain similarities, as well as differences, in anatomical structure and metabolism, which form the basis for the premise that using the results of a study in laboratory animals will predict a similar response in humans. There is general agreement among environmental scientists that laboratory-animal studies, despite some limitations, offer a necessary and useful means of assessing whether a given chemical may be hazardous to human health.

Not all chemicals cause adverse health effects in animals when administered in the doses and manner used by environmental scientists. In fact, most of the studies conducted by the National Toxicology Program yield negative results although this program focuses its studies on compounds that have the greatest theoretical potential for harm to humans because of their volume of use, exposure opportunities for people, or chemical structure or properties.

Scientists recognize the large degree to which individuals may vary in susceptibility to different toxic substances. The variations depend in part on differences in the way substances are metabolized in the body. For example, a drug may be more toxic to an older person than to a younger person, because older people generally do not "clear" or eliminate drugs as rapidly from the liver or kidneys. Also, people vary in the capacity of their immune systems to react to and protect against toxic substances.

An inherited increase in susceptibility may also affect whether an individual will develop a specific disease. Individuals with an inherited deficiency in the particular protein called alpha$_1$-antitrypsin are more likely to develop emphysema, a terminal lung disease. They also are more likely to develop the disease early—in their 30s and 40s. If people who are deficient in this protein also smoke cigarettes, the onset of emphysema may come even sooner, further shortening their life span.

In fact, choices in personal lifestyle—exemplified by the asbestos worker who chooses to smoke—are important in determining health risks from the environment. Communities influence their environmental quality by the ways in which they adopt and control technologies, permit the transport and storage of hazardous substances through and in the community, and dispose of hazardous waste. Individuals influence their health (and, in the case of pregnant women, the health of their unborn children) by specific choices about what they eat and drink, whether they smoke, how they live and work, etc. Far from being merely a passive recipient of environmental influences, the individual is often an active participant in making personal choices that may promote or jeopardize health.

Scientists now know more about which groups of people are at special risk for environmentally related health problems and how they can reduce their risks. Avoiding excessive exposure to sunlight, for example, is a personal choice that informed high-risk individuals can make to prevent disease. While prolonged, repetitive exposure to strong sunlight increases the risk of getting skin cancer, certain individuals are more susceptible than others. Fair-skinned individuals, especially those with red hair, are more likely to develop skin cancer. People with the rare illness *xeroderma pigmentosum*, a genetic condition involving impaired ability to repair sunlight-induced damage, are more likely to develop cancer when exposed to sunlight than the general population. If people with extremely fair skin or *xeroderma pigmentosum* avoid sunlight entirely, they usually avoid skin cancer.

Although the issues in environmental health sciences are growing more complex, there is every reason to think the challenges can be met and the problems ultimately solved. The primary cause for optimism comes from new knowledge and new technology, advances sometimes collectively referred to as "the new biology" and "the biological revolution."

The new biology is rapidly advancing our understanding of the basic nature of life. As the cell reveals more of its mysteries, a new blueprint of possibilities for ensuring human health and well-being emerges. Prominently displayed on that blueprint are new research directions made possible by advances in the field of basic genetics, including technology that allows scientists to define the most fundamental genetic component of the cell—the coiled ribbon of DNA that contains instructions for all the cell's vital functions.

Genes are composed of tight packets of DNA, located on the chromosomes, that instruct each cell how to carry out its functions, including protein synthesis. A better understanding of genes and how they work will suggest better ways in which environmental health scientists can identify environmental hazards and perhaps predict which people are most susceptible to them. This is the kind of information public health program planners need to begin to develop effective and measurable means for preventing, mitigating, or curing environmentally related illnesses.

A new understanding of genes has allowed scientists to produce highly specific proteins, called monoclonal antibodies, that act as "guided missiles" for certain target substances. The primary use of these antibodies will be to detect and quantify changes that result from environmental hazards and injury; and they may someday aid in the diagnosis and treatment of many illnesses.

The new biology has also yielded important knowledge about potentially cancer-causing oncogenes—tiny pieces of DNA that may be part of the normal genetic makeup of human cells. The riddle of why normal cells contain material that—when altered by environmental agents ranging from cigarette smoke to viruses—may initiate the cancerous process is still unsolved. But, as scientists move closer to solving that fundamental riddle, they are also closing in on the mysteries of the hundreds of diseases we know as cancer.

While some fear the biological revolution because it allows man increased abilities to affect basic natural processes in bacteria, viruses, plants, and certain animal species, new discoveries about the cell lie at the very heart of combatting diseases and protecting the health of all mankind. The understanding, prevention, and treatment of insidious inherited diseases by genetic means is moving from the stage of scientific dream to that of potentially practical problem solving. Within the next several decades, scientists may discover new preventive tools such as vaccines and may learn how to repair or replace abnormal genetic material in the cells of those who suffer from genetic illnesses. For example, researchers recently isolated a DNA clone (copy of a gene) containing the coding sequence for a specific unit of the enzyme beta-hexosaminidase. Mutations in this gene—and resultant defects in the enzyme unit—lead to Tay-Sachs disease, a rare, devastating genetic illness that affects primarily Jewish people of Eastern European extraction and that causes a build-up of fatty deposits in the brain, leading to early death. If scientists can learn more about mutations in this gene, they may eventually learn how to correct them and prevent Tay-Sachs disease.

The new biology has also yielded knowledge about important biochemical markers: signs in the body that serve as indicators of susceptibility to disease or as early signals of disease. By carefully analyzing body fluids, tissues, and cells to measure altered markers, it is now possible to detect the presence of potentially harmful chemicals or toxicological responses (such as mutations or chromosomal aberrations). Detecting and identifying these biochemical markers early may allow physicians to prevent or lessen the consequences of environmentally induced diseases.

For example, it was recently found that people with an inherited tendency to develop depression—a serious mental illness that afflicts 8 to 12 million Americans—tend to have in their skin cells increased numbers of receptors sensitive to the chemical acetylcholine which functions to transmit nerve impulses. In simple terms, people prone to depression have "hyperreactive skin cells" as detected in laboratory tests. This feature may eventually allow doctors to recognize people who are at risk for depression while they are young, and thus provide them with counseling and medical help early enough so they can avoid the impacts of environmental factors such as alcohol, drugs, and stressful settings which may compound the risks of depression and suicide (an estimated 75,000 Americans suffering from depression commit suicide every year). In this way, a basic scientific discovery may ultimately save many lives.

While the issues inherent in meeting the challenges of environmental health are complex, at no time in history has there been such promise that scientific research can be translated into practical benefits for all. Indeed, barriers to scientific progress seem to have been removed as more and more of life's biological mysteries are yielding their

11

riddles. In this world of promise, however, it must be remembered that environmental health sciences research is only as good as those who are trained to probe its mysteries. The complexity of environmental health problems requires well trained scientists and adequate modern research facilities and instrumentation.

A national commitment to environmental health sciences research is a serious and necessary commitment to preventing environmentally induced disease and improving the quality of life. The Report of the Third Task Force for Research Planning in Environmental Health Science represents an attempt to set research priorities enabling us to make that commitment as a nation.

The following brief summaries of the chapters in the report highlight some of the approaches recommended. Recommendations for research directions are made for the following broad categories:

- Molecular and Cellular Mechanisms of Environmental Injury
- Reproductive and Developmental Effects of Chemical Exposure
- Role of Immunological and Host Defense Mechanisms Genetics
- Dose and Species Extrapolation of Environmental Risks
- Differences Among Individuals in Responses to Environmental Stresses
- Pharmacokinetic Factors in Chemical Exposure
- Biochemical and Cellular Markers of Chemical Exposure and Preclinical Indicators of Disease
- Research Strategies for Prevention of Environmentally Provoked Disease
- Structure of Environmental Health Research in the United States
- Information Exchange in the Environmental Health Sciences

The recommendations in these sections identify approaches that can be used to develop additional preventive measures and strategies. For a fuller discussion of the issues and recommendations, the Task Force report should be consulted.

Summaries and Recommendations

I. Molecular and Cellular Mechanisms of Environmental Injury

The cell is the basic unit of life in all living organisms, and it is at the cell surface and within at the cell itself that environmental agents exert most of their toxic effects. For human beings to remain healthy, their cells, which regulate bodily functions and carry on all the often complex activities necessary to life, must be constantly supplied with essential nutrients and cleansed of wastes. In addition to many other mechanisms of control, cells are governed by DNA (deoxyribonucleic acid), the essential genetic "code" of instructions within each cell. For cells to function normally, their genetic code must remain intact.

Cells of different types vary in what and how they metabolize or biotransform chemicals and in their ability to resist and defend themselves against harmful agents. This cellular variability helps explain why a toxic chemical may have different effects on organisms of different species or even on different individuals within the same species. For example, the harmful substances in cigarette smoke may affect some smokers more than others; some people who are heavy smokers contract lung cancer, while others who are heavy smokers do not.

Important new knowledge in cellular and molecular biology is yielding promising new concepts and methods for studying the complexities of the cell's regulatory mechanisms, inherent weaknesses, and reactions to injury. It is now possible by using specific proteins called monoclonal antibodies to visualize more adequately structural details within cells. This microscopic visualization can help scientists determine the nature of cellular injuries caused by environmental agents. The current quickened pace of discovery provides new hope of solving the mysteries of how the cell does its work and how that work can be disrupted by environmental influences, leading to disease. This, in turn, may provide new strategies for disease prevention.

Among the recommendations of the Subtask Force on Molecular and Cellular Mechanisms of Environmental Injury were the following:

- The plasma membrane of the cell (a more or less fluid layer containing the proteins that mediate interactions between the internal and external environments of a cell) is a complex structure vital to the integrity of the cell. Thus studies should be directed to ways in which toxic chemicals affect the plasma membrane and alter its constituents.

- Studies need to be intensified on the internal structure of the cell, called the cytoskeleton. Specifically, exploration is needed on the mechanism by which environmental toxins alter the cytoskeleton, whether the cytoskeleton is a primary target of these toxins or is altered as a result of changes in cell metabolism, as well as on the functional significance of alterations in the cytoskeleton with respect to cell maintenance and survival. Additionally, more intensive studies are needed on how toxicants affect cellular organelles, such as mitochondria and lysosomes, and how organelles act to metabolize or secrete toxicants.

- More in-depth study needs to be made of the chronic development of fibrous tissue in response to environmental agents, such as mineral dust, in order to learn why healing or repair by fibrosis in tissues injured by some environmental toxins becomes chronic and sometimes fatal. This is in contrast to repair by fibrosis in surgical wounds, which is completed within several months, even though the same mechanisms presumably operate to stimulate repair for both types of injury.

- There should be investigation in much greater depth into the causes of cell death due to environmental insults and the complex adaptive changes that take place in cells that do not die of toxic insult.

- Advances in cellular and molecular biology should be combined with knowledge of recombinant DNA and sophisticated chemistry methods in studying the mechanisms of environmentally provoked diseases. It will take many well-educated people working in teams to mount the approaches and accomplish the tasks required.

- Scientists with doctoral degrees in molecular and cellular biology should be given opportunities for additional training in laboratories dedicated to the study of environmental disease.

- Grants should be made available to people interested in bridging disciplines as a means of studying illnesses linked to environmental factors, and for scientists who decide in mid-career to change direction in order to pursue research in environmental health.

II. Reproductive and Developmental Effects of Chemical Exposure

Human reproduction depends on the successful fertilization of an intact ovum (egg) and its subsequent transplantation, growth, and

14

development into a normal, healthy infant. It also depends on the transmission of accurate genetic information from one generation to the next. This process involves a complex series of inter-related functions, any one of which may be damaged by environmental agents. Problems in fertility and abnormalities in fetal growth and development are common. Today, the human population is exposed to a host of potentially toxic environmental chemicals, with some 500 to 1,000 new compounds being added every year. The effects that these chemical compounds may have on human reproduction and the development of healthy babies is a matter of increasing concern to scientists, physicians, and the public.

The male and female sex organs including the testes and ovaries serve an important dual function: they secrete the sex hormones which determine characteristics of masculinity and femininity, and they also produce the sperm and eggs which, when united, culminate in human reproduction. A healthy human baby is the result of a series of complex events requiring the right timing, hormonal regulation, successful fertilization, and a hospitable environment for the growing embryo and fetus and for its birth.

Any direct or indirect interruption or disturbance of the normal biological processes of the sex organs by a harmful chemical can result in reproductive dysfunction. If a toxic substance interferes with processes in the brain or in the pituitary gland that affect sex organ functioning, then the production of sperm, for instance, can decline. If the substance is highly toxic, sterility may result.

In addition to harmful effects on the sex organs, exposure of the developing fetus to any of more than 20 known toxic agents (ranging from the German measles virus to excessive alcohol consumption by the mother, or to such drugs as thalidomide and diethylstilbestrol [DES]) can result in an infant with physical or mental abnormalities. These problems may show up immediately—as the distinctive facial characteristics of babies with the fetal alcohol syndrome—or later as vaginal abnormalities in pubescent daughters whose mothers were prescribed DES to prevent miscarriage.

In light of the complex processes that make up human reproduction, the Subtask Force on Reproductive and Developmental Effects of Chemical Exposure recommended that researchers should:

- Pursue studies designed to find out more about basic mechanisms that regulate the central nervous system's role in normal reproduction and about the effects of chemicals on that role, because it is now recognized that disorders of brain function can profoundly affect reproductive activity.

- Undertake research to find out more about mechanisms by which sperm are formed and how their formation is affected by compounds that are toxic to the testes.

- Explore effects of toxic agents on hormonal mechanisms that control preparation of the endometrium (lining of the uterus) for implantation of the fertilized egg.

- Investigate characteristics of the menstrual cycle as a way of evaluating the function of ovaries in women who have been exposed to toxic agents.

- Evaluate in controlled studies the failure of contraceptives because it is recognized that some environmental exposures can increase fertility.

- Exploit recent advances in cellular and molecular biology to learn more about what happens during normal reproduction and development, so as to gain a better understanding of what is abnormal.

- Make further use of tests done both in intact animals and in the test tube, as well as of information about basic mechanisms of reproductive processes and toxicity, to identify harmful substances that may result in infertility, birth defects, or problems in subsequent development.

- Learn more about adaptive and repair processes that influence reproduction and development.

- Identify biological markers in the body that can help to detect evidence of reproductive problems.

- Develop new testing procedures to assess possible hazards that may be posed by exposure to various chemicals.

- Begin large-scale studies to define normal reproductive variations within the human population.

III. Role of Immunological and Host Defense Mechanisms

The term "immunity" refers to the ability of a living organism to ward off or protect itself against foreign substances, ranging from toxic chemicals to disease-causing bacteria or viruses. The immune system is a complex internal guardian that includes special types of cells designed to combat foreign substances. In the healthy immune system, a foreign substance, called an antigen, provokes the formation of protein substances called antibodies, which flow into the bloodstream and attack the antigen by binding and neutralizing it or by preparing it to be engulfed and broken down by specialized cells called macrophages. When this normal antigen-antibody response is weakened, the body becomes more susceptible to disease. When the immune system totally fails, as it does in the acquired immune deficiency syndrome (AIDS), death is almost always inevitable.

In the past 10 years, scientists have accumulated much evidence that exposure to toxic substances can modify the immune system in experimental animals. Similar observations have been made in human beings exposed accidentally or inadvertently to the same substances.

Apart from complete failure of the immune system, the system can turn upon and attack the body in which it resides—a phenomenon called autoimmune disease. The immune system can also be disturbed, so that it responds to antigens imperfectly. This kind of disturbed immune function is seen in the estimated 35 million Americans who have become allergic due to reactions to one or a number of foreign substances. People working in various industries are especially susceptible to this kind of hypersensitivity disease. Industrial workers with allergic reactions include: bakers reacting to flour, garment workers reacting to formaldehyde, textile workers sensitive to cotton dust, and metal-refining workers sensitive to platinum salts.

To bolster research on the role of the immune system in both healthy and disease states, the Subtask Force on the Role of Immunological and Host Defense Mechanisms recommended that scientists:

- Expand the base of knowledge on how chemicals interact with the immune system, to make possible sounder decisions on safe chemical usage and human hazard prevention.

- Determine to what extent immune function that has been affected in some way by exposure to chemicals alters the body's ability to express an immune response to viruses, bacteria, parasites, tumors, and the chemicals themselves.

- Study the relationship of chemically induced impairment of immune function to the development of autoimmune disease.

- Conduct research to attempt to provide better means of predicting, diagnosing, and treating hypersensitivity diseases resulting from allergic reactions to environmental substances.

- Exploit new immunologic techniques, particularly monoclonal antibody methodology (used to detect foreign substances in body fluids and tissues), for detecting and quantifying environmental contaminants in biological and environmental matrices.

- Expand efforts to define cellular and organ targets of immunotoxic chemicals in order to determine the immune cells sensitive to injury by chemicals. Because the immune system is regulated through multiple cellular and hormonal interactions, derangements in any component of the system can indirectly perturb other elements of the system.

- Incorporate more information about immunotoxicology in graduate and postgraduate medical education. Fellowships should be made available to train scientists in the subdisciplines of immunotoxicology.

IV. Genetics

For an organism to function normally, its genetic program must remain intact. This program is contained in genes, tiny biological units of heredity carried on thread-shaped structures called chromosomes. The genetic program is the essential biological blueprint that affects such factors as height, hair color, eye color and how an organism resists disease, digests food, and heals itself when injured.

The potentially harmful effects of environmental agents on genes are far reaching. If the environmental influence is powerful enough, it can damage genes or cause chromosomes to break and genes to be rearranged. These changes, which may go beyond the ability of the organism to repair, can have serious short-term and long term effects.

18

Important for the survival of the species is the fact that a deleterious mutation (significant and permanent change in hereditary material) in the genetic blueprint may be transmitted to future generations. Depending on the location or type as well as the severity of the mutation, offspring in future generations may suffer from serious disease. Any chemical or other agent that is capable of inducing mutations is called a mutagen.

Characterizing genetic damage is time-consuming and difficult work. In recent years, however, remarkable technical advances have given scientists better understanding of complex genetic mechanisms at the molecular level. Recombinant DNA techniques, for example, have allowed scientists to obtain specific genes in pure form and in large enough quantities to characterize them in detail. Recombinant DNA technology involves the process of modifying forms of life by taking heredity-controlling DNA from one cell or organism and splicing it into the DNA of another.

Because of advances in technical knowledge, the Subtask Force on Genetics saw the likelihood of major strides in this scientific area. The group therefore recommended the following directions, among others, for future research:

- Increased study of the molecular sites at which mutation-causing agents act, to determine whether there are genetic "hot spots" which are especially sensitive to the action of such mutagens.

- Establishment of reference banks of cells obtained from people who have been exposed to known mutagens to serve as an invaluable resource for future investigations as more powerful evaluation techniques become available.

- Investigation of the role of transposable elements (mobile sequences of DNA interspersed throughout chromosomes which play a major role in mutation processes) in mutation, transmission, and expression of genes, to understand how they contribute to the genetic diversity within and among species.

- Studies on some of the consequences of chromosomal breaks and rearrangements in human populations to facilitate assessment of the impact of environmental agents on gene expression.

- Studies of how the body repairs damage to cellular DNA to serve as a basis for beginning the study of defective repair.

- Studies to develop methods by which damage to the genetic material of human reproductive cells can be quantified to permit analysis of the genetic consequences of exposure to environmental chemicals.

- Development of new tests to screen chemicals for mutagenic properties, including research to improve the use and interpretation of data generated by such tests.

V. *Dose and Species Extrapolation of Environmental Risks*

An important way of learning how toxic chemicals may affect human beings is to test the substances in laboratory animals and then infer from the results what might happen in humans. This method of predicting risk is called extrapolation. To extrapolate from animal data to human beings in assessing hazards to health, toxicologists make predictions based on careful analyses of dose and metabolism of the chemical, comparisons of body size and weight, and other factors. The rationale for extrapolating from results in animals to predict risks for humans is based on the fact that all species of mammals, including humans, share many similarities, as well as differences, in structure and function, and that their responses to injury are similar in many ways. In general, substances that increase the risk of cancer in one species are presumed and often shown to increase the risk of cancer in other species, including humans.

Experiments in animals are conducted under rigidly controlled laboratory conditions, usually in strains of mice or rats which—because of selective interbreeding of animals with similar physical characteristics—are much alike in terms of life span, susceptibility to disease, and other factors. These similar animals are fed the same die every day, kept in atmospheres offering constant temperature and humidity, housed in uniform cages, and not used for normal reproduction. All this is in contrast to the human situation; so, in addition to obvious differences in size and weight, there are many variables that make extrapolation of animal data to humans challenging. Although such extrapolation requires careful analysis, scientists are reducing the inherent uncertainties through improved knowledge of comparative toxicology and better use of statistical methods.

In their consideration of dose and species extrapolation, this Subtask Force focused primarily on the evaluation of carcinogenic (cancer-causing) substances because mutagenic and teratogenic effects were dealt with in chapters 2 and 4 of the overall report. With regard to carcinogenesis testing, members postulated that the capacity of an environmental substance to produce cancer in both sexes of two or more species of laboratory animals suggests the chemical acts through mechanisms more likely to be present in other species (especially humans), making extrapolation more certain. The rationale for this line of reasoning is that the induction of tumors in more than one exposed group suggests sex-related differences, such as hormone levels, species-related differences in metabolism or disposition, or other intrinsic genetic differences, can be overridden by the effects of the chemical. In contrast, when a chemical induces tumors in only one sex of one species or at only one site, it may be that the action of the chemical is more idiosyncratic, possibly linked to some specific sex- or species-related characteristic.

The Subtask Force considered less costly and less time-consuming alternatives to animal testing, but noted that although progress has been made in these areas. Some animal testing of suspected high-risk substances will continue to be needed. In the long run, however, the Subtask Force was confident that relatively rapid tests performed on cells in culture (called *in vitro* testing) will help "pre-test" more of the large numbers of chemicals in the environment, as well as permit better understanding of why chemicals are toxic.

Among the recommendations made by the Subtask Force were the following:

- Further efforts should be made to refine mathematical methods for low-dose extrapolation from animal to human species.

- There should be more research on exposure regimens lasting less than the animal's lifetime, which more closely mimic common patterns of chemical exposure in humans.

- There is a need for more studies on interactions between toxic substances, because people often are exposed to multiple chemical substances which may interact with one another in the body. Interactions among toxic substances may produce additive effects, synergistic effects (the mixture causes an effect greater than the sum of the effects of the individual substances alone), or mutually antagonistic effects. Other than antibiotic combinations, few such interactions have been well studied thus far, with the result that the combined effects of multiple exposures cannot often be predicted.

21

- Because additional human data are necessary to validate the predictive reliability of animal models, epidemiologic studies should be expanded. Direct comparisons between epidemiologists and researchers should be encouraged to design studies that will maximize this possibility.

- To enhance the nation's ability to evaluate the environmental causes of disease in its citizens, a national clearinghouse for cataloging the nature and extent of environmental exposures should be established.

VI. Differences Among Individuals in Responses to Environmental Stresses

Not all people who are exposed to toxic substances react in the same way. Some may contract disease, but others may not. The reasons why one person will be harmed by an environmental exposure and another will not are still poorly known but fall into four broad categories. First, there are variations among individuals in the concentration of the substance in their immediate environment and in the other kinds of toxins and chemicals to which they have been exposed.

Second, there is a variation among individuals in pharmacokinetics: namely, those factors that govern the amount or concentration of the biologically active form of the toxic substance reaching target sites (places in the body where the substance is most active).

Third, there is a variation among individuals in pharmacodynamics: namely, those factors that govern the reaction of active forms of the toxic substance with the body's target sites.

Fourth, there is a variation among individuals in factors that govern the progression of the successive chemical and biological reactions caused by the toxic substance within the body, reactions that ultimately may result in reversible or irreversible disease processes.

At present, it is impossible to know the extent to which factors in the above categories may contribute to the total variation in human responses to any given environmental substance. Furthermore, if such information were known for one toxic substance, it would not necessarily be applicable to others.

The Subtask Force concentrated its efforts on variations caused by pharmacokinetic factors, especially genetic differences among people. It recommended the following approaches, among others, for additional research:

- The establishment of liver tissue banks—to include tissue specimens from normal and exposed individuals—to help researchers develop diagnostic tools for identifying changes in human liver cells exposed to different toxic substances.

- Increased emphasis on identifying and reporting unusual patterns of metabolism of foreign compounds by the human body. Such patterns should be searched for in clinical studies of commonly used drugs and new drugs being developed and should be reported even when not linked to any obvious disease problem.

- Further efforts to determine the extent to which abnormalities of drug metabolism are due to genetic variations or other causes.

VII. Pharmacokinetic Factors in Chemical Exposure

A basic goal of research on toxic substances is to provide a rational basis for determining the hazards and predicting the risks to human beings following exposure to different substances. Incorporating pharmacokinetic approaches (or study of the rate of absorption, distribution, metabolism, and excretion of substances from the body) in this research can add to the accuracy of such predictions.

As noted in the discussion of Differences Among Individual Subjects in Responses to Environmental Stresses, the toxicity of a chemical is related to the concentration of an active form of the chemical and the time during which it is present at its biological site of action. In making predictions of risk, scientists must consider not only the amount of chemical to which a person is exposed but also the amount that reaches a target organ; the body's handling of the chemical through the processes of absorption, distribution, metabolism, and excretion; and the kinds of effects resulting from the action of the chemical or its metabolites.

While the principles of pharmacokinetics have been used primarily in the design of new drugs in order to determine what kind of therapeutic effect a certain drug will have on a certain body system at a given dosage in a given form, these same principles can also be useful in predicting the effects of toxic substances (at given doses and sites of action) on the human body. For example, if it is known that a certain hazardous chemical is absorbed and distributed at a certain rate, acts primarily on the heart, and is metabolized and excreted at a certain rate, scientists can sometimes make predictions about the potential damaging effects of the chemical on the human body. Because the principles of pharmacokinetics may be useful in making such predictions, the Subtask Force made the following recommendations:

- More large-scale comparative studies of human and animal populations are needed to determine how accurately scientists can extrapolate from animal data to humans. Such studies have been shown to be useful in situations where human beings were exposed to a known toxic substances such as asbestos or cigarette smoke.

- Mathematical models based on anatomical, biochemical, and physiological effects of toxic substances in animals should be used more widely to predict (albeit not with complete certainty) what possible effects the substances will have in humans.

- Additional *in vitro* model systems should be developed as a means of predicting pharmacokinetic behavior, because it is impractical to test the pharmacokinetic properties of every substance in intact animals.

- Because the toxic effects of a given substance are studied and evaluated in laboratory animals generally at doses higher than those likely to be encountered in the human environment, continuing emphasis needs to be placed on consideration of dose-dependent factors when trying to estimate the effects of the substance at doses to which humans may be exposed. Studies predicting the pharmacokinetic behavior of toxic substances should be combined with studies on the mechanisms of their biological effects, including their interactions with enzymes, receptors, nuclei acids, cell membranes, and other biological structures. This would permit better understanding of the toxicological process(es) and, thus, more reliable hazard evaluations, risk assessments, and risk management actions.

VIII. Biochemical and Cellular Markers of Chemical Exposure and Preclinical Indicators of Disease

When a person is exposed to a potentially harmful substance, such as a toxic chemical, biological signs of this exposure or resulting damage may be detectable long before clinical illness becomes evident.

Such "markers" of exposure or "preclinical indicators" of disease are more readily detected now than before because of new laboratory tests.

One of the ultimate aims of identifying biological markers of early damage by chemicals is to be able to predict whether an affected person is at risk of possible illness, so as to be able to take steps to prevent or ameliorate the illness. The Subtask Force urged that the capacity of biochemical and cellular markers to predict illness be more thoroughly explored and validated. Among the Subtask Force's recommendations were the following:

- There should be more studies of cellular markers in population groups with defined exposures to known substances (patients undergoing cancer chemotherapy and industrial workers exposed to asbestos or benzene are suited for this type study). The principles so developed would be applicable to less obvious situations, so that once the markers were perfected, their use would be broadly transferrable.

- To amplify and reinforce the important process of extrapolation of data from animals to humans, parallel studies of cellular markers in animal and human population groups should be conducted.

- Future research should emphasize the development of methods (such as tests to determine changes in the immune system) for detecting the effects of toxicants at dose levels resulting from ambient exposure conditions—everyday conditions—in addition to methods for determining effects from higher levels of exposure such as are caused by accidents or other unusual conditions.

- Emphasis should be placed on the development of tests for environmentally induced mutations in cells from persons who have been exposed, as well as on the application of such tests in long-term studies to determine the extent to which mutations may lead to illnesses such as cancer.

- Work should continue on two promising approaches for detecting markers of environmentally provoked lung damage:
  1. laboratory analysis of fluids and cells extracted from the respiratory tract, a technique called bronchoalveolar lavage; and
  2. laboratory analysis of blood and urine for the presence of metabolic substances indicative of lung damage.

- Emphasis needs to be placed on developing and standardizing tests to detect environmentally provoked damage to the nervous system (for example, electrical techniques that can pinpoint damage to small nerve fibers).

- Work should continue on the wide array of tests that can be applied to sperm to detect early damage or impaired reproductive function resulting from exposure to harmful environmental agents. Such tests would be useful because they could measure the quantity and quality of the sperm and identify altered sperm forms; hence their results might be useful in detecting harmful exposure situations and in identifying those persons who have been so exposed.

IX. Research Strategies for the Prevention of Environmentally Provoked Disease

The main goal of research in environmental health sciences is to prevent environmentally related diseases. Health is better maintained by preventing the disease than by attempting to treat it after it has occurred. The Subtask Force on Research Strategies for the Prevention of Environmentally Provoked Disease identified two broad categories of preventive strategies by which scientists hope to reduce the toll from environmentally related diseases.

The first type of strategy, called primarily prevention, relies mainly on steps to reduce human exposure to harmful substances. These steps include premarket testing of chemicals for toxicity; setting of standards for limiting exposures of individuals to chemicals (within an industry, for example); development of engineering controls to prevent occupational exposure; dissemination of scientific and safety data on potentially harmful substances; labelling of chemicals for adverse effects; and educational programs with emphasis on safe handling and use of dangerous chemicals so as to prevent disease-producing exposures.

The second type of preventive strategy, called secondary prevention, consists of slowing down the progression of disease early enough in its development so that clinical signs and symptoms are largely averted, particularly before damage becomes irreversible. Secondary prevention calls for early identification of disease through medical screening. Such screening can often detect—through the biochemical and cellular markers discussed above, under section VIII—evidence of harm before it progresses into clinical disease. The term "secondary prevention" also encompasses therapies that can increase rates of detoxification of chemicals by increasing metabolism of them, and thereby lessen possible long-range disease consequences of harmful exposure. Obviously, primary prevention is preferable to secondary prevention.

Among the Subtask Force's recommendations were the following:

- Because there are gaps in data systems established for monitoring and surveillance of environmental exposure. Effort should be made to foster better linkage among existing systems.

- Existing data systems should be expanded to include biochemical and cellular indicators of early stages of disease.

- When a given substance is suspected of posing a risk to public health, full knowledge about the ways it produces its toxic effects may not be necessary for preventive intervention (Because proving cause, rather than association, may require the collection of extensive data over a long time period). Avoidance of exposure to the substance may be justified and should be considered even when it has been firmly established that a substance causes a particular health effect.

- The concept of prevention should be integrated into any legal and engineering strategies developed in the future to protect people from diseases caused by environmental exposures.

- Evaluation of the effectiveness of prevention strategies should be part of monitoring and disease surveillance techniques.

- The feasibility of having a uniform national system for labelling chemical substances should be explored. Such uniform labelling should warn of both the acute (immediate) and the chronic (late-occurring) hazards. There is also need for improving techniques for informing workers and members of the public who have been exposed to potentially harmful environmental substances that they may consequently be at increased risk of disease.

X. Structure of Environmental Health Research in the United States

The Subtask Force on the Structure of Environmental Health Research in the United States took on the challenging task of evaluating the scope and effectiveness of U.S. resources for environmental health research, including those in the university community, in government, in industry, in labor organizations, in voluntary agencies (including foundations), and in international institutions. The group found there is a need for more research and more systematic collection of data on the exposure of human populations to harmful substances. Reliable exposure data are necessary for assessing the probability that exposed populations will develop adverse health effects and the likelihood of success in intervening to reduce those risks.

The Subtask Force judged that a fruitful approach for enhancing U.S. environmental health research would be to foster joint research and training efforts on issues important to both environmental and occupational health. For example, joint long-term studies by environmental health and occupational health scientists could concern the health effects of occupational exposure of workers to chemicals that are also found in the general environment. Specifically, the Subtask Force recommended the following measures to enhance environmental research in the United States:

- Because most university laboratories lack the modern equipment and physical facilities needed for highly effective research programs in environmental and occupational health—because of the absence over several years of stable government funding—Congress should be encouraged to address this problem.

- Within universities, collaboration among researchers in different disciplines—engineering, biomathematics, cell biology, and genetics—must be encouraged and supported in order to solve crucial issues in environmental health.

- The unevenness in resources within the Federal government for funding different types of relevant research should be certified. Collaboration among researchers in different fields can help offset the disparity in funding for different research areas.

- In order for regulatory agencies to make informed decisions on substances that may pose hazards to human health, regulatory officials need to be given more scientific information and training to foster better basic understanding of the biological mechanisms of environmentally induced disease, better understanding of the relationship between exposure and risk, and improved ability to judge the relevance of short-term tests designed to determine risk.

- Industrial companies are an underused resource for important environmental health studies, and they should be encouraged to undertake research studies in addition to the pre-market testing of substances for meeting regulatory standards.

- Workers and union leaders need and should receive more and better information on the value of health research in worker populations in order that some of the barriers which often prevent such important research can be addressed.

- The resources of voluntary health agencies and private foundations have been scarcely tapped in this field, and such agencies and foundations need to be sensitized to the scope and impact of environmentally induced illness.

- Collaborative arrangements with international agencies in the environmental health field, such as the World Health Organization International Programme on Chemical Safety and the United Nations Environmental Programme, should be maintained; such collaborative efforts provide a unique and important forum for the exchange of data.

XI. Information Exchange in the Environmental Health Sciences

Scientists must cooperate in efforts to provide society with scientifically accurate and understandable information if the public is to make informed judgments about sound health habits and practices. Walking the line between information overload and quick-fix answers requires a delicate balance in communicating with the public.

The Subtask Force on Information Exchange in the Environmental Health Sciences considered the term "information exchange" to mean a two-way communication process. It also noted that knowledge gained from research is useless unless it is translated into information that can encourage productive changes, including those in attitude and behavior.

This Subtask Force, which was composed not of scientists but of science journalists, an attorney, and specialists in public policy, developed a series of guidelines for improving the credibility of communications with the general public, as well as a set of recommendations for specific projects to improve information exchange in the environmental health sciences.

Just as there is a need for more research on environmental health, so there is a need for more research in the field of communications to define what people know about environmental health and what they need or want to know. The communications process is especially challenging in the sciences because the uncertainties and complexities of science have to be conveyed to the public in understandable terms, and in statements that are properly qualified. The public needs to understand that a scientific development may not be a "cure," but an important step in the eventual development of a cure. This kind of distinction is essential in maintaining the general credibility of scientific information; when information is not properly qualified, public expectation may be greater than a scientific development warrants, and public disillusionment is thus inevitable.

Information must be conveyed in perspective (both scientific and social), so that the public will have some frame of reference for evaluating where the results of a new study fit into the complex fabric of scientific endeavor.

To improve the credibility and usefulness of information on environmental health sciences, the Subtask Force recommended that:

- In delivering information to the public, care should be taken to tailor presentations for special audiences with differing needs and educational levels.

- New communications technologies—such as home computers, computer software, videotapes on environmental health issues, and electronic billboards—should be exploited when appropriate for conveying information to the public.

- Information releases should identify all of the government agencies that have an interest in, or responsibility for, the material being disseminated, because agency collaboration often underlies projects in the environmental health sciences.

- Similarly, there should be joint communication (such as multiple press releases) of information by several government agencies and others with an interest in a scientific subject in order to be as coherent and comprehensive as possible.

- Government officials should strengthen their communication channels with labor, industry, trade associations, environmental groups, and professional organizations.

- Research studies in the communications field should be initiated to evaluate the success of efforts to improve information exchange in the environmental health sciences The issues and challenges facing scientists in environmental health are formidable. Yet a growing body of important knowledge in the basic sciences and recent rapid technological advances have given researchers more and better tools with which to do their work, and have opened doors to new paths of laboratory and field investigation.

- There is every reason to be optimistic that the goals and recommendations set forth in this summary and in the full report of the Third Task Force for Research Planning in Environmental Health Science can be accomplished.

- With the nation's philosophical commitment to better health for all U.S. citizens and with adequate and stable funding, environmental health scientists will be able to contribute substantially to a better understanding of environmental contributions to disease. This will provide directions to those people who want to decrease their risks of disease from environmental agents.

Chapter 2

The Environment: Our Mutual Concern

What Are Physicians Doing?

The quality of our global environment is deteriorating rapidly. As an Academy of over 9,200 physicians, we have a special responsibility to reverse this trend. The relationship between environmental factors and many diseases is well documented. We intend to take the following actions, through our Academy and as individuals, to improve environmental quality:

- Educate ourselves about pollution problems in our workplaces and communities.

- Help our patients understand and identify medical problems in the head, and neck region which are caused or aggravated by environmental pollutants.

- Use our medical and scientific expertise to take a leadership role in environmental protection and pollution prevention.

- Create environmental education programs for physicians and the public.

©1992 American Academy of Otolaryngology—Head and Neck Surgery, Inc. in cooperation with the Senior Environment Corps. Reprinted with acknowledgment.

- Work with the American Medical Association and other physician organizations to improve the environment.

- Support health officials, legislatures, and non-profit organizations in their national, state, and local environmental efforts.

- Cooperate with the National Institutes of Health in developing and fostering research on pollution-related medical disorders.

Noise Pollution

Hearing loss afflicts about 28 million people in the United States. The hearing loss of approximately 10 million is at least partially attributable to exposure to loud sound. More than 20 million Americans are regularly exposed to hazardous noise. Children are particularly vulnerable to excessive noise, which can permanently damage hearing.

In addition to loudness, the length of exposure and the proximity to the source increase damaging effects. For example, factory noise may not harm your hearing during the early period of employment, but exposure for eight hours a day for 10 or more years is likely to cause damage. Explosive sounds such as gun shots can cause hearing loss with a single exposure. Hearing loss caused by noise and the natural aging process is cumulative over a lifetime, so seniors (people over 50) are particularly impacted. Increased effort required for understanding speech leads to fatigue, anxiety and stress. Resulting isolation and loneliness are common feelings.

Most noise-induced hearing loss is preventable with proper use of protective ear devices and could be reduced by implementing broader preventive efforts. Labeling consumer products as to noise emission levels should be strengthened and enforced. Incentives are needed for manufacturers to design quieter industrial equipment and consumer goods. Regulations governing the maximum noise levels of consumer products, such as power tools, must be developed. Model community ordinances should control local environmental noise including noise levels at public events.

Air Pollution

Air pollution affects the nose, throat, sinuses, larynx (voice box), and the lungs.

Outdoor air pollution: Outdoor air pollution can cause postnasal drip, itching throat, sneezing, runny nose, recurrent sinusitis, shortness of breath chronic cough, voice problems (especially chronic hoarseness and laryngitis) and headache. Patients with asthma are particularly at risk. These pollutants also cause "acid rain" which kills life in lakes and streams, damages forests, and reduces crop yields.

Outdoor air pollution is caused mainly by burning fossil fuels (oil, gasoline, coal). Over 50 percent is caused by automobile exhausts, despite the positive results from auto pollution control devices and eliminating lead from gasoline. Pollution is increasing rapidly because the world fleet gains 19 million cars each year. The main components of smog from cars are ozone and carbon monoxide.

In 1986, 96 metropolitan areas (home to more than half of the nation's residents) failed to meet the U.S. Environmental Protection Agency's ozone safety standard, and 41 areas violated the carbon monoxide standard.

Indoor air pollution: Most Americans spend as much as 80 percent of their time indoors; seniors and infants likely spend more. Gas, oil and coal furnaces, gas ranges, wood-burning stoves and fireplaces, asbestos, radon, formaldehyde, lead (from lead-based paints), indoor pesticides, and tobacco smoke pollute indoor air.

The increased risk of cancer from smoking tobacco products was established conclusively several decades ago. Furthermore, tobacco usage causes changes in circulation (blood flow) that increase the death rate due to heart attack and stroke. It also contributes to bronchitis, pneumonia, and emphysema. Recently, medical research has associated passive tobacco smoke with lung cancer in non-smoking adults and increased risk of acute lower respiratory infections, middle ear fluid, and respiratory irritation in children. Our Academy has supported national legislation banning smoking in airplanes, public places and work areas. We are the first medical specialty to pass a resolution calling upon all members to provide a tobacco free office and offer advice on nicotine addiction. We also have a national "Through With Chew" campaign to educate the public about the health hazards of smokeless tobacco.

Taste and smell can be affected negatively by pollutants and chemicals in our environment too. Decrease in the ability to taste and smell may lessen desire to eat nutritious foods and decrease the pleasure from the aromas of flowers and foods. It can lower or completely eliminate the ability to detect air and water borne toxins.

Skin Cancers

Skin cancers are increasing at epidemic rates in the United States and around the world. Clearly, excessive exposure to ultraviolet sun rays is a major cause, and the impact on the skin is cumulative.

Otolaryngologist—head and neck surgeons frequently treat cancers of the head and neck including those on the skin. (Skin on the face and neck is more prone to exposure to the sun.)

Atmospheric scientists warn us that the ozone layer, which protects the earth from some of the cancer causing ultraviolet sun rays, is thinning in expanding areas over the Antarctic and potentially worldwide. This thinning can cause a further increase in skin cancers. It is caused by the reaction of manmade chemicals with the ozone layer—another example of human degradation to the environment. An international accord to phase out these chemicals illustrates that our actions can help solve pollution problems.

What Is Otolaryngology—Head and Neck Surgery?

Otolaryngology—head and neck surgery is a specialty concerned with the medical and surgical treatment of the ears, nose, throat and related structures of the head and neck. The specialty encompasses cosmetic facial reconstruction, surgery of benign and malignant tumors of the head and neck, management of patients with loss of hearing and balance, endoscopic examination of air and food passages and treatment of allergic, sinus, laryngeal, thyroid and esophageal disorders.

To qualify for the American Board of Otolaryngology certification examination, a physician must complete five or more years of post-M.D. (or D.O.) specialty training.

What Is the Senior Environment Corps?

The Senior Environment Corps is a recently established non-profit volunteer organization, which has as its primary concerns environmental education for seniors, the development of local senior teams for "hands-on" environmental activities, matching senior volunteers with specific skills to national, regional, state and local environmental organizations, as well as calling to public attention environmental health concerns specific to seniors.

Chapter 3

Environmental Assault on Immunity

Although scientists have known since the early 1900s that occupational exposure to certain chemicals can induce severe immune effects, recent chemical disasters of national and international prominence have renewed interest in the subject. It is generally agreed that human health is influenced by the environment and that many diseases are caused or enhanced by environmental factors, but effects on the immune system have been difficult to delineate. Researchers in the field of immunotoxicology, who study the adverse effects to immune function that result from occupational, inadvertent, or therapeutic exposure to environmental chemicals, biological materials, and drugs, debate if toxicants damage the immune system and to what extent. Some researchers contend that certain chemicals can affect immunity, significantly increasing an individual's susceptibility to disease, in some cases causing hypersensitivity reactions, autoimmunity, or immunosuppression. Others dispute this view, arguing that the evidence for immuno-toxicity in humans is greatly overstated.

The Immune System: To Serve and Protect

The immune system is the body's complex surveillance network whose mission is to recognize and destroy disease-causing or "foreign" agents. It contains millions of highly specialized cells in the bloodstream and various tissues designed for this purpose. When the body

NIH Publication *Environmental Health Perspectives*, Volume 103, Number 3, March 1995.

is invaded by foreign substances such as viruses and bacteria, the appropriate immune cells respond by destroying the foreign matter or rendering it harmless. When parts of the immune system are damaged, the body cannot fight its adversaries and conditions and diseases ranging from allergies to AIDS may result.

In order to perform its safeguarding duties, the immune system has developed a number of important attributes. Each individual's immune system is distinctive. This causes enemy agents and immune cells to interact differently from person to person, thanks to a unique set of molecules on the surface of immune cells called antigens. The healthy immune system can discriminate the body's own antigens, known as "self," from foreign antigens, known as "nonself." Not only can the immune system detect millions of nonself antigens, it can produce armies of cellular and chemical mediators to launch an initial attack against a foreign substance and manufacture great numbers of specialized cells in the process. The immune system is able to "remember" foreign antigens once the attack is over so that immune responses are activated more rapidly if exposure to a particular antigen recurs. This rapid recall is the basis for protection against antigens by vaccination.

Cells designed to develop into immune cells are produced in the bone marrow in a process called lymphopoiesis. These immune cells, called leukocytes or white blood cells, include a variety of specialized cells: macrophages, eosinophils, natural killer (NK) cells, plasma cells, and T- and B-lymphocytes. The development of these various cell types is directed by chemicals called cytokines. Some lymphocytes cluster in immune organs including the thymus, spleen, lymph nodes, tonsils, and adenoids, while others flow continuously throughout the body in the blood and through a network of lymphatic vessels. The vessels carry lymph to the lymph nodes, the small bean-shaped organs that store lymphocytes and other immune cells. In the lymph nodes, antigens are filtered out and handed over to immune cells and lymph flows back into the bloodstream to monitor organs and tissue for foreign antigens. Lymphoid tissues are also present in local groups known as bronchus-, gut-, and skin-associated lymphoid tissue.

Immune cells manufacture a wide variety of chemical messengers that instruct and control other immune cells or help to attack and destroy foreign antigens. These chemicals include antibodies, which are protein molecules capable of combining with a foreign substance, cytokines such as interferon and interleukins, and complement, which consists of proteins that act in concert with antibodies.

The responses of the immune system to the presence of foreign agents are divided into innate and acquired responses. Innate immune responses can be thought of as the first line of defense against foreign bodies carried out by all-purpose immune cells such as particle-eating cells like macrophages and neutrophils. NK cells are also part of the innate response destroying any cells containing tumor or viral antigens. Acquired immune responses develop to attack specific infectious agents, tumor cells, or allergens. Macrophages do play a role in acquired immunity when they process and present antigens to T-lymphocytes or T-cells, that work to destroy specific antigens. There are different types of T-cells that play different roles when the body is under attack. For example, cytotoxic T-cells recognize and kill cells containing viral or tumor antigens and suppressor T-cells decrease the immune response when needed.

B-lymphocytes or B-cells, also multiply in the presence of a specific antigen often with the assistance of T-cells. B-cells differentiate into plasma cells that produce antibodies that specifically bind to the antigens of the invading foreign body. These antibodies may also assist macrophages in engulfing foreign bodies, rupture bacterial cells, neutralize viruses, and facilitate the cytotoxic activities of NK cells.

Who Is Susceptible?

According to Michael Luster head of the Environmental Immunology and Neurobiology Section of the NIEHS, age, gender pre-existing disease, lifestyle, diet, drugs or stress may compound the effects of chemical exposures to further compromise immune function and increase the chance of disease. Most of the evidence for this interaction comes from animal studies, but there is evidence from human observations as well. About 10 percent of the U.S. population has a genetic tendency to develop allergies. Studies have shown that parents with allergies have a higher proportion of children with allergies. In one study, children born to allergic parents had a 50 percent chance of being allergic; with only one allergic parent, the chances were still 30 percent. Normal immune response depends on the collaboration of more than 60 genes.

It is thought that some immunologic disorders surface even under ordinary environmental conditions, while others appear only after toxic challenges from the environment that act to invoke a previously, detected genetic condition. Genetic studies have demonstrated the existence of a receptor, called the Ah receptor for aromatic hydrocarbon responsiveness, in some animals and humans that binds to halogenated aromatic hydrocarbons, or HAHs. This binding of an HAH may cause toxicity to immune cells, the liver, and DNA and increase cancer risk.

Children and the elderly may be especially susceptible to reductions in immune function. It is well known that the developing immune system is vulnerable to chemical injury. Infants are born with only passive immunity; that is, they are protected for a short period by maternal antibodies that they receive through the placenta and later from breast milk. Although studies of long-term, low-level exposures to environmental toxicants have not been done in the elderly, it is probable that some of the health problems in this population may be associated with reductions in immune function.

Certain therapeutic drugs may also damage immunity. Vitamins, antibiotics, antifungal agents, replacement hormones, diphenylhydantoin and lithium are a few of the drugs associated with immunologic changes. Abused substances, including alcohol, cocaine, and opioids, may be immuno-toxic as well.

Do Chemicals Injure Immunity?

Many immuno-toxicologists say that exposures to certain chemicals can have a significant effect on immune function. Studies have shown that chemical exposures can affect immunity in two major ways: by causing hypersensitivity reactions, including allergy, which can be harmful to organs and tissues autoimmunity, in which immune cells attack self; or by causing immunosuppression, a reduction in the responses and activities of the immune system.

Hypersensitivity

Luster has written that 35 million Americans suffer from allergies, of which 2 to 5 percent are due to occupational chemical exposure. In some individuals, certain substances can aggravate the immune system and cause it to overreact. The first time that an allergy-prone person is exposed to an allergy-causing antigen (an allergen), the matching B-cells generate the class of antibody called immunoglobulin E (IgE). These IgE antibodies attach to the surfaces of other immune cells known as mast cells and basophils, which are found in the lungs, skin, tongue, nose, and intestinal tract. Upon second exposure to the allergen, IgE antibodies on mast cells or basophils signal the release of chemicals such as histamine, which is largely responsible for the intense itching, watery eyes, and runny noses that are commonly associated with allergies.

Some people have more severe allergic reactions than others. Many chemicals cause serious allergic responses beyond the ordinary mild reactions. For example, exposure to toluene diisocyanate (TDI), used in the production of plastics and resins, can result in both contact dermatitis and asthma. Workers in the paint and plastic industries exposed to trimetallic anhydrides had antigen-mediated asthma and rhinitis, late respiratory systemic syndrome, and pulmonary disease anemia.

Other agents induce different types of hypersensitivities. Metals can cause the development of autoimmunity, in which the immune system identifies self as nonself, and mounts an aberrant assault. The result can be an autoimmune disease of the joints and kidneys, such as rheumatoid arthritis, glomerulonephritis, and interstitial nephritis, all of which have been associated with exposures to mercury, gold, or lead. Other organ systems such as the gastrointestinal tract, blood and blood vessels, the central nervous system, and the thyroid, may be targeted for chemically induced autoimmunity.

Exposure to beryllium, a metal used in the manufacture of copper alloys and in the aerospace, nuclear, and electronics industries, is associated with delayed hypersensitivity, in which the immune system reacts to antigen in an immune cell that cannot be cleared or digested. T-cells are then activated to release substances called lymphokines, which cause inflammation due to the influx of immune cells and lymphocytes to the site. With repeated exposures, cells gather at the site of the metal and form masses known as granulomas. When granulomas collect in the lungs, the chronic lung disease known as berylliosis sets in. Short-term, high-concentration beryllium exposure can also lead to dermatitis and sensitization to beryllium.

Immunosuppression

Immunosuppression is normally associated with drugs used to treat autoimmune diseases and increase the survivability of an organ transplant. No matter how closely an organ donor matches an organ recipient, the new organ will have some different antigens that may be perceived by the immune system as foreign bodies. Because the activities of the immune system have been reduced, immuno-suppressed patients are more susceptible to infections and cancers.

A number of human studies cite evidence that immunosuppression also occurs in individuals exposed to environmental agents. In the late 1970s, a group of dairy farmers living in a small town in Michigan who were affected by Hodgkin's disease was also found to have been exposed to polybrominated biphenyls. Children exposed to industrial chemical-contaminated drinking water in the 1980s were reported to have a higher incidence of leukemia and recurrent infections, and their family members had increased levels of T-cells, antibodies directed against self antigens, and repeated rashes. Taiwanese individuals who ingested rice oil contaminated with polychlorinated biphenyls (PCBs) and dibenzofurans exhibited increased sino-pulmonary infections and altered T-cell functions. Other researchers have reported incidence of "toxic oil syndrome," an immunosuppressive disease that appears to also involve autoimmunity, in Spanish residents who consumed rape-seed oil containing imidazolidethion. Evidence also shows that exposure to ultraviolet radiation and ozone suppresses immune responses in humans.

While the mechanism of chemically induced immunosuppression is not completely understood, it appears that in some cases hemotoxicity, direct damage to the organs and progenitor immune cells, is partially responsible. Specifically, environmental chemicals can affect the process of hematopoiesis, the production and maturation of blood cells, including immune cells. Environmental agents can target stem cells, reducing the number of cells available for maturation; affect the marrow itself, rendering it nonfunctional; or damage specific types of immune cells, causing imbalances among cell types.

Organic solvents are well known for their destructive effect on hematopoiesis. Used in the paint and other industries, benzene exposure can lead to abnormalities in the numbers of blood cell types, including leukopenia, and bone marrow hyperplasia. In the past, exposures to heavy metals, in particular lead, were thought to only affect red blood cells. Recently, studies have shown that lead accumulates in the bone marrow, reducing the number of stem and other types of cells. Another chemical, dimethylnitrosamine, is a potent inhibitor of antibody production.

HAHs such as 2,4-dichlorophenoxyacetic acid (2,4-D) and 2,4,5-trichlorophenoxylacetic acid, the active ingredients in Agent Orange, have multiple effects on immune functions. TCDD(2,3,7,8-tetrachlorodibenzo-p-dioxin) is an HAH considered to be the prototype dioxin. Dioxins affect antibody production and immune cell activities. They may also cause immuno-suppression and decreased resistance to disease.

The Debate

The controversy over immunity focuses mainly on the questions of whether environmental and chemical agents can suppress the immune system in the general population and, if so, if this reduction in the immune function can result in clinical disease. While animal toxicology data clearly demonstrate such effects, many researchers and clinicians in the field of immunotoxicology believe that current evidence is not sufficient to support the notion that immunologic damage to humans occurs as the result of chemical exposures. Epidemiologic studies demonstrating such immuno-toxic effects have come under fire from researchers who criticize, among other things, lack of a complete or firm immunodeficiency diagnosis, small patient group sizes, and the inability to establish actual exposure levels. These are problems that have plagued epidemiology and toxicology for decades, making it difficult to evaluate the magnitude of health problems associated with occupational exposures or the effects on the population at large.

Some point out that the immune system, like every physiological system, probably has "reserve capacity," that is, an overlap in functions that small amounts of injury are anticipated and absorbed. While the possibility exists that high-dose toxic exposures could cause significant changes, "the immune system is resilient," says Jack Dean, president of the research division of Sanofi-Winthrop. "You need a lot of injury before you can see an effect. There are very few cases where the two can be linked," says Dean. In a number of studies, immune function was normal in individuals exposed to high levels of immuno-toxic chemicals including heavy metals and TCDD. Another example is the Bhopal disaster, in which individuals exposed to methyl isocyanate, an intermediate chemical produced in the manufacture of carbamate pesticides were found to have increases in numbers of T-cells and decreases in cell activity following exposure to methyl isocyanate but no clinical immunologic diseases were reported. Neighbors of the Michigan dairy farmers who were exposed to polybrominated biphenyls had no immune changes at all. Even in factory workers exposed to benzene and other organic solvents, the clinical relevance of immune system changes is unclear.

Luster admits that the question of whether environmental agents can decrease immune function is difficult to answer because the types of immunologic effects one might expect in the general population are probably subtle. "There is a lot of immunologic variability between individuals, it would be hard to establish a 10 to 15 percent reduction immune function," he says. To sort out the effects of environmental agents, researchers agree that further clinical studies using well-defined sub-populations and the development of sensitive tests are needed. But opinions on what the best approaches might vary widely.

The value of animal models for collecting data on immuno-toxicity is even questioned, despite the fact that the majority of data on immuno-toxic chemicals comes from such studies. In the past, some animal studies were criticized because the doses used were well beyond what humans might be exposed to except in cases of accidents, but most researchers have recognized this problem and adjusted their studies. The problem of how to extrapolate animal results to humans still remains an issue. "The challenge for risk assessment is to extrapolate from immuno-toxicity testing, which is usually a measure of cellular effects in animals, to human health effects at the population level," says Mary Jane Selgrade, Chief, Health Effects Research Laboratory of the EPA Immunotoxicology Branch. "We can do this qualitatively but not quantitatively."

Research in animals has confirmed the results of accidental exposures. The immune systems of several laboratory animals are similar to that of humans in organization, function, and responsiveness, including those of mice and rats. Monkeys chronically exposed to a mixture of PCBs equivalent to that found in the environment became immuno-suppressed: they had aberrant ratios of T-cell types and lowered antibody responses. Moreover, immuno-suppression was seen in the offspring that were exposed perinatally. These immunological effects were similar to those reported in individuals from Taiwan who were exposed to PCB-contaminated rice oil.

Selgrade has developed a mouse model to examine the relationship between chemical suppression of natural killer cells (which are nonspecific) and susceptibility to cytomegalovirus infection. She administered eight chemicals in various doses and found that a significant correlation was observed between chemical suppression of natural killer cell activity against the virus and an increased number of deaths due to viral infection. Selgrade and others have done similar studies with bacterial infections and their effect on lung immune cells, specifically suppression of alveolar macrophages in which phagocytosis correlates with susceptibility to streptococcus infection in the lung. In situations where comparisons are possible between effect of environmental agents on human and mouse immune responses, she has found that "the mouse has predicted pretty well what happens in humans."

Nancy Kerkvliet, associate professor in the Department of Agricultural Chemistry at Oregon State University, cites another problem with animal studies: most examine the spleen after exposure, whereas in humans, blood tests are used to measure immune impairment. "We need more comparable models," says Kerkvliet. Measurements of toxic effects to immunity in humans rely on the use of standard clinical tests, which include measures of antibody levels, the ability of lymphocytes to proliferate, and responses of immune cells to antigens. In a few cases, such assays are accepted as indicative of exposure. Clinical evidence of beryllium exposure is strongly associated with immune activity against the metal by T-lymphocytes obtained from bronchoalveolar lavage or peripheral blood, for example. However, these types of tests may not be sensitive enough to assess immuno-toxic problems due to most low-level chemical exposures. "You expect these effects to be more subtle; we really can't depend on the standard tests," says Michael Holsapple, Research Associate of Dow Chemical, who conducted a number of TCDD studies in animals. Others would go one step further in questioning the validity of such tests for immunotoxicology. Says Dean, "It is not clear how much of a change in functional assay signals a difference in the immune system."

It may be that the small changes observed in the laboratory are often blown out of proportion, according to Kerkvliet. In addition, she says, little attention is paid to the chemical exposures that appear to increase immune system activity. "Except in cases of autoimmunity and allergy, the negative interpretations for this boost in immunity may not necessarily be valid." But immuno-toxic damage in both humans and animals happens "against a back ground of other factors," says Selgrade. "Immunocompetence in the general population probably is a bell-shaped curve. The concern in immuno-toxicity is most likely those individuals that fall on the lower end of the curve," she says. Most immuno-toxicologists would agree that there is a need for more well-controlled epidemiology studies in humans. Holsapple suggests that better ways to assess risk might be to look more closely at chemical-exposed populations. For instance, the administration of a flu vaccine to a dioxin-exposed population would give direct information on how these individuals handle direct antigenic challenge. Selgrade is involved in collaborative research in which humans are exposed to ozone by inhalation in order to quantify alveolar macrophage responses and compare them to the animal responses she has studied. Similarly, following controlled human exposures to ultraviolet radiation, EPA studies have demonstrated immune suppression that is similar to that observed in mice. Says Holsapple: "We need to ask more and more analogous questions in humans to take advantage of what we've learned in animals." Immunologists continue to struggle with these issues in attempts to aid the risk assessment process in a way that is meaningful for human health.

— by Janet Glover-Kerkvliet

Janet Glover-Kerkvliet is a freelance journalist from Cockeysville, Maryland.

Chapter 4

Healing Environmental Harm: Is There a Doctor in the House?

The ideological battle between nurture and nature aside, an unhealthy environment generally evokes greater rates of morbidity, mortality, and disability in a population. Given that, it would seem to follow that environmental medicine would be among the dominant forces in the world of medicine. But in practice, environmental medicine boasts only a small following in the international medical community. Not surprisingly, the training of primary care physicians in occupational and environmental medicine has traditionally been inadequate at every level of medical education. Yet the prognosis for environmental medicine isn't entirely grim: in recent years, improvements have been made and the trend is toward continuing to expand the field of environmental medicine.

"Public health and preventive medicine has been a neglected wing of medicine in the U.S. and environmental and occupational medicine has been a part of that wing," observes Rosemary Sokas, associate professor of medicine and health care sciences at George Washington University in Washington, D.C. As a result, fewer resources have historically been dedicated to environmental medicine, and its knowledge base has been left wanting—not only in the research arena but among individual doctors and the public as well. "The tragedy is that traditional medicine has given environmental medicine the back seat—partly due to money and partly status," Sokas says.

The historic disregard of environmental medicine is bumping up against the modern realization that primary care physicians are the

NIH Publication *Environmental Health Perspectives* Volume 104, Number 2, February 1996.

main protection citizens have against environmental illness and effects. "There isn't too much else out there," says James P. Keogh, associate director of the Occupational Health Project at the University of Maryland Medical School.

The picture isn't looking any brighter in terms of what type of environmental hazards people will be exposed to in the future either. "Communities will be in greater jeopardy....As community standards go down, the health of the community will, too," says Annette Kirshner, a program administrator in the Division of Extramural Research and Training at the NIEHS.

Defining the Field

A leading obstacle to the acceptance of environmental medicine by the mainstream medical community has been the ambiguity and mutability of its definition. While most people instantly know what a cardiologist or a radiologist is, even some in the health care business are often confused by the term environmental physician.

Different experts describe varying components when attempting to define environmental medicine. "Traditional medicine has been very disease oriented. Environmental medicine really requires a slightly different focus—though it's a more nebulous focus—and it also requires taking a different history [of the patient]," explains Kirshner. Yet another school of thought believes the field encompasses a more global definition, whose parameters only seem to expand with the research's knowledge base. Scientists and doctors in this group would include everything from health effects experienced from exercising on a day when air pollution is particularly bad, to the symptoms described as Gulf War syndrome, to the relation of climate change to malaria in the bailiwick of environmental medicine.

"Some people get kind of manic about it, but I kind of like thinking about it [in a global way]," says Sokas. Many doctors who are specialists in other fields actually practice environmental medicine on a daily basis, says Sokas, citing tropical medicine or infectious disease experts as examples. Accordingly, she says, such overlapping specialties should be included when inventorying environmental medicine.

A committee of the National Academy of Sciences' Institute of Medicine came up with a working definition—which acknowledges environmental medicine's broad parameters—in a 1995 report on the subject titled *Environmental Medicine: Integrating a Missing Element into Medical Education*. "Environmental medicine refers to diagnosing and caring for people exposed to chemical and physical hazards in their homes, communities, and workplaces through such media as contaminated soil, water, and air," the report states. The definition excludes diseases caused by lifestyle factors such as tobacco and alcohol use and diet, as well as environmental conditions such as violence.

Clearly, there is dissension within the medical and scientific community as to what environmental medicine embraces. And in practice, what is considered environmental medicine usually depends on the physician. Generally speaking, however, environmental medicine refers to the prevention and treatment of diseases related to the environment, as opposed to occupational medicine which is concerned with the prevention and treatment of work-related injuries and illnesses. But even this distinction is blurred. Many people still tend to confuse the two specialties or view them as "merged at the hip," as Sokas puts it, because environmental medicine got its start in occupational medicine departments at many medical schools. In addition, environmental medicine's traditional origins in occupational medicine "have given it a slightly litigious quality," Kirshner says, that may detract from its credibility.

Another twist in the evolution of the field is that contemporary society itself is blurring the lines between home and office, further clouding the distinction between occupational and environmental medicine. For example, some people bring their children into the workplace, while others work at home. Meanwhile, most departments of occupational medicine have been changing their names to environmental and occupational medicine in recognition of the broader context that is evolving. Just the same, the NIEHS's Kirshner says "we view occupational medicine as a subset of environmental medicine."

Currently, occupational medicine is the only specialty of the two that is recognized by the American Board of Specialties. A physician can be board-certified in preventive medicine in one of three categories: occupational medicine, public health and general preventive medicine, and aerospace medicine. In the next year, medical management may be added to this list. Also, there is talk of changing the occupational medicine specialty to "environmental and occupational medicine," but a formal push has not been launched with the board.

Second Class Citizenship

No matter how they define it, most experts agree that environmental medicine has not been awarded the respect it deserves in the medical community. A 1991 survey of more than 100 medical schools published in the *American Journal of Public Health* found that, for the most part, occupational and environmental health issues continue to be overlooked by most medical schools. According to a 1994 report in the *American Journal of Public Health* of a 1991 survey, about 68 percent of schools teach environmental and occupational medicine with an average of six hours of the curriculum being spent on environmental and occupational health. And these numbers are an improvement. A similar survey in 1977, reported in the same journal article, found that only half of U.S. medical schools taught occupational and environmental health and when they did, spent an average of only four hours on the unit.

The way the medical system is structured has also been a stumbling block in the evolution of environmental medicine. Medical school curricula are crowded and their departmental structures tend to be very hierarchical and highly competitive. "So much depends on the public health sector, but for medical centers [environmental medicine] has traditionally not been a moneymaker and has suffered from the fact that it can't pay its own way," explains Kirshner. The effect of this attitude within the medical profession has been that environmental medicine is viewed as far less glamorous than other specialties. Sokas notes, "People don't make TV shows about environmental physicians, they make them about ER doctors."

In addition, doctors generally get promoted in a discipline on the basis of how specialized and focused their practice is, and greater focus typically brings more publicity and more grant money. "That's the scientific model. You don't get points for being interdisciplinary," says Sokas.

Practice

One obstacle to the advancement of environmental medicine has been the frustrations physician encounter when trying to practice it clinically. First, research in environmental medicine lags far behind other more traditional medical specialties. In environmental medicine, Sokas explains, researchers are still figuring out what the questions are. Thus, the level of uncertainty that environmental physicians must work with can be far greater than for more established areas of medicine. Second, resources available to environmental physicians to help them understand the complex interactions of factors such as video display terminals (VDTs), toxic emissions, and genetics in human systems are often lacking. Third, physicians are usually reluctant to become involved in the bureaucracy of worker's compensation cases, debates between environmentalists and industry, or the legal ramifications that may accompany a diagnosis of an adverse environmental health effect. "Often when contamination occurs in a community, physicians back off," Sokas says.

In short, Sokas says, "Training is very important, but beyond training the way people practice medicine has to include population-based information and also have the research to back it up."

Industry Influences

Since the early days of occupational and environmental medicine, industry has been a key player in how these disciplines have evolved and are perceived. Traditionally, occupational physicians employed by industry have generally practiced in a health care setting. But in the past decade, in light of regulations, liability, and mounting health care costs, the business world has shifted its emphasis beyond the traditional clinical settings to in-house assessment of the ramifications of its operations. In fact, strategic guidance in regulatory areas has become increasingly necessary for businesses to stay competitive. The chemical industry, for one, has been at the forefront of addressing this need.

"Environmental medicine was really noticed by the business world about five years ago," says Elizabeth E. Gresch, currently an occupational physician consultant for General Motors. The change, she says, is due partly to media attention, partly to lawsuits, and partly to the reality that American businesses have to compete with countries where the wages are one-tenth of those in the United States.

"Businesses are generally concentrated inward on making a profit," says Gresch, a past president of the American College of Occupational and Environmental Medicine. Companies simply haven't had the resources in the past to address many of these concerns, according to Gresch, who has worked for Dow Chemical and other large companies. Moreover, Gresch says the challenges of occupational medicine are not limited to the United States. "It's a worldwide issue," Gresch says.

In the near future, most experts predict the need for environmental medicine consultants will increase as consciousness about the effects of work on health, law suits, and government rules and regulations increase. About one-third of environmental and occupational medicine residents were planning to look to industry for employment immediately after finishing training, according to the 1991 survey reported in the May 1994 issue of the *American Journal of Public Health*. However, over the long haul, about 40 percent said they would prefer consulting positions like those enjoyed by Stephen Dawkins, owner of Occupational Health International in Atlanta (which consults to Coca-Cola and the Cable News Network) and Richard Cohen, who oversees the health and safety of workers at Varian Associates Inc., a manufacturer of equipment and systems for communications in the scientific, medical, and industrial markets, in Palo Alto, California. Gresch predicts that environmental medicine will play an even larger role in business in the future.

Regardless of impending budget cuts, the federal government will continue to be a large employer of environmental physicians in the future. Experts say that some of the leading career opportunities in this area will continue to be found in the federal sector at agencies such as the Centers for Disease Control and Prevention, the Department of Energy, the Environmental Protection Agency, and the Food and Drug Administration. There is also room for environmental physicians in science-oriented professional associations and environmental organizations like the World Watch Institute or the Canadian-based MotherRisk Program.

Training

A major reason for the lack of environmental physicians, some experts charge, is due to a fundamental problem in the way that medical schools train doctors. On the whole, the medical profession has been "abysmally ignorant" about environmental medicine, Kirshner says. Keogh says that often physicians will treat symptoms without a real handle on what the cause of an illness is. Moreover, says Sokas, "The focus [of training] is too heavily on treatment and not prevention, and when it does focus on prevention it focuses only on the patient in front of [a physician]." Sokas argues that medical students need to learn to look at both individual patients and larger groups of potential patients. "Not many students take a population view of health care," she says.

Experts from all walks seem to agree that changing the way physicians are trained is the best way to ensure the future of environmental medicine. While past attempts to reform medical curricula have largely been hindered by entrenched opposition to change within the medical establishment, a push is on to change not only the content but also the structure of medical education. And many medical educators are looking to incorporating environmental medicine in the medical school curriculum as a part of future reforms.

An ongoing study by the Institute of Medicine is assessing how to change environmental medicine education, among other things. David P. Rall, chairperson of the IOM Committee on Curriculum Development in Environmental Medicine, writes in the 1995 IOM report, "The committee is confident that integrating environmental medicine into medical education will substantially enhance the competence of tomorrow's physicians in addressing the growing environmental health concerns of their patients and communities."

In an effort to keep up, many medical schools are working to incorporate some sort of training in environmental health into their curricula. Rather than segmenting out new blocks or courses in an already crowded and often territorial curriculum, a concerted effort is being made to integrate environmental medicine into current courses, internships, and other areas, according to the IOM report. This approach is in keeping with the idea that environmental medicine is a continuum that extends across the gamut of medical practice.

In the past year, about 180 occupational and environmental medicine residents were enrolled in the 40 accredited occupational and environmental medicine residencies in the United States and Canada. In a recent survey of these residents published in the *Journal of Occupational and Environmental Medicine*, the majority of residents opted to go into this type of training after they had already begun working professionally. In fact, only 11 percent made up their minds to pursue an occupational and environmental medicine residency before or during medical school. The survey also found that only 16 percent learned about occupational and environmental medicine in medical school and 11 percent were first exposed to the specialty during residency training.

In its 1995 report, the IOM committee recommends that graduating medical students have the following basic competencies in environmental medicine: they should understand the influences of the environment and its agents on human health on the basis of knowledge of relevant epidemiological, toxicological, and exposure factors; they should be able to recognize the signs, symptoms, diseases, and sources of exposure relating to common environmental agents and conditions; they should be able to elicit appropriately detailed environmental exposure history, including a work history from all patients; they should be able to identify and access the informational, clinical, and other resources available to help address patient and community environmental health problems and concerns; they should be able to discuss environmental risks with their patients and provide understandable information about risk-reduction strategies in ways that exhibit sensitivity to patients' health beliefs and concerns; and they should be able to understand the ethical and legal responsibilities of seeing patients with environmental and occupational health problems or concerns.

A variety of groups are interested in broadening the role of environmental medicine in medical education, and "ours is one of them," says Kirshner, who considers the programs supported by the NIEHS to be some of the most progressive approaches to altering medical school curricula. In 1990, the NIEHS launched a grant program to help schools develop their curricula to incorporate environmental and occupational health. Currently 17 medical schools have been granted five-year Environmental Occupational Medical Academic Awards, which range from $92,000 to $188,000 a year. The University of Maryland, George Washington University School of Medicine, Yale University School of Medicine, Mount Sinai School of Medicine, Harvard Medical School, and the University of Rochester School of Medicine are among the recipients.

Although they have the common goal of integration, exactly how the programs are set up to accomplish this is left to the individual medical schools. The NIEHS hopes that the environmental medicine elements of the curricula will continue even after the grants run out.

Keogh says his goal at the University of Maryland is to educate physicians in environmental medicine "enough to play a positive role in the community." Sokas agrees, noting that primary care physicians need to be able to recognize an environmental problem in an exposure case. "If they don't have the information on hand, they need to know what type of problem they could be looking at. They don't have to learn everything—just know when they don't know."

The NIEHS also makes Environmental Health Sciences Center Awards to schools to conduct interdisciplinary research in environmental health, has set up Basic Research and Education Programs to fund research on the prevention of adverse health effects from hazardous substances, and has established Hazardous Waste Worker Health and Safety Training Awards and Programs to develop training programs for health and safety workers and supervisors.

But there are other types of programs that also accomplish some of these same goals, Kirshner acknowledges. Many schools that did not receive NIEHS funds are working to expand medical students' exposure to environmental medicine. The ATSDR and NIOSH have joined forces to set up a project called EPOCH-Envi, which works to introduce occupational and environmental medicine curricula into primary care residency programs. In addition, the ATSDR offers a self-study series: Case Studies in Environmental Medicine, and supports state and county programs that help health departments develop environmental medicine educational materials and activities for health care professionals. The American College of Occupational and Environmental Medicine also offers continuing education.

For the most part, the field of environmental medicine is being led by doctors who chose it as a second career or who received training after completing their medical degrees. More and more programs are cropping up around the nation to make this possible.

One of the more innovative programs is located in the Medical College of Wisconsin, which allows doctors to earn a master's degree in public health by computer. The program, which began enrolling students in 1986, now has 500 active students and has graduated about 165 to date, according to William Greaves, director of the Master of Public Health Programs in the Department of Preventive Medicine at the Medical College of Wisconsin in Milwaukee, who was instrumental in getting the program off the ground.

"The program was started to meet the needs of physicians to become more competent in environmental medicine while continuing to work full-time as a physician," Greaves says. All a doctor needs is a computer and a modem to enroll, so he or she doesn't have to quit practicing and lose his or her income while retraining. Students go to Milwaukee about once a year for testing.

"Compared to quitting practice it is cheap," observes Gresch. Wisconsin enrolls 50 licensed physicians three times a year on a first come-first served basis in the program. The tuition costs about $14,400 for the ten-course program, which on average takes three years to complete, though a couple of students have finished in a year's time, Greaves says. Wisconsin's program is the first long-distance education concept applied to environmental medicine that has no formal classes. A similar program is in the works at Duke University.

Long-distance commuting programs have also been successful. A prime example is the "On the Job—On Campus" program at the University of Michigan's Medical School in Ann Arbor. The two-year program allows physicians to keep their jobs while studying environmental medicine during weekend courses.

Bright Future

By all indications, experts from many interested sectors—industry, academia, government, private practice—agree that better training at all levels, while not a panacea, is an excellent starting point for pushing environmental medicine into the next century. And indeed progress has been seen in recent years.

"The situation is changing," Kirshner says. Just 30 years ago, most Americans gave little thought to the environment. But in recent years, the environment has become a key health issue in some parts of the country. Signs are indicating that the limits which once defined occupational medicine and more recently environmental medicine are continuing to expand to include increasingly interdisciplinary areas of science and medicine that may come to include everything from global change to the psychological impact of the environment. Says Sokas, someday physicians may even come to more widely recognize that the environment can be a healing place.

—by Julie Wakefield

Chapter 5

What Is Environmental Medicine?

The specialty in medicine in which doctors assist patients in uncovering the cause and effect relationship between their environment and their ill-health, and help them learn to avoid those inciting factors is called Environmental Medicine.

The term "allergy" was created to describe an abnormal response to substances that your system recognizes as foreign which do not cause reactions in most people. Substances which cause allergies include pollens, danders, mold, dust, foods, chemicals, drugs, air pollution, and perfumes. These substances are called "allergens" or "antigens." Allergy can produce symptoms in almost every organ of the body and often masquerades as other diseases. Allergy can affect your skin, eyes, ears, nose, throat, lungs, stomach, bladder, vagina, muscles, joints, and your entire nervous system, including your brain.

Heredity: The ability to have an allergic reaction appears to be hereditary. Somewhere in your family somebody slipped you some allergic genes. The more people, and the more severe the allergies, the earlier you are likely to experience allergic manifestations. In childhood, more boys than girls have allergies. In adults, the ratio is reversed and more women have allergies, especially beginning at age thirty and lasting until menopause. After that the incidence is about the some for men and women. For some people there is a hormonal component. By the way, parents and children may be allergic to different things.

Extracted from *What is Environmental Medicine* and *Practice Guidelines*. American Academy of Environmental Medicine^{SM.} Reprinted with permission.

Infection: It is possible to develop allergic sensitivities after a bout of severe infection: viral, bacterial or fungal.

Chemical Exposure: Heavy exposure to pesticides or other petrochemicals can lead to the development of allergic reactions.

Stress: An increased stress load, whether emotional or physical, positive or negative, can play a role in allergies. Getting married or having a baby are happy events, but they are stressful.

Nutrition: Poor nutritional habits contribute to the development of allergies as well as other illnesses.

In many cases the allergies have existed for a while, but gradually become worse until you are forced to do something about them. Your ability to adapt to these stresses finally runs out.

Practice Guidelines

Clinical Indicators

History. Patients may present with many types of disorders that result at least in part from adverse reactions to any combination of a multitude of environmental or internal substances (for example, biologic inhalants, venoms, foods, and chemicals).

The manifestations of these disorders may be quite diverse. They are individually specific from patient to patient and are modified by individual susceptibility, genetics, functional nutritional status, and specific adaptation. The patient may often be able to identify environmental and/or dietary factors that contribute to the symptoms, but this is not always the case. Symptoms may variably involve any one or more organs or systems over time. Symptoms may be acute, chronic, or recurrent, with or without fluctuations, and may sometimes have seasonal variations.

An appropriately detailed chronological history should be developed for each organ or system that seems to be involved with each patient's illness. This history should attempt to identify known presenting patterns that are seen when adverse reactions to environmental substances are occurring over time. Other aspects of each patient's history should also be obtained as indicated. Examples would include reviews of one or more of the following:

- the patient's home, occupational, and recreational environments;
- a dietary history;
- the medical, dental, surgical, educational, psycho-social, and occupational history;
- and family history.

Physical Examination. An appropriate physical examination is indicated for every patient. Each organ or system should be examined as indicated by the history.

Diagnostic Techniques. After an appropriate history has been obtained and a physical examination performed, if a provisional diagnosis has been made that may involve adverse reactions of the above type to environmental substances, various diagnostic techniques are appropriate to corroborate and clarify this possibility.

An appropriate work-up to evaluate for other possible medical, surgical, and/or psychological conditions that may not involve the types of adverse reactions noted above is also appropriate if indicated by the history or physical examination. This work-up may also involve various laboratory tests, medical imaging studies, and/or surgical procedures.

Biologic Inhalant and Venom Hypersensitivity

DIAGNOSTIC TECHNIQUES.

Examples of biologic inhalant groups might include: tree, grass and weed pollens, various dust components, airborne molds, and animal danders. Other biologic substances might include Hymenoptera venoms.

Skin Testing. Intradermal Serial Dilution Endpoint Titration and Provocation/Neutralization Testing (Intradermal or Sublingual) are the preferred techniques to aid in the evaluation of biologic inhalants suspected to be contributing to this type of illness.

Screening for up to twenty of the most common biologic inhalants in the patient's geographic area is appropriate, as indicated by the history. If significant sensitivity to any of the above groups is found, then testing for additional members of the incriminated group(s) in the patient's geographic area may be appropriate. Total additional testing should rarely exceed thirty more substances except in highly complicated patients.

Serial Dilution Endpoint Titration is also appropriate as part of the evaluation for Hymenoptera venom allergy.

In-Vitro Blood Testing. When evaluating for IgE-mediated reactions, initial screening of biologic inhalants may also be accomplished by using serum measurements of antigen-specific IgE antibodies. Further testing based on positive screen results may also be appropriate. Various techniques are available that offer quantitative levels of IgE for each antigen tested. The appropriate number of antigens tested would be the same as for the skin testing techniques above.

This technique is also appropriate in the evaluation of IgE-mediated Hymenoptera venom allergy. In the case of severe Hymenoptera venom allergy, it may by appropriate to perform, both skin tests and in-vitro tests.

Duplicating both skin testing and in-vitro testing for the same antigens is not indicated in the routine case. Using one or the other technique for different antigens where the IgE mechanism is suspected may be appropriate. However, some highly complicated cases may require both skin testing and in-vitro techniques for the same antigens. These cases may be dealt with on an individual basis.

Finally, before starting immunotherapy with extracts based solely upon in-vitro testing, it is appropriate to use the treatment extracts to perform skin tests to assess the exacts' safety. This is not to be considered duplicate testing.

TREATMENT

Patient Education. Proper education about how to identify and avoid environmental sources of incriminated biologic inhalants and venoms is the treatment of choice where possible and practical.

Immunotherapy. Immunotherapy for appropriate biological mechanisms that respond to Serial Dilution Endpoint Titration, Provocation/Neutralization Testing, or appropriate In-Vitro testing is efficacious and appropriate where strict avoidance of incriminated biologic inhalants is either not possible or is impractical. Treatment doses may be administered either subcutaneously or sublingually and may be given by the physician/staff or patient as deemed appropriate.

Immunotherapy based on Serial Dilution Endpoint Titration and In-Vitro Testing is appropriate in the long term treatment of severe

Hymenoptera venom allergy. Treatment doses should be administered subcutaneously.

The dose sizes and the intervals between doses must be individualized in each patient to achieve optimal results.

Nutritional Supplements. Micronutrients (vitamins, minerals, amino acids, and essential fatty acids) and other nutritional supplements administered orally or parenterally may be indicated in cases where functional deficiencies of these substances have been found by laboratory assessments or suspected on appropriate clinical grounds.

Drug Therapy. Symptom-relieving medications found to be safe and efficacious for the patient's particular symptoms may be an appropriate adjunct to therapy where indicated.

Food Hypersensitivity

DIAGNOSTIC TECHNIQUES

Dietary History. An appropriate dietary history should be obtained on each patient.

Oral Elimination/Challenge Feeding Tests. Various elimination/challenge feeding tests are an appropriate modality to use in the assessment for food susceptibilities. After completely avoiding the food(s) for four to seven days, the oral challenge part of the test may be performed in the physician's office or in the patient's home, as deemed appropriate by the patient's history.

Any number of suspected foods may be evaluated by these procedures. Some of the common variations of this technique would include the single food elimination/challenge diet, the "cave man" diet, the rare food diet, the oligoantigenic diet, and the total elimination/challenge diet (diagnostic fasting).

Provocation/Neutralization Testing. Intradermal or sublingual forms of this procedure are appropriate to aid in the evaluation of food susceptibilities where the biologic mechanisms detected by this technique are suspected to be playing a role in the patient's symptoms.

An initial evaluation for the average patient may include testing for the commonly eaten hidden foods such as baker's and brewer's yeast, milk, egg, corn, wheat, soy, coconut, cane sugar, and beet sugar.

Other frequently eaten foods may also be tested as indicated by the patient's diet diary and history.

The average adult patient can usually be adequately worked up by testing twenty or less foods, while all but the most severe cases may usually be adequately evaluated with thirty or less foods. Infants and young children who have more limited diets may need fewer foods tested.

In-Vitro Blood Testing. Testing large numbers of foods by any single in-vitro technique has not been proven to be consistently clinically efficacious in diagnosing food susceptibilities in the routine patient, due to the potentially large number of biological mechanisms that may simultaneously be playing a role in causing each patient's food-related symptoms. However, IgE in-vitro techniques may be useful in assisting to evaluate for severe IgE-mediated reactions to specific foods suspected from the history. Also, in children, screening up to ten commonly eaten foods for antigen-specific IgE may be useful in evaluating for significant IgE-mediated reactions. The clinical significance of any related in-vitro IgE screening test should be confirmed by appropriate elimination diet trials, oral elimination/challenge feeding tests, and/or provocation/neutralization tests, as deemed appropriate from the patient's history.

At this time, in routine cases, measurements for other types of antigen-specific antibodies of other classes of immunoglobulins, immune complexes, other mediators of immunity, and live cell analyses may be considered on an individual basis.

TREATMENT

Patient Education. Proper education about how to correctly identify and avoid sources of incriminated foods is the treatment of choice where avoidance is possible and practical. Dietary information about alternative food sources and recipes should be provided as needed.

The Rotary Diversified Elimination Diet technique should be taught to all patients, who may use it as indicated. Use of the techniques may be therapeutic, diagnostic, and preventive.

All diet regimens should accommodate general guidelines required to satisfy overall good nutrition.

Immunotherapy. Immunotherapy for appropriate biological mechanisms that respond to Provocation/Neutralization Testing is efficacious and appropriate where strict avoidance of incriminated foods is either not possible or impractical. Treatment doses may be administered either subcutaneously or sublingually and may be given by the physician/staff or patient as deemed appropriate. The dose intervals and dietary intake of treated foods must be individualized in each patient to achieve optimal results.

Nutritional Supplements. Micronutrients (vitamins, minerals, amino acids, and essential fatty acids) and other nutritional supplements administered orally or parenterally may be indicated where functional deficiencies of these substances have been found by laboratory assessments or suspected on appropriate clinical grounds.

Drug Therapy. Symptom-relieving medications found to be safe and efficacious for the patient's particular symptoms may be an appropriate adjunct to therapy where indicated.

Chemical Hypersensitivity

DIAGNOSTIC TECHNIQUES

Inhalant Elimination/Challenge Testing. Susceptibility to various volatile chemicals may be evaluated through use of appropriate inhalant elimination/challenge techniques.

In-vivo chemical testing should be done in a setting as free as possible from exposures to potential environmental excitants, under appropriate supervision, and the patient should be in a non-adapted state to the test substance, if possible. This non-adapted state may be achieved by careful avoidance of the test substance for four to seven days before the challenge test.

Provocation/Neutralization Testing. Intradermal or sublingual forms of this technique are appropriate to assist in the evaluation for susceptibility to various inorganic, organic, and petrochemical compounds, as well as other chemical substances such as various mediators, neurotransmitters, hormones, and infectious organisms, when the biological mechanisms detected by this technique are thought to be involved with the patient's symptoms.

Epidermal Patch Testing. This technique is often helpful as an aid in diagnosing contact chemical sensitivities.

Contamination Profiles. Quantitative and qualitative measurements of pesticides, hydrocarbons, and other externally derived chemical substances in blood, various body fluids, bone, exhaled breath, hair, and fat may prove useful when evaluating for chemical susceptibilities.

Chemical Hypersensitivity

TREATMENT

Patient Education. Proper education about how to identify and avoid incriminated environmental chemicals is the treatment of choice where possible and practical. This may be achieved indoors by environmental control of home and occupational indoor air pollution by improving ventilation, various air cleaning systems, various protective devices, and by use of less toxic substitutes via changes in lifestyle and manufacturing techniques. Outdoor ambient air may be improved through the use of appropriate technology to clean the air. A pure as possible water supply should be used whenever possible.

Immunotherapy. Immunotherapy for appropriate biological mechanisms that respond to Provocation/Neutralization Testing is efficacious and appropriate where strict avoidance of incriminated chemicals is either not possible or impractical. Treatment doses may be administered either subcutaneously or sublingually, depending on the toxicity of the chemical, and may be administered by the physician/staff or patient, as deemed appropriate. The dose intervals must be individualized in each patient to achieve optimal results.

Nutritional Supplements. Micronutrients (vitamins, minerals, amino acids, and essential fatty acids) and other nutritional supplements administered orally or parenterally may be indicated when functional deficiencies of these substances have been found in laboratory assessments or suspected on appropriate clinical grounds.

Drug Therapy. Symptom-relieving medications found to be safe and efficacious for the patient's particular symptoms may be an appropriate adjunct to therapy where indicated.

Detoxification. Appropriately supervised chemical detoxification by physical therapy.

Additional Diagnostic Techniques

In each case, other diagnostic techniques may also be appropriate if indicated by the history or physical examination. These techniques may include (but are not necessarily limited to) the following:

- **Metabolic Assessments:** in-vitro and in-vivo analyses of absorption, digestion, excretion, xenobiotic detoxification systems, and other metabolic functions.

- **Immune System Assessments:** In-vitro and in-vivo analysis of various immune system functions.

- **Endocrine System Assessments:** Measurement of auto-antibodies to different components of various endocrine glands, as well as in-vitro and in-vivo hormone analysis.

- **Nutritional Assessments:** Qualitative and functional in-vitro and in-vivo analyses of various nutrients (for example, vitamins, minerals, proteins, carbohydrates, and fats) are appropriate in the overall evaluation where functional nutritional deficiencies or excesses are suspected to be contributing to the patient's illness.

- **Environmental Assessments:** Qualitative and quantitative measurements of environmental contaminants in ambient, domiciliary, and occupational air, food and water, and in the other environments where the patient is known to be symptomatic.

- **Comprehensive Environmentally Controlled Inpatient Hospital Care:** The great majority of cases where illnesses are contributed to by these types of adverse reactions to environmental substances may be safely and effectively worked up in an outpatient setting. However, there may be certain complex and/or severe cases where evaluation and treatment may need to be initiated in a specialized inpatient Environmentally Controlled Unit (ECU) where all environmental and dietary exposures are carefully controlled.

Treatment Outcome Criteria

1. Significant reduction or elimination of acute and/or chronic symptoms in any organ or system.

2. Improvement of measured functions in any organ or system.

3. Improvement in the ability to carry out the tasks of daily living.

4. Improvement in psychological well-being.

5. Improvement in the ability to sustain gainful employment.

6. Improvement or correction of incriminated environmental exposures.

7. Improved tolerance to environmental stressors that previously caused symptoms.

8. Through appropriate patient education, improvement in the ability to follow treatment protocols and to prevent the development of new illnesses.

For more information contact:

American Academy of Environmental Medicine
4510 West 89th Street
Prairie Village, KS 66207
(913) 642-6062
fax (913) 341-6912

The AAEM provides referrals for environmental medicine physicians to those seeking assistance. It holds two instructional meetings per year (open to the public as well as medical personnel) and produces a quarterly newsletter as well as quarterly journal. It also makes available resource information (networking groups, information regarding attorneys that handle environmental cases, sources for products/services, and approximately 100 books available to any interested party.

Chapter 6

Clinical Ecology: Unproven and Under Fire

Clinical ecology is a relatively new medical specialty based on the theory that many common symptoms are triggered by hypersensitivity to common foods and chemicals. Clinical ecologists consider their patients to be suffering from "environmental or ecological illness," "cerebral allergy," "total allergy syndrome," or "20th century disease," the later of which can mimic almost any other illness.

The signs and symptoms of this condition are said to include depression, irritability, mood swings, inability to think clearly, poor memory, fatigue, drowsiness, diarrhea, constipation, sneezing, running or stuffy nose, wheezing, itching eyes, skin rashes, headaches, muscle and joint pain, urinary frequency, pounding heart, swelling of various parts of the body, and even schizophrenia.

Clinical ecologists speculate that hypersensitivity develops when the total load of physical and psychological stresses exceeds what a person can tolerate. According to proponents, potential stressors include practically everything that modern humans encounter, such as urban air, diesel exhaust, tobacco smoke, fresh paint or tar, organic solvents and pesticides, certain plastics, newsprint, perfumes and colognes, medications, gas used for cooking and heating, building materials, permanent press and synthetic fabrics, household cleaners, rubbing alcohol, felt-tip pens, tap water, and electro-magnetic forces.

To diagnose ecologically related diseases, practitioners take a history that emphasizes dietary habits and exposure to environmental chemicals they consider harmful. A physician examination and certain laboratory tests may be performed mainly to rule out other causes of disease. Standard allergy test results are usually normal.

Various nonstandard tests are also used. The main test, called provocation and neutralization, consists of the patient reporting symptoms that develop after various concentrations of suspected substances are administered under the tongue or injected into the skin. If any symptoms occur within 10 minutes, the test is considered positive and lower concentrations are given until a dose is found that "neutralizes" the symptoms. Elimination and rotation diets are used with the hope of identifying foods that cause problems.

In severe cases, patients may spend several weeks in environmental control units designed to remove them from exposure to airborne pollutants and synthetic substances that might cause adverse reactions. After fasting for several days, the patients are given "organically grown" foods and gradually exposed to environmental substances to see which ones cause symptoms to recur.

Treatment requires avoidance of suspected substances and involves lifestyle changes that can range from minor to extensive. Patients are usually instructed to modify their diet and to avoid such substances as scented shampoos, aftershave products, deodorants, cigarette smoke, automobile fumes, and clothing, furniture, and carpets that contain synthetic fibers. Extreme restriction can involve staying at home for months or avoiding physical contact with family members. In many cases, patients' lives become centered around their treatment.

Critical Reports and Studies

Given the expense, time, and effort involved in such sweeping treatments, the question must be asked, Are they worth it? Are environmental factors really the cause of these problems? What does the mainstream medical community think about clinical ecology?

During the past few years, three prominent scientific panels have explored these question, concluding that clinical ecology is speculative and unproven.

- The California Medical Association Scientific Board Task Force on Clinical Ecology conducted an extensive literature review and held a hearing at which proponents testified. The task force concluded that "clinical ecology does not constitute a valid medical discipline." The task force also expressed concern that unproven diagnostic tests can lead to misdiagnosis that results in patients becoming psychologically dependent, believing themselves to be seriously and chronically impaired.

- The Ad Hoc Committee on the Environmental Hypersensitivity Disorders established by the Minister of Health of Ontario, Canada, received submissions, heard testimony from a large number of professionals and laypersons, observed practitioners at work, and issued a 500-page report. An expert panel then reviewed this report and concluded that "scientific support for the mechanism that have been proposed to underlie the wide variety of dysfunctions are at best hypothetical. Moreover, the majority of techniques for evaluating the patients and the treatments espoused are unproven."

- The American Academy of Allergy and Immunology, which is the nation's largest professional organization of allergists, published a position statement based on an extensive literature review and comments by its members. The statement said, "The idea that the environment is responsible for a multitude of human health problems is most appealing. However, to present, such ideas as facts, conclusions, or even likely mechanisms without adequate support is poor medical practice."

Independent studies of both diagnostic and treatment methods used in clinical ecology have likewise been critical:

- Abba I. Terr, MD., an allergist affiliated with Stanford University Medical Center, has reported on 50 patients who had received treatment from one or more of 16 clinical ecologists for an average of two years. Although all had received diagnosis of an environmental illness, Dr. Terr could find no unifying pattern of symptoms, physical findings, or laboratory abnormalities. Among other things, 14 of the patients had been advised to move their homes to rural areas, and a few were given vitamin and mineral supplements, gamma globulin, interferon, female hormones, and/or oral urine. Eight of the patients had not gotten their symptoms until after they had consulted the clinical ecologist because they had been worried about exposure to a chemical at work. Despite treatment, 26 patients reported no lessening of symptoms, 22 were clearly worse, and only two improved. Dr. Terr concluded that although exposure to chemicals can cause disease, it is unlikely that the diagnostic and treatment methods of clinical ecology are effective. He also concluded that its methods and theories appear to cause unnecessary fears and lifestyle restrictions. In 1989, he reported similar observations in 90 patients, including 40 from his previous report. More than one out of three had been diagnosed as suffering from candidiasis hypersensitivity, a controversial diagnosis discussed in the November 1990 issue of *Healthline*.

- Caroll M. Brodsky, M.D., Ph.D., professor of psychiatry at the University of California (San Francisco) School of Medicine, made similar observations after studying eight people who had filed claims for injury caused primarily by airborne substances after these injuries were diagnosed by clinical ecologists. He concluded that they became "adherents of physicians who believed that symptoms attributed by orthodox physicians to psychiatric causes are in fact due to common substances in air, food, and water."

- Donna E. Stewart, M.D., Associate Professor of Psychiatry and of Obstetrics and Gynecology at the University of Toronto, assessed 18 "20th century disease" patients referred to the university's psychiatric consultation service. She concluded that "virtually all had a long history of visits to physicians, and their symptoms were characteristic of several well-known psychiatric disorders."

How the Specialty Has Fought Back

Rejection by the scientific community has not dampened the enthusiasm of clinical ecologists, about 400 of whom belong to the American Academy of Environmental Medicine. This group, which holds meetings and publishes a quarterly journal, is composed mainly of medical doctors and osteopaths. Two years ago the journal announced that the paper on which it is printed had been changed because several readers had complained that the old paper had made them ill. Many doctors who treat "environmental illness" believe that they themselves have it.

Another advocacy group is the Human Ecology Action League (HEAL), formed in 1976 and composed of mainly laypersons. HEAL has chapters and support groups in about 100 cities. It distributes physician referral lists and publishes *The Human Ecologist*, a quarterly magazine of news and advice for patients and their families.

One major agenda item of proponents is trying to convince insurance companies to pay for their treatment, which can be quite expensive. In 18 cases reported to the Canadian committee, patients bore an average annual cost of $4,463 with a range from $400 to $12,378, most of which was not covered by insurance companies or government programs. In the United States, many suits have been filed by "ecologically ill" patients seeking reimbursement from insurance companies, but the scientific community's skepticism may mean that clinical ecology treatments continue to be considered speculative or unproven by insurance companies as well.

Too Many Questions

The number of people under the treatment of clinical ecologists is unknown. Nor can it be determined what percentage of them are being helped or harmed as a result. With these fundamental questions unanswered and with what data are available, I believe we must assume environmental illness is an imaginary condition, and patients who rely on its proponents may be risking misdiagnosis, mistreatment, and delay of proper medical care. Aggressive action by health educators and state licensing boards must be taken to alert the public and help protect them from these risks.

—by Stephen Barrett, M.D.

Dr. Barrett, a practicing psychiatrist and consumer advocate, edits *Nutrition Forum Newsletter* and is co-author/editor of 25 books including *Vitamins and "Health" Foods: The Great American Hustle*. In 1984, he received the FDA Commissioner's Special Citation Award for Public Service in fighting nutrition quackery.

Part Two

Outdoor Air Pollution

Chapter 7

Air Pollution and Your Health

Is Air Pollution Still a Problem?

Despite years of effort and some improvements, air pollution still clogs our nation's skies. Millions of tons of harmful gases and particles are released into the air each year. Smoke, smog and the murky "brown cloud" that blots out the sun in many cities are the air pollutants we see. Just as hazardous are other widespread pollutants and chemical poisons we can't see in the air.

Almost every major city in America is polluted, and air pollution problems have spread to smaller cities and even to rural areas. The U.S. Environmental Protection Agency (EPA) lists many areas of the nation, home to millions of Americans, where air pollution is so bad it exceeds federal health standards.

Polluted air can make healthy people cough and wheeze. For people who are already sick or especially sensitive, air pollution may mean discomfort, limited activities, increased use of medications, more frequent visits to doctors and hospitals, and even a shortened life. And a growing body of scientific studies suggests that air pollution has long-term effects on the lung's ability to function and on the development of lung disease.

Air pollution comes from power plants, factories, cars, trucks, and buses. It also comes from off-road vehicles such as farm and construction equipment, as well as from sources in our homes.

Air pollution costs us billions of dollars every year in health care and lost productivity. So even the fortunate Americans who are not breathing polluted air pay a price for it.

The level of risk posed by air pollution depends on several factors, including the amount of pollution in the air, the amount of air we breathe in a given time, the amount of air our lungs can accept, and our overall health.

The lung's natural defense system helps to protect against some of the air pollutants we breathe. And people respond differently to pollution. But, no matter where you live, chances are your lungs have been exposed to air pollution.

How Does Air Pollution Hurt the Body?

Air pollution hurts the body both by directly inflaming and destroying the lung tissue and by weakening the lung's defense against contaminants. Our bodies have ways of protecting us from breathing dust, pollen, and germs. Air pollution is an additional stress on the body's defenses.

A sticky substance called mucus lines our air passages. It traps germs and particles before they can enter the lungs. Then cells with tiny, waving hairs called cilia, push the mucus up and out of the body. Air pollution can paralyze or even destroy the cilia. That allows dirt and germs to build up in the mucus, leaving our bodies more vulnerable to disease.

Our bodies also defend themselves against pollution by trying to breathe less. Air passages tighten temporarily and breathing becomes harder. Air pollution can make your eyes water, irritate your nose, mouth and throat, and make you cough and sneeze.

Air pollution can make the effects of lung diseases like asthma, bronchitis and emphysema worse. High levels of carbon monoxide can add to the chest pain of people with heart disease, and may affect unborn and newborn children. It can make breathing harder, and can contribute to the premature death of people with heart and lung disease.

Smoking also harms the body's defenses, making the body more vulnerable to pollution and disease. It can make the effects of air pollution much worse.

What Are the Problem Pollutants?

Almost all chemicals find their way into the air. But many are released in such small amounts that they are not a health concern. Some substances are so common and widespread they build up in the air

76

and become a hazard to human health. The U.S. Environmental Protection Agency has developed health-based national air quality standards for six pollutants. They are:

- **Carbon monoxide (CO)** is an odorless, colorless, poisonous gas that comes mainly from motor vehicles and other combustion exhaust. Carbon monoxide interferes with the blood's ability to carry oxygen to the brain, heart and other tissues, and it is particularly dangerous for people with existing heart disease, and unborn or newborn children.

- **Ozone (O_3)** is the major harmful ingredient in smog. It is not emitted directly into the air but produced in the atmosphere when gases or vapors of organic chemicals called hydrocarbons combine with nitrogen oxide compounds in the presence of sunlight. Ozone reacts with lung tissue. It can inflame and cause harmful changes in breathing passages, decrease the lungs' working ability and cause both coughing and chest pains. Ozone air pollution, found at unhealthful levels in nearly all of the nation's major urban areas, may particularly affect millions of otherwise healthy Americans who, for currently unknown reasons, are especially sensitive to it. People who exercise also are more vulnerable to the effects of ozone, suffering symptoms and a reduced ability to breathe at relatively low ozone levels.

  Organic hydrocarbon gases, one of the raw ingredients of ozone, are released from a variety of sources related to human activities. Major sources include refineries, gas stations and motor vehicles, chemical plants, and paints and solvents.

  Harmful ozone in the lower atmosphere should not be confused with ozone in the upper atmosphere which protects us from ultraviolet radiation.

- **Nitrogen dioxide (NO_2)** and related nitrogen oxides (NO_x) are produced when fuel is burned, especially in power plants and motor vehicles. These oxides of nitrogen compounds contribute to ozone formation, and are a health problem themselves. NO_2 also changes in the atmosphere to form acidic particles and liquid nitric acid. Both may threaten human health. Nitrogen dioxide seems to act on the body like both ozone and sulfur dioxide.

- **Sulfur dioxide (SO_2)** is created when sulfur-containing fuel is burned, primarily in power plants and diesel engines. Like NO_2, it can also change in the atmosphere into acidic particles and into sulfuric acid.

Sulfur dioxide constricts air passages, making it a problem for people with asthma and for young children whose small lungs need to work harder than adult lungs. Even brief exposure to relatively low levels of sulfur dioxide can cause an asthma attack.

- **Particulate matter** includes microscopic particles and tiny droplets of liquid. These particles come from the burning of fuels by industry and diesel vehicles and from earth-moving activities such as construction and mining.

  Larger particles can be stopped in the nose and upper lungs by the body's natural defenses. The smallest particles escape the body's defenses and go deep into the lungs, where they may become trapped. Exposure to particulate pollution can cause wheezing and other symptoms in people with asthma or sensitive airways.

- **Lead** has been known as a poisonous substance for many years. The lead fumes in our urban air have come mostly from vehicles that use lead-containing gasoline. Lead poisoning can reduce mental ability, damage blood, nerves and organs, and raise blood pressure. Lead accumulates in the body, so repeated small doses can be harmful. In recent years, large reductions in the amount of lead in gasoline have resulted in a significant drop in public exposure to outdoor lead pollution. Remaining sources include incineration of lead batteries, burning lead-contaminated waste oil and exposure to old lead-containing paint.

In addition to these six pollutants for which air quality standards have been met, **toxic air pollution**, also referred to as hazardous air pollution, consists of those substances in the air which are known or suspected to cause cancer, genetic mutation, birth defects or other serious illnesses in people even at relatively low exposure levels. Toxic and cancer-causing chemicals can be inhaled directly or carried by small particles into the lungs. Millions of pounds of these chemicals are emitted into the air over our nation every year by motor vehicles and by both large and small industry. Exposure to these toxic contaminants is regulated by requiring the use of pollution controls on these sources, rather than by air quality standards. Your local American Lung Association has more information on these toxic pollutants.

What Is the Evidence Against Air Pollution?

Scientists study the effects of air pollution through animal experiments, by using human volunteers, and by examining hospital records and other health data from community surveys and testing of lung function.

Air pollution's harm has been documented in all three kinds of studies. Air pollution can kill, especially when several kinds of pollution work together. In London, a "killer fog" in 1952, polluted with sulfur and particles, took an estimated 3,500 lives. People with lung and heart diseases were particularly vulnerable.

Closer to home, a Harvard University study estimated that about 5 percent of deaths in the typical polluted American city each year are linked to acidic particles in the air. Another study of particulate pollution estimates that 60,000 premature deaths each year can be attributed to this type of air pollution.

Smog and sulfur pollution have been linked to increases in emergency room visits by asthma victims and others with lung problems.

Pollution is a serious problem even at relatively low levels. Studies of children and people with asthma have related coughing, wheezing and other signs of lung distress to pollution levels.

How Can I Protect Myself Against Air Pollution?

On days when weather forecasters or pollution control agencies report that air pollution levels are high, avoid exercise or strenuous activity outdoors. The elderly, people with heart or lung disease, and children should remain indoors and avoid exposure to outdoor air. Athletes should reschedule exercise for times when levels are lower.

What Can You Do about Air Pollution?

Actively support strong federal, state and local laws and regulations requiring effective control of air pollution. Public support is vital to the success of our nation's air pollution control efforts. Your own decisions about transportation and as a consumer of energy and products also makes a difference.

To find out more about air pollution and your health and how you can fight air pollution, contact your local American Lung Association today!

American Lung Association
475 H Street, N.W.
Washington, D.C. 20001

Chapter 8

Measuring Air Quality: The Pollutant Standards Index

The Pollutant Standards Index (PSI) has been developed by the Environmental Protection Agency (EPA) to provide accurate, timely, and easily understandable information about daily levels of air pollution. The Index provides EPA with a uniform system of measuring pollution levels for the major air pollutants regulated under the Clean Air Act. Once these levels are measured, the PSI figures are reported in all metropolitan areas of the United States with populations exceeding 200,000.

Index figures enable the public to determine whether air pollution levels in a particular location are good, moderate, unhealthful or worse. In addition, EPA and local officials use the PSI as a public information tool to advise the public about the general a health effects associated with different pollution levels, and to describe whatever precautionary steps may need to be taken if air pollution levels rise into the unhealthful range.

The EPA uses the Pollutant Standards Index to measure five major pollutants for which it has established National Ambient Air Quality Standards under the Clean Air Act. The pollutants are particulate matter (soot, dust, particles), sulfur dioxide, carbon monoxide, nitrogen dioxide and ozone.

Ozone at the ground level can be a health and environmental problem, but ozone is beneficial in the stratosphere (6-30 miles above the Earth) where it shields the Earth from the sun's harmful ultraviolet radiation. EPA has programs to reduce chlorofluorocarbons

EPA publication #451/K-94-001, February 1994.

and related substances to protect the stratospheric ozone layer. The PSI relates only to ground-level ozone, a major component of smog.

For each of these pollutants, EPA has established air quality standards protecting against health effects that can occur within short periods of time (a few hours or a day). For example, the standard for sulfur dioxide—that is, the allowable concentration of this pollutant in a community's air—is 0.14 parts per million measured over a 24-hour period. Air concentrations higher than 0.14 parts per million exceed the national standard. For ozone, the hourly average concentration permitted under the standard is 0.12 parts per million (ppm).

The PSI converts the measured pollutant concentration in a community's air to a number on a scale of 0 to 500. The most important number on this scale is 100, since that number corresponds to the standard established under the Clean Air Act. A 0.14 ppm reading for sulfur dioxide or a 0.12 ppm reading for ozone would translate to a PSI level of 100. A PSI level in excess of 100 means that a pollutant is in the unhealthful range on a given day; a PSI level at or below 100 means that a pollutant reading is in the satisfactory range.

The intervals and the terms describing the PSI air quality levels are as follows:

From 0 to 50	good
From 50 to 100	moderate
From 100 to 200	unhealthful
From 200 to 300	very unhealthful
Above 300	hazardous

The intervals on the PSI scale relate to the potential health effects of the daily concentrations of each of these five pollutants.

Each value has built into it a margin of safety that, based on current knowledge, protects highly susceptible members of the public.

EPA determines the index number on a daily basis for each of the five pollutants; it then reports the highest of the five figures for each major metropolitan area, and identifies which pollutant corresponds to the figure that is reported. For example, if EPA reports a PSI level of 90 for ozone for a given metropolitan area, residents of the area would know that the ozone level for the region is at the high end of the moderate range; they would also know that ozone is the pollutant with the highest PSI reading for the day, and that all other pollutants are therefore in the good or moderate range. On days when two or more pollutants exceed the standard (that is, have PSI values greater than 100), the pollutant with the highest index level is reported, but information on any other pollutants above 100 may also be reported.

Levels above 100 may trigger preventive action by State or local officials, depending upon the level of the pollution concentration. This could include health advisories for citizens or susceptible individuals to limit certain activities and potential restrictions on industrial activities. The 200 level is likely to trigger an "**Alert**" stage. Activities that might be restricted by local governments, depending upon the nature of the problem, include incinerator use, and open burning of leaves or refuse. A level of 300 on the PSI will probably trigger a "**Warning**," which is likely to prohibit the use of incinerators, severely curtail power plant operations, cut back operations at specified manufacturing facilities, and require the public to limit driving by using car pools and public transportation. A PSI level of 400 or above would constitute an "**Emergency**," and would require a cessation of most industrial and commercial activity, plus a prohibition of almost all private use of motor vehicles. If air pollution were to reach such extremely high levels, death could occur in some sick and elderly people, and even healthy people would likely experience symptoms that would necessitate restrictions on normal activity. Before determining which stage is to be called, officials examine both current pollutant concentrations and prevailing and predicted meteorological conditions.

The following identifies health effects associated with different levels of air pollution, along with the cautionary statements that would be appropriate if air pollution in a community were to fall into one of the "unhealthful" categories on the PSI scale:

General Health Effects and Cautionary Statements

Up to 50, Good. No general health effects for the general population. No cautionary statements required.

50 to 100, Moderate. Few or no health effects for the general populations. No statements required.

100 to 200 Unhealthful. Mild aggravation of symptoms among susceptible people, with irritation symptoms in the healthy population. Persons with existing heart or respiratory ailments should reduce physical exertion and outdoor activity. General population should reduce vigorous outdoor activity.

200 to 300 Very Unhealthful. Significant aggravation of symptoms and decreased exercise tolerance in persons with heart or lung disease; widespread symptoms in the healthy population. Elderly and persons with existing heart or lung disease should stay indoors and reduce physical activity. General population should avoid vigorous outdoor activity.

Over 300 Hazardous. Early onset of certain diseases in addition to significant aggravation of symptoms and decreased exercise tolerance in healthy persons. At PSI levels above 400, premature death of ill and elderly persons may result. Healthy people experience adverse symptoms that affect normal activity. Elderly and persons with existing diseases should stay indoors and avoid physical exertion. At PSI levels above 400, general population should avoid outdoor activity. All people should remain indoors, keeping windows and doors closed, and minimize physical exertion.

In most communities in the United States, PSI levels generally fall between zero and 100; readings in excess of 100 are likely to occur only a few times a year, if at all. Only 1.4 percent of all readings in the U.S. exceeded 100 during calendar years 1990 and 1991. Several metropolitan areas in the U.S. have more severe air pollution problems, and may often experience PSI levels in excess of 100. However, even in these areas, PSI readings in excess of 200 are quite rare. During calendar years 1990 and 1991, for example, just one-tenth of 1 percent of the PSI readings exceeded 200, and only 0.003 of 1 percent exceeded 300. (Urban areas outside the U.S. with dense population centers and large numbers of uncontrolled pollution sources frequently report PSI levels in excess of 250.)

Significant seasonal variations can occur in PSI-reported values. In winter, carbon monoxide is likely to be the pollutant with the highest PSI levels, because cold weather makes it much more difficult for automotive emission control systems to operate effectively. In summer, the chief pollutant in many communities is likely to be ozone, since emissions of volatile organic compounds and nitrogen oxides form ozone much more rapidly in the presence of heat and sunlight.

The PSI places maximum emphasis on acute health effects occurring over very short time periods—24 hours or less—rather than chronic effects occurring over months or years. By notifying the public when a PSI value exceeds 100, citizens are given an adequate opportunity to react and take whatever steps they can to avoid exposure.

The approach EPA follows is conservative, because (1) each standard has built into it a margin of safety that is designed to protect highly susceptible people, and (2) the public notice is triggered as soon as a single sampling station in the community records a PSI level that exceeds 100.

Use of the PSI allows for flexible reporting. A typical television or radio announcement might read: "The pollution index reported at noon today is 150, and the air is considered unhealthful. The pollutant causing this problem is ozone, which, along with other components of smog, can cause eye, nose and throat irritation, as well as chest pain. We expect the concentration of ozone to diminish this afternoon. People with respiratory ailments and heart disease should reduce physical exertion and outdoor activity at this time. The forecast for tomorrow calls for no change in the index." A more detailed account could be provided by recorded telephone reports or newspapers. For example, listeners can be informed that ozone normally peaks in the afternoon so that later PSI reports will show the index declining, unless there is a significant episode taking place that would cause ozone to continue to build throughout the day. Likewise, if carbon monoxide is the pollutant of concern, the PSI report could add that carbon monoxide is usually only a problem during morning or evening rush hours with acceptable air quality expected during the rest of the day.

Although it is uniform across the country, the PSI cannot be used as the sole method for ranking the relative healthfulness of different cities—a variety of factors in addition to PSI levels would have to be considered. For example, the number of people actually exposed to air pollution, transportation patterns, industrial composition, and the representativeness of the monitoring sites would also need to be taken into account in developing an accurate ranking of metropolitan areas.

Moreover, the PSI does not specifically take into account the damage air pollutants can do to animals, vegetation, and certain materials, like building surfaces and statues. There is, however, likely to be a correlation between increased PSI levels and increased damage to the overall environment, and a local regulatory agency might choose to point out the impact that an elevated PSI value is likely to have on agriculture and property in the region.

Finally, the PSI does not take into account the possible adverse effects associated with combinations of pollutants (synergism). As more research is completed in the future, the PSI may be modified by EPA to include such effects. The following material highlights the sources, health effects, and significant harm levels for the five air pollutants for which the PSI currently applies: carbon monoxide, ozone, nitrogen dioxide, sulfur dioxide, and particulate matter. This information will be revised over time as EPA analyzes newly available scientific studies.

Carbon Monoxide

Sources. Carbon monoxide (CO) is an odorless, colorless gas that is a by-product of the incomplete burning of fuels. Industrial processes contribute to CO pollution levels, but the principal source of CO pollution in most large urban areas is the automobile. Cigarettes and other sources of incomplete burning in the indoor environment also produce CO. CO is inhaled and enters the blood stream; there it binds chemically to hemoglobin, the substance that carries oxygen to the cells, thereby reducing the amount of oxygen delivered to all tissues of the body. The percentage of hemoglobin inactivated by CO depends on the amount of air breathed, the concentration of CO in air, and length of exposure; this is indexed by the percentage of carboxyhemoglobin found in the blood.

Health effects. CO weakens the contractions of the heart, thus reducing the amount of blood pumped to various parts of the body and, therefore, the oxygen available to the muscles and various organs. In a healthy person, this effect significantly reduces the ability to perform physical exercises. In persons with chronic heart disease, these effects can threaten the overall quality of life, since their systems are unable to compensate for the decrease in oxygen. CO pollution is also likely to cause such individuals to experience angina during exercise. Adverse effects have also been observed in individuals with heart conditions who are exposed to CO pollution in heavy freeway traffic for one to two hours or more.

In addition, fetuses, young infants, pregnant women, elderly people, and individuals with anemia or emphysema are likely to be more susceptible to the effects of CO. For these individuals, the effects are more pronounced when exposure takes place at high altitude locations, where oxygen concentration is lower. CO can also affect mental function, visual activity, and alertness of healthy individuals, even at relatively low concentrations.

Air quality levels. The air quality standard for CO, which is designed to protect public health with an adequate margin of safety, is

9 ppm, averaged over eight hours. EPA is required to issue a public alert when CO levels reach 15 ppm, a public warning when CO levels reach 30 ppm, and a public declaration of emergency at the level of 40 ppm. The significant harm level, at which serious and widespread health effects occur to the general population, is 50 ppm of CO.

Ozone

Sources. Ozone (O_3), a colorless gas, is the major constituent of smog. It is produced by the chemical reaction of nitrogen dioxide with reactive organic substances—such as hydrocarbons in automobile exhaust or vapors from cleaning solvents in the presence of sunlight. This type of pollution first gained attention in the 1940s as Los Angeles "smog." Since then, photochemical smog has been observed frequently in many other cities as well. [Note: In the upper atmosphere, naturally occurring ozone is beneficial in protecting us from the harmful solar rays.]

Health effects. Ozone and other photochemical oxidants such as peroxyacyl nitrates and aldehydes are associated with health effects in humans. Peroxyacyl nitrates and aldehydes cause the eye irritation that is characteristic of photochemical pollution. Ozone has a greater impact on the respiratory system, where it irritates the mucous membranes of the nose, throat and airways; 90 percent of the ozone inhaled into the lungs is never exhaled. Symptoms associated with exposure include cough, chest pain, and throat irritation. Ozone can also increase susceptibility to respiratory infections. In addition, ozone impairs normal functioning of the lungs and reduces the ability to perform physical exercise. For example, healthy individuals who exercise heavily for brief periods (one to two hours) may experience respiratory symptoms at levels exceeding the national standard (0.12 ppm). Recent studies also suggest that even at lower ozone concentrations some healthy individuals engaged in moderate exercise for six to eight hours may experience symptoms. All of these effects are more severe in individuals with sensitive respiratory systems, and studies show that moderate levels may impair the ability of individuals with asthma or respiratory disease to engage in normal daily activities.

The potential chronic effects of repeated exposure to ozone are of even greater concern. Laboratory studies show that people exposed over a six to eight hour period to relatively low ozone levels develop lung inflammation. Animal studies suggest that if exposures are repeated over a long period (e.g., months, years, lifetime), inflammation of this type may lead to permanent scarring of lung tissue, loss of lung function, and reduced lung elasticity.

Air quality levels. The air quality standard for ozone, which is designed to protect public health with an adequate margin of safety, is 0.12 ppm, hourly average. EPA is required to issue a public alert when ozone levels reach 0.20 ppm, a public warning when ozone levels reach 0.40 ppm, and a declaration of public emergency at 0.50 ppm. The significant harm level, at which serious and widespread health effects occur among the general population, is 0.60 ppm of ozone, averaged over two hours.

Nitrogen Dioxide

Sources. Nitrogen dioxide (NO_2) is a light brown gas that can become an important component of urban haze. Nitrogen oxides usually enter the air as the result of high-temperature combustion processes, such as those occurring in automobiles and power plants. NO_2 plays an important role in the atmospheric reactions that generate ozone. Home heaters and gas stoves also produce substantial amounts of NO_2.

Health effects. Healthy individuals experience respiratory problems when exposed to high levels of NO_2 for short durations (less than three hours). Asthmatics are especially sensitive, and changes in airway responsiveness have been observed in some studies of exercising asthmatics exposed to relatively low levels of NO_2. Studies also indicate a relationship between indoor NO_2 exposures and increased respiratory illness rates in young children, but definitive results are still lacking. Many animal studies suggest that NO_2 impairs respiratory defense mechanisms and increases susceptibility to infection.

Several studies also show that chronic exposure to relatively low NO_2 pollution levels may cause structural changes in the lungs of animals. These studies suggest that chronic exposure to NO_2 could lead to adverse health effects in humans, but specific levels and durations likely to cause such effects have not yet been determined.

Air quality levels. The air quality standard for NO_2, which is designed to protect public health with an adequate margin of safety, is 0.053 ppm, annual average. EPA is required to issue a public alert when NO_2 reaches 0.6 ppm on a one hour average, a public warning when NO_2 reaches 1.2 ppm, and a declaration of public emergency at the level of 1.6 ppm. The significant harm level, at which serious and widespread health effects occur to the general population, is 2.0 ppm of NO_2.

Sulfur Dioxide

Sources. Sulfur dioxide (SO_2) is a colorless reactive gas that is odorless at low concentrations, but pungent at very high concentrations. It is emitted primarily when fossil fuels and ores that contain sulfur are burned or processed. Major sources of SO_2 are fossil-fuel-burning power plants and industrial boilers.

Health effects. Exposure to SO_2 can cause impairment of respiratory function, aggravation of existing respiratory disease (especially bronchitis), and a decrease in the ability of the lungs to clear foreign particles. It can also lead to increased mortality, especially if elevated levels of particulate matter (PM) are also present. Groups that appear most sensitive to the effects of SO_2 include asthmatics and other individuals with hyperactive airways, and individuals with chronic obstructive lung or cardiovascular disease. Elderly people and children are also likely to be sensitive to SO_2.

Effects of short-term peak exposures have been evaluated in controlled human exposure studies. These studies show that SO_2 generally increases airway resistance in the lungs, and can cause significant constriction of air passages in sensitive asthmatics. These impacts have been observed in subjects engaged in moderate to heavy exercise while exposed to relatively high peak concentrations. These changes in lung function are accompanied by perceptible symptoms such as wheezing, shortness of breath, and coughing in these sensitive groups.

The presence of PM appears to aggravate the impact of SO_2 pollution. Several studies of chronic effects have found that people living in areas with high PM and SO_2 levels have a higher incidence of respiratory illnesses and symptoms than people living in areas without such a synergistic combination of pollutants.

Air quality levels. The air quality standard for SO_2, which is designed to protect public health with an adequate margin safety, is 0.14 ppm, averaged over 24 hours. EPA is required to issue a public alert when SO_2 levels reach 0.30 ppm on hour average, a public warning when SO_2 levels reach 0.60 ppm on a 24-hour average, and a declaration of public emergency at the level of 0.80 ppm. The significant harm level, at which serious and widespread health effects occur to the general population, is 1.0 ppm of SO_2.

Particulate Matter.

Sources. Particulate matter (PM) is solid matter or liquid droplets from smoke, dust, fly ash, or condensing vapors that can be suspended in the air for long periods of time. It represents a broad class of chemically diverse particles that range in size from molecular clusters of 0.005 micrometers (μm) to coarse particles of 50-100 μm in diameter (100 μm is about the thickness of an average human hair). PM results from all types of combustion. The carbon-based particles that result from incomplete burning of diesel fuel in buses, trucks and cars are of particular concern. Another important combustion source is the burning of wood in stoves and fireplaces in residential settings. Also of concern are the sulfate and nitrate particles that are formed as a byproduct of SO_2 and NO_2 emissions, primarily from fossil fuel-burning power plants and vehicular exhausts.

The U.S. national ambient air quality standard was originally based on particles up to 25-45 μm in size, termed "total suspended particles" (TSP). In 1987, EPA replaced TSP with an indicator that includes only those particles smaller than 10 μm, termed PM_{10}. These smaller particles cause most of the adverse health effects because of their ability to penetrate deeply into the lungs.

Health Effects. The observed human health effects of PM include breathing and respiratory symptoms, aggravation of existing respiratory and cardiovascular disease, alterations in the body's defense system against inhaled materials and organisms, and damage to lung tissue. Groups that appear to be most sensitive to the effects of PM include individuals with chronic lung or cardiovascular disease, individuals with influenza, asthmatics, elderly people, and children.

Marked increases in daily mortality have been statistically associated with very high 24-hour concentrations of PM_{10}, with some increased risk of mortality at lower concentrations. Small increases in mortality appear to exist at even lower levels. Risks to sensitive individuals increase with consecutive, multiday exposures to elevated PM concentrations. The research also indicates that aggravation of bronchitis occurs with elevated 24-hour PM_{10} levels, and small decreases in lung function take place when children are exposed to lower 24-hour peak PM_{10} levels. Lung function impairment persists for 2-3 weeks following exposure to PM.

Air quality levels. The air quality standard for PM_{10}, which is designed to protect public health with an adequate margin of safety, is 150 micrograms per cubic meter (μm^3), averaged over 24 hours. EPA is required to issue a public alert when PM_{10} levels reach 350 μm^3 on a 24-hour average, a public warning when PM_{10} levels reach 420 μm^3 on a 24-hour average, and a declaration of public emergency at the level of 500 μm^3. The significant harm level, at which serious and widespread health effects occur to the general population, is 600 μm^3 of PM_{10}.

Chapter 9

Declining Air Quality Triggers More Attacks of Asthma

Breathing is something that most people take for granted. Without giving it a thought, we pull an invisible stream of gases, aerosols, particles, microbes, pollen, and dust into our lungs with every breath. But not everyone breathes easily. For the more than 14 million Americans with asthma, breathing becomes difficult when sensitive airways are inflamed and constricted. The number of people with asthma increased by 42 percent in the last decade, according to a recent report by the Centers for Disease Control. Not only is asthma becoming more prevalent, but it is also more severe. According to the National Heart, Lung, and Blood Institute, the number of people who die of asthma jumped 58 percent between 1979 and 1992. Emergency room visits and hospital admissions for asthma are increasing. Children, ethnic minorities, and the urban poor are at the greatest risk. Researchers suspect that a variety of factors such as air contaminants and heightened exposure to aero-allergens in airtight homes trigger bouts of asthma or cause chronic airway inflammation that may lead to permanent lung dysfunction.

What could be making a respiratory disease, triggered by an allergic response and aggravated by a multitude of factors, more common, more acute, and potentially more fatal?

The rising number of asthmatics might be attributed to increased awareness among physicians, said Gale Weinman of the National Heart, Lung, and Blood Institute (NHLBI). "Physicians may now be

NIH Publication, *Environmental Health Perspectives* Volume 104, Number 1, January 1996.

recognizing ailments previously diagnosed as a cold or bronchitis as the long-term, chronic illness of asthma. However, increased diagnosis of asthma cannot [totally] explain the rise in its prevalence," she said.

"We're looking at a disproportionate rise in the incidence and mortality of asthma in ethnic minorities and those living in poverty," said Darryl Zeldin, a clinical investigator of asthma in the NIEHS Laboratory of Pulmonary Pathobiology. "Most researchers believe that there must be some environmental component to that. In the lower socioeconomic groups, individuals are being exposed very early in life to allergens. Once sensitized, repeated exposure to these allergens leads to chronic airway inflammation and asthma. But most likely there are multiple factors."

More Common, More Deadly

When people with asthma encounter allergens, environmental irritants, cold air, or viral infections, a complex cascade of events leads to airway inflammation and constriction. As air is forced past smaller and constricted openings, asthmatics develop an audible wheeze, shortness of breath, chest pain, and often coughing. Long-term exposure to irritants without medical intervention can lead to permanent reductions in lung function, damage to lung tissue, severe breathing discomfort, and lower resistance to infection, according to the American Lung Association (ALA).

For the 70 to 75 percent of asthmatics who have allergic asthma, their respiratory systems have developed a very specific response to a specific allergens. Nonallergic asthmatics, on the other hand, may wheeze after exercising or taking aspirin, and show little sensitivity to allergens. Asthma and allergies appear to be inherited separately, but they are mysteriously associated. Most asthmatics can name at least one person in their family who has asthma or allergies. At least half of the people with asthma have allergic rhinitis, or inflammation of the nasal membranes, and 35 percent have atopic dermatitis, known as eczema.

Asthma is a more manageable disease than it was three decades ago. "The philosophy of asthma management has changed," said Peter Gergen, director of the Office of Epidemiology and Clinical Trials at the National Institute of Allergy and Infectious Diseases. "The role of inflammation in asthma became more accepted. The use of anti-inflammatory drugs and the monitoring of peak-flow [a measurement of the ability to exhale air from the lungs] has been increasing through the 1980s." Rather than focussing on asthma attacks already on progress, physicians emphasize prevention of wheezing and maintenance of optimal lung function, said Gergen. The National Asthma Education Program, sponsored by the NHLBI, has provided physicians and patients with guidelines for treating asthma and helped change their understanding and management of the disease.

Still, during the last three decades, asthma prevalence and morbidity in the United States has been rising. "The paradox of asthma is that we've had good treatment and quite adequate medications, and yet we're still having this problem," said Gergen. From 1982 to 1992, the number of people 5 to 34 years old who were afflicted with asthma increased by 52 percent, according to a recent CDC report. This seems to follow an earlier trend found by Gergen and associates in the 1970s, when asthma prevalence among 6 to 11 year-olds increased by 58 percent.

The increase in asthma is not unique to the United States. Asthma appears to be growing worse in other economically developed countries as well. In Great Britain, deaths and hospital admissions due to asthma doubled between 1979 and 1985. In Finland, the proportion of military recruits with asthma increased 20-fold between 1961 and 1989. Sweden and Denmark also saw increasing death rates from asthma through the 1970s. Health statistics are only one measure of asthma's high cost.

Health care expenses for asthma reach $6.2 billion per year, or nearly 1 percent of all U.S. health care expenses in 1985, according to a 1992 study by Kevin Weiss, director of research at the Rush Presbyterian St. Luke's Medical Center in Chicago, published in the *New England Journal of Medicine*. Of that amount, $1.6 billion was spent for inpatient hospital costs.

Asthma exacts an equally significant personal cost. Asthma is the number one cause of absenteeism for schoolchildren and a common reason for adult absenteeism from work. In 1985, adults with asthma lost nearly three million work days, at a cost of $285 million, according to an analysis by Weiss.

Though death from asthma is relatively rare, it is becoming more frequent. Asthma mortality in the United States declined by nearly 8 percent per year during the 1970s, but by 1977, the trend reversed, and the number of deaths due to asthma began to climb steadily, increasing about 6 percent per year. Asthma killed 1,674 Americans in 1977, but by 1991 the death rate had risen to 5,106 (from 0.8 to 2.0 per 100,000 people). Although most asthmatics who die of the disease are over 50 years old, rates of asthma death have increased in almost all age groups, according to Michael Sly, chairman of Allergy and Immunology at the Children's National Medical Center in Washington, D.C..

Most asthma deaths occur in urban areas. In 1985, 21 percent of asthma deaths among 5 to 34 year olds occurred in New York City and Cook County, Illinois (which includes Chicago), where only 6.8 percent of the U.S. population in this age group resided, according to Weiss. David Lang and Marcia Polansky of the Hahnemann University Hospital reported in a 1994 study in the *New England Journal of Medicine* that a disproportionate number of the asthma deaths in Pennsylvania occurred in Philadelphia, where mortality was clustered in poorer neighborhoods.

Although some evidence suggests that asthma's death toll could be leveling off, the rising rate of hospital admissions and emergency room and doctor's office visits for asthma suggests the disease is becoming more severe. Between 1965 and 1983, hospitalization rates for asthma increased by 50 percent in adults and over 200 percent in children. Approximately 4.5 percent more children were hospitalized for asthma each year from 1979 to 1987, Gergen and Weiss found.

Disproportionate Risk

Blacks, Hispanics, and people living in urban environments seem to be at the greatest risk for asthma. Using data on the U.S. population between 1976 and 1908 from the National Health and Nutrition Examination Survey, Gergen and co-workers found that asthma occurs more frequently in black children than in white, and more often in urban areas than rural ones. The prevalence of asthma in these groups was not associated with gross family income, education level of the head of household, poverty index ratio, or crowding, the researchers found. In the 1980s, three times as many black children as white children under four were hospitalized because of asthma. Blacks 5 to 34 years of age are five times more likely to die of asthma than whites.

As depicted in a recent *New York Times* article about inhaler use in the South Bronx, Puerto Ricans in the United States suffer from asthma far more frequently than other ethnic groups. One in every five (20.1 percent) Puerto Rican children (6 months to 11 years) in the United States had asthma in 1982 to 1984, compared to 4.5 percent of Mexican-American, 8.8 percent of Cuban, 9.1 percent of black, and 6.5 percent of white children. Researchers have proposed that the high prevalence of asthma among Puerto Ricans could result from a possible genetic predisposition, or from the high rate of smoking among Puerto Rican women of childbearing age.

Blacks and Hispanics in Philadelphia had higher rates of death from asthma, but only in areas with higher poverty rates, according to Lang and Polansky. A study by Lawrence Wissow and colleagues at the Johns Hopkins University Hospital suggests that black children in Maryland are more likely to be hospitalized for asthma, but this tendency may be more strongly related to poverty than to race. The hospitalization rate for asthma in Maryland increased three times faster for blacks than for whites during the 1979 to 1982 period, but when poverty was considered as a factor, many of the racial differences in hospitalization rates disappeared. A higher proportion of children on Medicaid, or with no health insurance, were hospitalized for asthma than children with private health insurance.

These findings raise important questions about why the economically disadvantaged are at greatest risk of dying from asthma. "Poverty is associated with all sorts of diseases," said Gergen. "Poor people in the United States die more than the rich of all causes, and the gap is widening. General health is poorer, as well as access to medical care. Exposure, environmental quality of life, stress, and social factors all play a role," said Gergen.

Environmental Culprits

Spurred by the alarming statistics, researchers are focusing on direct exposures to allergens indoors where people are spending more of their time. Allergen levels are thought to be higher in less well-ventilated homes, where moisture accumulates, allowing mildew and molds to grow. Research shows that cumulative exposure to dust mites, which live in bedding, upholstery, and carpets, causes some people to develop allergic sensitivity, including asthma and airway hyper-responsiveness. The levels of cockroach antigen generally found in suburban homes are too low to sensitize individuals, but the 10-fold higher levels found in inner-city dwellings are enough to cause sensitization and appear to be associated with asthma.

"We're also concerned about second-hand tobacco smoke," said Alfred Munzer, pulmonary specialist at Washington Adventist Hospital and former president of the ALA. "There is increasing evidence that childhood exposure to environmental smoke can be a predisposing factor to developing asthma." The Harvard Six Cities Air Pollution Health Study demonstrated that in families where parents smoke, the frequency of coughing and wheezing in their children is increased by up to 30 percent. A 1986 study reported in the *American Review of Respiratory Diseases* that was conducted in Tecumseh, Michigan, showed parental smoking was associated with increased prevalence and risk of asthma in children.

Infants of women who smoke have higher levels of the antibody immunoglobin E (IgE) in umbilical cord blood compared to infants of nonsmokers, indicating an immune reaction. Whether children born to smoking mothers develop asthma pre- or post-natally, is an unanswered question. The increase in asthma prevalence in western countries is correlated with more women of childbearing age smoking, according to a 1990 British study in the *British Medical Journal.*

Increasing asthma incidence cannot totally be explained by smoking in the United States, however. Between 1965 and 1990, cigarette smoking in the United States declined by 40 percent. Though the greatest number of smokers are 25 to 44 years of age, poorly educated, and live below the poverty level, according to statistics from the CDC's Office on Smoking and Health, the proportion of smokers in this group is also following a downward trend.

The National Inner City Asthma Study (NICAS), underway in seven U.S. cities, sponsored by the National Institute of Allergy and Infectious Diseases (NIAID), may soon add to our understanding of the disease. During the first phase of NICAS, begun in 1991, health researchers surveyed people with asthma in selected cities to identify factors in their lives most strongly associated with asthma. These included access to medical care, the patient's understanding of the disease and its potential severity, and factors in the home that exacerbate asthma. Results are still being analyzed, but initial conclusions indicate that cockroach antigen is a more prevalent allergen in inner-city households than dust mite antigen.

In the second phase of NICAS, co-sponsored by the NIEHS, researchers will intervene to reduce allergen exposure inside inner-city residences. George Malindzak of the NIEHS is an administrator for the second phase, scheduled to begin this winter. "We know that some components of indoor air have a definite provocative effect on asthma," Malindzak said. "We're now looking into things that people with asthma can do for themselves to alleviate asthma episodes."

The NIEHS is involved in recommending ways to reduce dust mites and cockroaches as well as evaluating allergy symptoms and lung function in children who are susceptible to recurrent wheezing. NICAS data should provide some insight into the soaring asthma rates among the poor and minorities in inner cities.

Other studies are exploring the influence of a child's surroundings during the vulnerable first weeks and months of life. It is precisely during this period, scientists believe, that the environment of a child with a genetic predisposition can tip the scales toward developing a full-fledged allergy.

"Sensitization is the critical point," said Harvard School of Public Health researcher Douglas Dockery, who is working on another study funded by NIAID. "You have to have a combination of genetic factors which puts you at risk but also a challenge via environmental exposure that sensitizes you," said Dockery. Indeed, evidence suggests that increased exposure to dust mites in early life is associated with increased allergic responses and asthma.

Using a sample of newborn children whose parents have a history of asthma and allergies, Dockery and co-workers will follow the infants' health while monitoring their home exposure to dust mites, cockroaches, and other antigens. "Asthma is clearly a multifactorial process," said Dockery. "A lot of things could be contributing. I believe nutritional factors are important. There is also the whole maintenance issue and the need for empowerment of these people who have asthma and need appropriate clinical support."

In some urban areas, more than half of the children with asthma may receive all their medical care at the emergency room, and many are never diagnosed. "The fact that many inner-city asthmatics end up in the hospital shows that something is wrong with the treatment," said Gergen. The uninsured have poor access to long-range care programs that would provide help in managing the disease and preventing acute episodes.

Increasing awareness of asthma and improving treatment are the aims of the National Asthma Education Program, a major effort of the NHLBI since 1989. In addition to training professionals about asthma management, the program is working with communities and organizations to educate people about asthma, including school staff, teachers, and coaches.

Breathing Bad Air

"The consensus seems to be that the environment is playing a tremendous role in the increasing prevalence of asthma," said Munzer. In addition to the provocation of asthma by allergens, he says, "air pollution is a big factor."

The nation's air has improved dramatically in the past 25 years. Emissions of soot and smog-forming volatile organic compounds have decreased significantly in the United States since 1970 despite crowded highways where more vehicles are driven twice as many miles. Release of sulfur oxide has decreased by 30 percent since 1970. Between 1988 and 1993, overall industrial emissions of toxic compounds decreased by 39 percent.

The distribution of asthma in other countries also fails to implicate pollution as an aggravating factor. Some of the highest asthma mortality rates occur in Australia and New Zealand, which have excellent air quality. Asthma is more prevalent in rural areas of the Scottish highlands, which have some of the lowest ozone concentrations in the world, than in more urban and polluted parts of the United Kingdom, according to a recent report.

Several U.S. studies of air quality and respiratory disease have also come up empty-handed in linking asthma to air pollution. In a comparison of schoolchildren in the Six Cities Study, measurements of lung function and asthma prevalence did not differ significantly between cities in relation to air quality. Philadelphia's soaring numbers of asthma deaths from 1978 to 1991 were starkly contrasted with the city's declining average annual air pollutant levels in the study by Lang and Polansky.

In spite of overall improvements in air quality, many Americans are not breathing risk-free air, according to EPA Administrator Carol Browner. Almost 100 million people live in areas where the air does not meet national air quality standards. Eighty percent of Hispanics and 65 percent of blacks live in "non-attainment areas" for air standards. For more sensitive populations, like those with asthma, polluted air presents a daily challenge.

"It is clear that for people with asthma, episodes of air pollution will aggravate that preexisting condition, resulting in more symptoms, more use of medications, and more hospital visits," said Dockery. "We can show that it is related to day-to-day variations in air quality."

In the Six Cities Study, scientists found that the odds of having bronchitis increased with greater concentrations of fine particulates (particles less than 15 micrometers in diameter). Moreover, the 10 percent of children with asthma or persistent wheeze accounted for 42 percent of the bronchitis episodes.

Another study by Dockery and Harvard researcher C.A. Pope substantiated these findings. When fine particle concentrations reached the current air quality standard of 150 micrograms per cubic meter

(μg/m^3), schoolchildren experienced increased respiratory symptoms, and those with asthma doubled their use of asthma medications.

The question remains whether small particles in the atmosphere provoke asthma episodes. In Seattle, Washington, a study by Joel Schwartz of the Harvard School of Public Health and co-workers showed that the PM$_{10}$ level (number of particles less than 10 micrometers in diameter) on the previous day was a significant predictor of the number of emergency room visits for asthma. At 30 μg/m^3—the mean concentration of PM$_{10}$ in Seattle during the study period—PM$_{10}$ exposure appeared to be responsible for approximately 12 percent of the emergency visits for asthma, according to Schwartz.

Higher PM$_{10}$ levels in other communities also present a serious concern. In 1992, nearly one-fifth of Americans with asthma lived in areas where PM$_{10}$ levels exceeded the national standard of 150 μg/m^3, and nearly one-half were exposed to levels exceeding 55 μg/m^3, according to the ALA.

No one understands why small particles may provoke asthma. "Larger particles get trapped by our defense mechanisms, but these fine particles behave almost like a gas, going very deep into the lungs," said Munzer.

"It is puzzling that we observed the same effects: mortality, hospital admissions, aggravation of asthma, and reduced pulmonary function, associated with particles in Los Angeles, Philadelphia, and Steubenville, Ohio," said Dockery. "Clearly, the particles in these cities have a different chemical makeup, but all of the particles in the different communities come from combustion, whether from automobile engines, as in Los Angeles, from industry and power plants in Philadelphia, or from steel mills in Steubenville," he said.

In 1993, the ALA sued the EPA for failing to follow the Clean Air Act requirement to review the PM$_{10}$ standard five years after its establishment in 1987. The EPA, now performing a review under a court-ordered schedule, is required to make recommendations by the end of January 1997. "If EPA tightens the current particulate standards, as recent scientific evidence suggests it should, potentially tens of thousands of hospitalizations, respiratory problems, and premature deaths can be avoided each year," said Ronald H. White, ALA director of environmental health.

Mark Utell, of the University of Rochester Medical Center and a member of the EPA's Clean Air Scientific Advisory Committee, which reviews EPA staff recommendations and PM$_{10}$ criteria documents, believes that the toxicity of particulates should be more completely understood before standards are lowered. "There is no real toxicological basis for understanding how PM_{10} is linked with the epidemiological results. We need a stronger framework for understanding associations that occur with PM_{10}, at concentrations as low as 30 micrograms per cubic meter," said Utell.

The ALA also sued the EPA for failing to review the federal ozone standard. The ALA estimates that the health of two million children under age 18 who have asthma is potentially at risk because they live in high-smog areas (ozone is the main component of smog). EPA staff scientists concede that a more stringent standard is needed to protect public health. In the second staff paper of the review, the agency has recommended that the old standard of 0.12 ppm be lowered to an average concentration of 0.07 to 0.09 ppm over an 8-hour period, with one to five exceedances allowed per year.

Ozone is a powerful oxidant and respiratory irritant. Studies in recent years have linked ozone levels well below current U.S. health standards to a decline in lung function, respiratory symptoms, and increased hospital admissions and emergency room visits for respiratory problems. Other pollutants, such as sulfur dioxide, the main component of acid aerosols, and nitrogen dioxide, an indoor pollutant from gas stoves, dearly exacerbate asthma. Results of the Six Cities Study associated acid aerosols with respiratory symptoms, changed pulmonary function, and mortality.

"An important question is whether pollutant gases can enhance a person's susceptibility to being sensitized [to allergens]," said Paul Nettesheim, chief of the Laboratory of Pulmonary Pathobiology at the NIEHS. Animal studies have shown that ozone, sulfur dioxide, and components of diesel exhaust fumes irritate cells lining the airways and increase an animal's sensitivity to inhaled allergens. Irritation of the bronchi by pollutants like ozone could make it easier for antigens to penetrate the airway lining and reach lymphocytes and other cells involved in the allergic response, Nettesheim said.

David Peden, an investigator at the Center for Environmental Medicine and Lung Biology of the University of North Carolina at Chapel Hill School of Medicine, has examined how ozone exposure might exacerbate the response of people who are allergic to dust mites when they are in contact with the allergen. His results suggest that ozone would worsen the asthmatic response. But whether ozone exposure increases the likelihood of developing allergies in general, is still open to question.

One study showed people with asthma to be more sensitive to ragweed pollen when they were exposed to substantial amounts of ozone.

"One could say . . . if not for ozone, these people with asthma could make it all the way through the ragweed season without trouble," said Jane Koenig of the University of Washington School of Public Health, a co-author of the paper with Schwartz. "Then you have to ask, how does one decide what your main stimulus is to control? Ragweed would be hard to control. Ozone might be a little easier."

While many factors that provoke asthma, such as air pollution and cigarette smoking, are decreasing, the disease is becoming more prevalent. Its increasing severity is concentrated in urban pockets where children live under poor conditions, are frequently exposed to allergens and air pollution episodes, and have sporadic medical care. Research suggests that education, controlling exposure to antigens in the indoor environment, and improving urban air quality could improve the quality of life for these children.

—by Elaine Friebele

Chapter 10

Chemical Air Pollutants and Otorhinolaryngeal Toxicity

Introduction

Air pollution and the specific issue regarding the impact of airborne chemical agents to human health are familiar topics to most members of the environmental health science and environmental medicine communities. Some aspects, however, have received relatively less attention. Much has been published regarding the impact of air pollutants on the human upper and lower respiratory system, including interaction with the rhinologic (nasal) system. Relatively fewer data have been published, however, regarding the potential impact of air pollutants in reference specifically to the otologic (auditory and vestibular) and the laryngeal (larynx) system. Adverse impact to the ears, nose and throat, referred to as the "otorhinolaryngeal system," warrants attention as an important environmental health issue. Toxic interactions from exposure to many chemical air pollutants not only cause potential respiratory irritation and lung disease, but can also result in impaired hearing, balance, sense of smell, taste, and speech due to interaction with related target systems. This may be significant to environmental health risk assessment of chemical air pollutants if multi-target site models are considered.

The major modes for foreign or exogenous chemical agents entering the human body are inhalation, ingestion, and dermal absorption. Although debatable, inhalation of chemical aerosols, gases, and vapors is considered by many to be the primary mode of exposure to chemical agents. Exposure to chemical air pollutants is a concern because many can interfere toxicologically with specific and multiple biochemical and physiological processes of the human body and, in turn, cause illness or dysfunction. Environmental risk assessments must consider both short term and long term effects to multiple target sites relative to duration, intensity, and frequency of exposure to airborne chemical agents.

Air pollution and the specific issue regarding the impact of airborne chemical agents to human health are familiar topics to most members of the environmental health science and environmental medicine communities. Some aspects, however, have received relatively less attention. For example, much has been published regarding the impact of air pollutants on the human upper and lower respiratory system, including interaction with the rhinologic (nasal) system and lungs, respectively. Until recently, however, relatively few data have been published regarding the potential impact of air pollutants specifically in reference to the otologic (auditory and vestibular) and the laryngeal (larynx) systems. Adverse impact to the ears, nose, and throat, hereafter referred to as the "otorhinolaryngeal system," should be an important environmental health concern. Toxic interactions from exposure to chemical air pollutants not only cause potential irritation and lung disease, but can also result in impaired hearing, balance, sense of smell, taste, and speech. Accordingly, the objectives of this chapter are to initially provide an overview of major aspects of chemical air pollution and, subsequently, to provide a summary of the potential impact to the otorhinolaryngeal system.

Characteristics of Chemical Air Pollutants

Sources of air pollutants in the ambient or outdoor setting include mobile sources (i.e., automobiles, aircraft, water craft) and stationary sources (i.e., industries, homes, agricultural lands, volcanic eruptions, fires). Industrial sources alone generate chemical air contaminants at a rate of two to three billion pounds a year. Major settings for indoor exposures to air pollutants are the workplace, recreational and public facilities, and residential dwellings. Sources of chemical agents in indoor air include manufacturing processes, incomplete combustion (e.g., smoking, cooking, heating), evaporation of chemical products (solvents, cleaners, paints), mechanical processes, building materials, and cleaning processes.

Any chemical molecule in air other than nitrogen, oxygen, water, carbon dioxide, and trace noble gases can be considered an air contaminant. Chemical contaminants are physically characterized as solid, liquid, and gaseous matter in the form of aerosols, gases, and vapors. Aerosols are solid or liquid particulates generated from mechanical disturbance of solids and liquids, sublimation of solids, condensation of gases or vapors, and incomplete combustion of solids, liquids, and gases (see Table 10.1). Common classes of aerosols include: solid spheroid dust, solid fibrous dust, solid carbonaceous smoke, solid fume, and liquid mist. Gases and vapors are physically identical to each other except true gases which are present in a gaseous state at normal temperature and pressure (NTP; $25°$ C and 760mmHg), while vapors are generated from materials which are solids or liquids at NTP.

State of Matter	Classification	Examples	
Solids	Aerosols	Dusts:	Metals, Plastics, Wood
		Fibers:	Asbestos
		Smoke:	Hydrocarbon
		Fumes:	Metallic Oxides
Liquids	Aerosols	Mists:	Corrosives, Organic Solvents
Gases	True Gases	Oxides of Carbon, Nitrogen, Sulfur	
	Vapors	Organic Solvents	

Table 10.1. *Physical States and Classes of Chemical Air Pollutants*

Airborne contaminants are chemically characterized as organic and inorganic. The distinction is based on the presence (organics) versus the absence (inorganics) of carbon as the foundation element of the molecules. As air pollutants, chemicals are further classified as primary and secondary. This distinction is based on the form in which the pollutant exists at the time and point of generation. The original molecular form generated is referred to as the "primary" pollutant. Several primary pollutants, however, are chemically (i.e., photochemically) transformed into new molecules after they are discharged into the air, whether indoor or outdoor. These contaminants are called "secondary" pollutants. When inhaled, both primary and secondary pollutants exhibit the capacity to adversely impact human systems, including the otorhinolaryngeal system.

Nitrogen dioxide (NO_2) and sulfur dioxide (SO_2) are major primary pollutants generated into the ambient atmosphere. These contaminants interact with atmospheric water and electromagnetic energy from the sun and are photochemically converted into secondary pollutants predominantly as nitric acid (HNO_3) and sulfuric acid (H_2SO_4), respectively. Nitrogen dioxide can also interact with electromagnetic radiation and molecular oxygen (O_2) to form nitric oxide (NO) and ozone (O_3) as secondary pollutants. Photochemical smog is produced from the transformation of primary organic compounds to free radicals (R•), which in turn, combine with molecular oxygen and nitrogen dioxide to form secondary pollutants called peroxyacetyl nitrates (PAN).

Vapors from volatile organic solvents and constituents of building materials, dusts from various mechanical processes, in addition, smoke and nitrogenous and carbonaceous gases from incomplete combustion are major indoor air pollutants. Air pollutants can be concentrated indoors due to a combination of excess generation and inadequate ventilation. This condition has been linked with occupational illnesses among workers, including those in offices, exposed to chemical compounds. In addition, indoor environments of residential dwellings also can be significant sources of exposure to toxic air pollutants. The terms "Building Related Illness" and "Sick Building Syndrome" have been coined to describe illnesses thought to be associated with occupancy in contaminated indoor environments. This source is significant given the fact that humans spend more time indoors.

Research data has shown that various airborne pollutants—whether organic or inorganic, primary or secondary, indoor or outdoor—can indeed cause adverse effects to the otorhinolaryngeal system. The impact is both inflammatory and neurological. Examples of major irritants include: aldehydes, alkaline dusts and mists, ammonia, acids, bromine, cyanide salts, chlorine, chlorine oxides, ethylene oxide, fluorine, hydrogen chlorine, hydrogen cyanide, hydrogen fluoride, iodine, isocyanates, nitrogen oxides, ozone, sulfur dioxide, sulfur trioxide, and sulfur chlorides.

Chemical Aerosols, Gases, and Vapors

Assuming light activity and an average respiration rate of five lpm, approximately 7.2 m^3 of air is inhaled daily by an average human. The adverse toxic impact of chemical aerosols, gases, and vapors contained in this air is classified as a "local effect" if the toxic interaction occurs at the site of contact with tissue. This includes local irritation of upper and lower respiratory tissues plus a variety of lung diseases which have been associated with exposure to chemical air pollutants. A "systematic effect" can occur, however, if the contaminant absorbs into the blood and is distributed to a target site, such as the nervous system, liver, or kidneys.

The fate of aerosols, gases, and vapors following initial inspiration is dependent upon several factors. Exposure to aerosols is influenced mostly by particle size and water solubility. Gas and vapor exposures, however, are influenced mainly by water solubility since particle size is essentially non-existent for these classes of molecules.

Aerosols with aerodynamic diameters less than 10 microns are considered respirable. Non-respirable aerosols are trapped in the nose and eliminated via sneezing and drainage. In general, aerosols with an aerodynamic diameter of 5 to 30 microns are mainly deposited via impaction and interception in the nasopharyngeal region. This means that respirable aerosols can pass through the nasal passages bypass the nasal turbinates, and enter the lungs. Theoretically, the smaller the particle size, the deeper the penetration to the alveolar region is. Estimates indicate that approximately 25 percent are deposited in the lower respiratory tract. Non-respirable aerosols are not necessarily innocuous. These contaminants can cause local effects such as irritation at the site of deposition.

Gases and vapors either directly interact with tissue at the site of contact or are absorbed into the circulatory system. Gases and vapors can adsorb to the surface of the mucociliary lining of the respiratory system.

The conducting airways and gas exchange regions of the upper and lower respiratory system are lined with epithelial cells. The cells provide a defense against the potential impact from deposited aerosols and adsorbed gases and vapors. The architecture of the arrangement of epithelial cells consists of tight junctions which decrease accessibility of airborne contaminants to underlying nerve cells. In addition, the cells generate secretions of mucous. When inhaled contaminants contact the sticky mucous, they may become inhibited from additional transport down into the lungs and, eventually, into the systemic circulation. Instead, hair-like cilia which project from the surface of the epithelial cells sweep upwardly to transport the contaminants for elimination via sneezing, wiping the nose, or expectorating in a process called "mucociliary escalation and clearance." If the cleared contaminants are not expectorated, they are commonly swallowed and, unfortunately, reintroduced into the body via the gastrointestinal system. Immunologic defense mechanisms are also present which can respond to the inhaled chemical aerosols, gases, and vapors.

Toxicity to the Auditory and Vestibular Systems (Ototoxicity)

It has long been recognized that excessive sound levels can damage the auditory system and adversely affect hearing in humans. Relatively recent reports of animal and epidemiological research data have shown that chemical air pollutants (see Table 10.2) can also adversely affect the auditory system. The air contaminants consist of organic solvents, inorganic gases, inorganic metals, and organometallics.

Rats exposed via inhalation to the organic solvent butyl nitrite exhibited an acute decrease in auditory sensitivity at frequencies of 10 kHz and 40 kHz following systemic doses of 50 and 70 μl/100g. Sensorineural loss at elevated frequencies in rats and humans has been associated with airborne exposure to the solvents carbon disulfide, styrene, toluene, trichloroethylene, and xylene.

Workers exposed to varying concentrations of carbon disulfide ranging from 30 to 900 mg/m^3 exhibited an increased incidence of sensorineural lesions. In addition, workers simultaneously exposed to noise levels of 86 to 89 da and 89.92 mg/m^3 of carbon disulfide demonstrated increased hearing loss after three years of exposure, suggesting a synergistic effect. A review of case studies suggested that other organic solvents, such as those present in oil-based paints, interact synergistically with noise to cause increased hearing loss in humans. Toluene damaged cochlear hair cells in rats exposed to O.5 to 1 ml/kg for 21 days. Workers exposed to trichloroethylene and exhibiting internal absorption based on urinalysis (trichloroacetic acid metabolite >40 mg/L), demonstrated increased hearing loss related to duration of exposure of one to more than 15 years. A study involving rats exposed to airborne levels or xylene isomers and styrene at concentrations ranging from 800 to 1200 ppm, 14 hr/day for three to six weeks exhibited increased hearing loss. Additional studies involving rats suggested that the ototoxicity of xylenes and styrene is greater than that caused by toluene. Carbon monoxide gas has been associated with both acute and chronic sensorineural deafness in humans at elevated frequencies and appears to disrupt the cochleus and potentiate loss of hair cells.

Toxic Effect	Class of Chemical Air Pollutant	Examples
Sensorineural Loss[1]	Fumes and Dusts Gases Vapors	arsenic, lead, manganese, tin carbon monoxide butyl nitrite, carbon disulfide, mercury, styrene, toluene, trichloroethylene, xylene
Conductive Loss[2]	Vapors	carbon disulfide
Abnormal Brain Auditory Evoked Response[3]	Fumes and Dusts Gases Vapors	lead, manganese, tin carbon monoxide carbon disulfide, styrene, toluene, trichloroethylene, xylene
Retrocochlear Lesions[3]	Fume Vapor	mercury
High Frequency Loss	Fumes and Dust Gases Vapors	lead, manganese, mercury, tin carbon monoxide butyl nitrite, carbon disulfide, mercury, styrene, toluene, trichloroethylene, xylene
Low Frequency Loss	Fumes and Dusts Vapor	arsenic, manganese, mercury, tin mercury
Cohlear Lesions[4]	Fume and Dust Vapor	mercury, tin mercury
Hair Cell Damage[5]	Fume and Dust Gas Vapors	arsenic, mercury, tin carbon monoxide mercury, toluene
Demyelination[6]	Fume and Dust Vapors	lead, mercury mercury
Synergistic with Noise	Fume and Dust Gas Vapors	manganese carbon monoxide carbon disulfide, toluene

Table 10.2. Examples of Potential Oxytoxic Chemical Air Pollutants

Exposure to metals, such as arsenic, lead, manganese, mercury, and tin also can cause sensorineural hearing loss in humans. An epidemiology study of children exposed environmentally to airborne arsenic from a power plant exhibited statistically significant hearing loss, especially at lower frequencies. Blood lead levels in children have been shown to be statistically related to increased hearing loss based on elevated hearing thresholds at 500, 1000, 2000, and 4000 Hz. In addition, lead exposure has been associated with elevated frequency thresholds in humans plus demonstration of demyelination of the eighth cranial nerve in guinea pigs, indicative of toxicity to the inner ear. Manganese exposures may cause loss at both low and high frequencies in humans and appears to interact synergistically with noise. Epidemiologic data from environmental exposure to mercury have suggested possible increased inner ear lesions in humans. The metal has also been associated with damage to labyrinthine blood vessels, damaged endothelial cells, and mitochondrial swelling in guinea pigs exposed systemically to 2.5 to 7.5 mg/kg/day for one to 16 days. Systemic exposure of rats to 8 mg/kg trimethyltin for one to 18 days resulted in neural damage to the cochlea which, in turn, can cause sensory hearing loss.

The central and peripheral nervous systems in humans and research animals are particularly vulnerable to toxic effects from exposure to certain types of exogenous chemical compounds. Numerous organic chemical solvents, including several already mentioned above, which are utilized in the home as components of various commercial products, in the workplace for manufacturing and production, and those eventually released into the ambient environment have been classified as potentially neurotoxic. One particularly susceptible component of the central nervous system appears to be the vestibular system. The vestibular ("equilibrium") system controls balance. Effective exposure of the human vestibular system to organic solvents can cause symptoms such as vertigo, unsteadiness, and dizziness. These symptoms are indicative of vestibular dysfunction. The dysfunction, in turn, may be attributable to neurochemical and/or morphological alterations of the vestibulo-cerebellar system.

Toxicicity to the Nose and Sinuses (Rhinotoxicity)

Based on the anatomical structure of the nasal and sinus passages, inhaled air comes into direct contact with the mucosal lining and epithelial cilia. Toxic aerosols, gases, and vapors (see Table 10.3) can interact with nasal and sinus tissues when in contact. Chemical air pollutants can be odiferous and cause irritation of the nasal mucosa, suggesting stimulation of the olfactory (odor detection) and trigeminal (irritation detection) nerves. Human subjects exposed to a mixture of volatile organic compounds associated with indoor air quality at a concentration of 25 mg/m³ for 2.75 hours demonstrated increased signs of discomfort, including nose and throat irritation. Compounds such as sulfur dioxide and cigarette smoke cause increased nasal resistance to airflow in humans. In addition, humans exposed to particulates such as environmental tobacco smoke, paper dust, cotton

Toxic Effect	Class of Chemical Air Pollutant	Examples
Mucosal Irritation	Dusts	cadmium, nickel, wood
	Fibers	fiberglass
	Smoke	tobacco
	Mists	solvents (hair spray, paint)
	Gases	freon, ozone, sulfur dioxide
	Vapors	formaldehyde, solvents
Decreased Mucociliary Escalation	Dusts	cadmium, nickel, wood
	Smoke	tobacco
	Mists	solvents (hair spray, paint) (?)
	Gases	ozone, sulfur dioxide
	Vapors	formaldehyde (?), solvents (?)
Benign Tissue Changes	Dusts	cadmium (?), nickel, wood
	Smoke	diesel, tobacco (?)
	Mists	solvents (paint)
	Gases	ozone, sulfur dioxide
	Vapors	formaldehyde, solvents (paint)
Malignant Tissue Changes	Dusts	cadmium (?), nickel, wood
	Smoke	diesel (?), tobacco (?)
	Gases	ozone (?), sulfur dioxide (?)
	Vapors	formaldehyde (?)

Table 10.3. Examples of Potential Rhinotoxic Chemical Air Pollutants

dust, cadmium dust, and wood dust may exhibit irritation and rhinorrhea. Many of these responses may be associated with hyper-sensitivity or allergic responses. Human subjects exposed via inhalation of 2 to 6 mg newspaper dust exhibited nasal symptoms suggestive of hyper-reactivity. Organic solvent vapors and mists from aerosol pro-pellants such as hair-sprays and paints can also cause irritation. In-deed, irritation can extend from the nasal region to the pharynegeal and laryngeal tissues.

Mucociliary clearance can also be adversely affected due to alter-ation of secretions and disturbance of nasal cilia. This occurs via breakdown of mucous barrier covering cilia or compounding of cilia, that is, two or more cilia are incorporated into a single membrane. As a result, upper respiratory defense mechanisms can be compro-mised due to exposure to rhinotoxic compounds.

Cellular and tissue changes in the nose and sinuses can also re-sult from excessive exposure to air pollutants. These changes include deviated septa in humans from agents such as arsenic and acids and formation of premalignant cells and tumors from agents such as hy-drocarbon particulates from combusted fuel emissions. Human nasal carcinomas are linked to exposure to some materials, including treated woods, nickel and the irritant, formaldehyde. Numerous chemical air pollutants can stimulate the olfactory chemosensory tissue and be detected as an odor. Unfortunately, many of the chemical contami-nants can result in alterations of olfactory function. Indeed, exposure to several metallic and nonmetallic inorganics plus a variety of or-ganic compounds, such as solvents, can reduce olfactory sensitivity.

Toxicicity to the Throat and Larynx (Laryngeotoxicity)

There is also a suggested link between human inhalation of air pollutants and adverse impact to the laryngeal system. The impact can include changes in voice quality such as hoarseness, voice fatigue, or neoplasms. Common agents reported in the literature which can potentially adversely affect the laryngeal tissue include smoke, vari-ous dusts and fibers, ozone, sulfur dioxide, nitrogen dioxide, and or-ganic solvents. Note that these irritants were also listed in Table 10.3 as nasal and sinus irritants.

The vocal cords may be indirectly affected from the stimulation of the cough reflex during exposure to irritants. Coughing can cause vocal fold injury, including mucosal disruption and vocal fold hemor-rhage. In addition, it is clear that air pollutants which alter pulmonary function may have an adverse effect on the larynx. Thus, research literature indicates that if the lungs are adversely affected, then secondary impact can manifest as voice change due to compensatory muscular tension dysphonia (speaking difficulty or pain), voice fatigue, hoarseness, and vocal nodules. It is uncertain, however, whether interaction of contaminants with the laryngeal system adversely affects the surface integrity, mucous viscosity, or surface tension of the larynx or impacts neurologic control mechanisms.

Conclusions

Published research data regarding human toxicity of chemical air pollutants indicate that the scope of adverse effects and target systems involved are broader than commonly known. While the traditional foci of toxicological research and emphasis have been centered mainly on the adverse impact to the general upper and lower respiratory tract, a review of the literature has revealed impact to a spectrum of target sites specific to the otorhinolaryngeal system. This is important to environmental health professionals when considering the scope of potential local and systemic effects caused by human exposure to chemical air contaminants. In addition, this may be significant to environmental health risk assessment of airborne chemical agents if multi-target site models are considered.

Unfortunately, there is a relative paucity of research data from investigations of human exposure to chemical agents and associated otorhinolaryngeal toxicity, especially impact to the auditory, vestibular, and laryngeal systems. Accordingly, additional research is needed to qualitatively identify chemical agents which are potentially and actually associated with otorhinolaryngeal toxicity in relation to the quantitative doses. Epidemiological research of otorhinolaryngeal toxicity, including quantitative assessment of human exposure to airborne chemicals, is needed to generate data which are necessary for risk characterization and establishing indoor and outdoor exposure limits for chemical air contaminants.

—by Michael S. Bisesi, Ph.D., RS, CIH
and Allan M. Rubin, M.D., Ph.D.

Part Three

Water Pollution

Chapter 11

Keeping Track: National Water Quality Inventory, 1994 Report to Congress

Background

The National Water Quality Inventory Report to Congress is prepared every two years under Section 305(b) of the Clean Water Act. The 1994 Report is the tenth in its series.

The Clean Water Act gives States the responsibility to monitor and assess their waters and report the results to EPA. EPA provides technical assistance and guidance on monitoring and reporting, and summarizes the results of the state assessments in this report to Congress.

This 1994 Report is based on water quality assessments submitted by 61 States, territories, interstate Water Commissions, the District of Columbia, and American Indian Tribes (hereafter collectively referred to as States, Tribes, and other jurisdictions). These State, Tribe, and other jurisdiction assessments describe water quality conditions during 1992-1993.

Rivers, lakes, estuaries, wetlands, coastal waters, Great Lakes, and ground water are all covered in this report. The full report also contains information on public health and aquatic life concerns, water quality monitoring, and state and federal water pollution control programs.

States measure water quality by determining if individual waters are clean enough to support uses such as fishing, swimming, and drinking. These uses are part of the state water quality standards, are set by the States, and are approved by EPA.

Adapted from United States Environmental Protection Agency, Office of Water (4503F) EPA841-F-96-002, 1996. http://earth1.epa.gov/305b/execsum.html.

How Many of Our Waters Were Surveyed for 1994?

- Rivers and Streams—615,806—17 percent surveyed—Total miles: 3,548,738.

- Lakes, Ponds, and Reservoirs—17,134,153—2 percent surveyed—Total acres: 40,826,064.

- Estuaries—26,847—78 percent surveyed—Total square miles: 34,388 Excluding estuarine waters in Alaska because no estimate was available.

- Ocean Shoreline Waters—5,208—9 percent surveyed—Total miles: 58,421 miles, including Alaska's 36,000 miles of shoreline.

- Great Lakes Shoreline—5,224—94 percent surveyed—Total miles: 5,559.

National estimates of the total waters of our country provide the foundation for determining the percentage of waters surveyed by the States, Tribes, and other jurisdictions and the portion impaired by pollution. For the 1992 reporting period, EPA provided the States with estimates of total river miles and lake acres derived from the EPA Reach File, a database containing traces of waterbodies adapted from 1:100,000 scale maps prepared by the U.S. Geological Survey. The States modified these total water estimates where necessary. Based on the 1992 EPA/State figures, the national estimate of total river miles doubled in large part because the EPA/State estimates included non-perennial streams, canals, and ditches that were previously excluded from estimates of total stream miles.

Estimates for the 1994 reporting cycle are a minor refinement of the 1992 figures and indicate that the United States has:

- More than 3.5 million miles of rivers and streams, which range in size from the Mississippi River to small streams that flow only when wet weather conditions exist (i.e., "non-perennial" streams)

- Approximately 40.8 million acres of lakes, ponds, and reservoirs

- About 34,388 square miles of estuaries (excluding Alaska)

- More than 58,000 miles of ocean shoreline, including 36,000 miles in Alaska

- 5,559 miles of Great Lakes shoreline

- More than 277 million acres of wetlands such as marshes, swamps, bogs, fens, including 170 million acres of wetlands in Alaska.

Pollutants and Processes That Degrade Water Quality

Where possible, States, Tribes, and other jurisdictions identify the pollutants or processes that degrade water quality and indicators that document impacts of water quality degradation. The most widespread pollutants and processes identified in rivers, lakes, and estuaries are presented in Table 11.1. Pollutants include sediment, nutrients, and chemical contaminants (such as dioxins and metals). Processes that degrade waters include habitat modification (such as destruction of streamside vegetation) and hydrologic modification (such as flow reduction). Indicators of water quality degradation include physical, chemical, and biological parameters. Examples of biological parameters include species diversity and abundance. Examples of physical and chemical parameters include pH, turbidity, and temperature.

Following are descriptions of the effects of the pollutants and processes most commonly identified in rivers, lakes, estuaries, coastal waters, wetlands, and ground water.

Low Dissolved Oxygen

Dissolved oxygen is a basic requirement for a healthy aquatic ecosystem. Most fish and beneficial aquatic insects "breathe" oxygen dissolved in the water column. Some fish and aquatic organisms (such as carp and sludge worms) are adapted to low oxygen conditions, but most desirable fish species (such as trout and salmon) suffer if dissolved oxygen concentrations fall below 3 to 4 mg/L (3 to 4 milligrams of oxygen dissolved in 1 liter of water, or 3 to 4 parts of oxygen per million parts of water). Larvae and juvenile fish are more sensitive and require even higher concentrations of dissolved oxygen.

Many fish and other aquatic organisms can recover from short periods of low dissolved oxygen availability. However, prolonged episodes of depressed dissolved oxygen concentrations of 2 mg/L or less can result in "dead" waterbodies. Prolonged exposure to low dissolved oxygen conditions can suffocate adult fish or reduce their reproductive survival by suffocating sensitive eggs and larvae or can starve fish by killing aquatic insect larvae and other prey. Low dissolved oxygen concentrations also favor anaerobic bacterial activity that produces noxious gases or foul odors often associated with polluted waterbodies.

Rank	Rivers	Lakes	Estuaries
1	Bacteria	Nutrients	Nutrients
2	Siltation	Siltation	Bacteria
3	Nutrients	Oxygen-Depleting Substances	Oxygen-Depleting Substances
4	Oxygen-Depleting Substances	Metals	Habitat Alterations
5	Metals	Suspended Solids	Oil and Grease

Figure 11.1. *Five Leading Causes of Water Quality Impairment. Source: Based on 1994 Section 305(b) reports submitted by States, Tribes, Territories, Commissions, and the District of Columbia*

Oxygen concentrations in the water column fluctuate under natural conditions, but severe oxygen depletion usually results from human activities that introduce large quantities of biodegradable organic materials into surface waters. Biodegradable organic materials contain plant, fish, or animal matter. Leaves, lawn clippings, sewage, manure, shellfish processing waste, milk solids, and other food processing wastes are examples of "oxygen-depleting" organic materials that enter our surface waters.

In both pristine and polluted waters, beneficial bacteria use oxygen to break apart (or decompose) organic materials. Pollution-containing organic wastes provide a continuous glut of food for the bacteria, which accelerates bacterial activity and population growth. In polluted waters, bacterial consumption of oxygen can rapidly outpace oxygen replenishment from the atmosphere and photosynthesis performed by algae and aquatic plants. The result is a net decline in oxygen concentrations in the water.

Toxic pollutants can indirectly lower oxygen concentrations by killing algae, aquatic weeds, or fish, which provides an abundance of food for oxygen-consuming bacteria. Oxygen depletion can also result from chemical reactions that do not involve bacteria. Some pollutants trigger chemical reactions that place a chemical oxygen demand on receiving waters.

Other factors (such as temperature and salinity) influence the amount of oxygen dissolved in water. Prolonged hot weather will depress oxygen concentrations and may cause fish kills even in clean waters because warm water cannot hold as much oxygen as cold water. Warm conditions further aggravate oxygen depletion by stimulating bacterial activity and respiration in fish, which consumes oxygen. Removal of streamside vegetation eliminates shade, thereby raising water temperatures, and accelerates runoff of organic debris. Under such conditions, minor additions of pollution-containing organic materials can severely deplete oxygen.

Nutrients

Nutrients are essential building blocks for healthy aquatic communities, but excess nutrients (especially nitrogen and phosphorus compounds) overstimulate the growth of aquatic weeds and algae. Excessive growth of these organisms, in turn, can clog navigable waters, interfere with swimming and boating, out-compete native submerged aquatic vegetation (SAV), and lead to oxygen depletion. Oxygen concentrations can fluctuate daily during algal blooms, rising during the day as algae perform photosynthesis, and falling at night as algae continue to respire, which consumes oxygen. Beneficial bacteria also consume oxygen as they decompose the abundant organic food supply in dying algae cells.

Lawn and crop fertilizers, sewage, manure, and detergents contain nitrogen and phosphorus, the nutrients most often responsible for water quality degradation. Rural areas are vulnerable to ground water contamination from nitrates (a compound containing nitrogen) found in fertilizer and manure. Very high concentrations of nitrate (>10 mg/L) in drinking water cause methemoglobinemia, or blue baby syndrome, an inability to fix oxygen in the blood.

Nutrients are difficult to control because lake and estuarine ecosystems recycle nutrients. Rather than leaving the ecosystem, the nutrients cycle among the water column, algae and plant tissues, and the bottom sediments. For example, algae may temporarily remove all the nitrogen from the water column, but the nutrients will return to the water column when the algae die and are decomposed by bacteria. Therefore, gradual inputs of nutrients tend to accumulate over time rather than leave the system.

Sediment and Siltation

In a water quality context, sediment usually refers to soil particles that enter the water column from eroding land. Sediment consists of particles of all sizes, including fine clay particles, silt, sand, and gravel. Water quality managers use the term "siltation" to describe the suspension and deposition of small sediment particles in waterbodies.

Sediment and siltation can severely alter aquatic communities. Sediment may clog and abrade fish gills, suffocate eggs and aquatic insect larvae on the bottom, and fill in the pore space between bottom cobbles where fish lay eggs. Silt and sediment interfere with recreational activities and aesthetic enjoyment at waterbodies by reducing water clarity and filling in waterbodies. Sediment may also carry other pollutants into waterbodies. Nutrients and toxic chemicals may attach to sediment particles on land and ride the particles into surface waters where the pollutants may settle with the sediment or detach and become soluble in the water column.

Rain washes silt and other soil particles off of plowed fields, construction sites, logging sites, urban areas, and strip-mined lands into waterbodies. Eroding stream banks also deposit silt and sediment in waterbodies. Removal of vegetation on shore can accelerate streambank erosion.

Bacteria and Pathogens

Some waterborne bacteria, viruses, and protozoa cause human illnesses that range from typhoid and dysentery to minor respiratory and skin diseases. These organisms may enter waters through a number of routes, including inadequately treated sewage, stormwater drains, septic systems, runoff from livestock pens, and sewage dumped overboard from recreational boats.

Because it is impossible to test waters for every possible disease-causing organism, States and other jurisdictions usually measure indicator bacteria that are found in great numbers in the stomachs and intestines of warm-blooded animals and people. The presence of indicator bacteria suggests that the "waterbody" may be contaminated with untreated sewage and that other, more dangerous organisms may be present. The States, Tribes, and other jurisdictions use bacterial criteria to determine if waters are safe for recreation and shellfish harvesting.

Toxic Organic Chemicals and Metals

Toxic organic chemicals are synthetic compounds that contain carbon, such as polychlorinated biphenyls (PCBs), dioxins, and the pesticide DDT. These synthesized compounds often persist and accumulate in the environment because they do not readily break down in natural ecosystems. Many of these compounds cause cancer in people and birth defects in other predators near the top of the food chain, such as birds and fish.

Metals occur naturally in the environment, but human activities (such as industrial processes and mining) have altered the distribution of metals in the environment. In most reported cases of metals contamination, high concentrations of metals appear in fish tissues rather than the water column because the metals accumulate in greater concentrations in predators near the top of the food chain.

pH

Acidity, the concentration of hydrogen ions, drives many chemical reactions in living organisms. The standard measure of acidity is pH, and a pH value of 7 represents a neutral condition. A low pH value (less than 5) indicates acidic conditions; a high pH (greater than 9) indicates alkaline conditions. Many biological processes, such as reproduction, cannot function in acidic or alkaline waters. Acidic conditions also aggravate toxic contamination problems because sediments release toxicants in acidic waters. Common sources of acidity include mine drainage, runoff from mine tailings, and atmospheric deposition.

Habitat Modification/hydrologic Modification

Habitat modifications include activities in the landscape, on shore, and in waterbodies that alter the physical structure of aquatic ecosystems and have adverse impacts on aquatic life. Examples of habitat modifications include:

- Removal of streamside vegetation that stabilizes the shoreline and provides shade, which moderates in-stream temperatures

- Excavation of cobbles from a stream bed that provide nesting habitat for fish

- Stream burial

- Excessive suburban sprawl that alters the natural drainage patterns by increasing the intensity, magnitude, and energy of runoff waters.

Hydrologic modifications alter the flow of water. Examples of hydrologic modifications include channelization, dewatering, damming, and dredging.

Other pollutants include salts and oil and grease. Fresh waters may become unfit for aquatic life and some human uses when they become contaminated by salts. Sources of salinity include irrigation runoff, brine used in oil extraction, road deicing operations, and the intrusion of sea water into ground and surface waters in coastal areas. Crude oil and processed petroleum products may be spilled during extraction, processing, or transport or leaked from underground storage tanks.

Sources of Water Pollution

Sources of impairment generate the pollutants that violate use support criteria. Point sources discharge pollutants directly into surface waters from a conveyance. Point sources include industrial facilities, municipal sewage treatment plants, and combined sewer overflows. Non-point sources deliver pollutants to surface waters from diffuse origins. Non-point sources include urban runoff, agricultural runoff, and atmospheric deposition of contaminants in air pollution. Habitat alterations, such as hydromodification, dredging, and streambank destabilization, can also degrade water quality.

Table 11.2 lists the leading sources of impairment related to human activities as reported by States, Tribes, and other jurisdictions for their rivers, lakes, and estuaries. Other sources cited include removal of riparian vegetation, forestry activities, land disposal, petroleum extraction and processing activities, and construction. In addition to human activities, the States, Tribes, and other jurisdictions also reported impairments from natural sources. Natural sources refer to an assortment of water quality problems:

- Natural deposits of salts, gypsum, nutrients, and metals in soils that leach into surface and ground waters

- Warm weather and dry conditions that raise water temperatures, depress dissolved oxygen concentrations, and dry up shallow waterbodies

- Low-flow conditions and tannic acids from decaying leaves that lower pH and dissolved oxygen concentrations in swamps draining into streams.

Rank	Rivers	Lakes	Estuaries
1	Agriculture	Agriculture	Urban Runoff/ Storm Sewers
2	Municipal Sewage Treatment Plants	Municipal Sewage Treatment Plants	Municipal Sewage Treatment Plants
3	Hydrologic/Habitat Modification	Urban Runoff/ Storm Sewers	Agriculture
4	Urban Runoff/ Storm Sewers	Unspecified Nonpoint Sources	Industrial Point Sources
5	Resource Extraction	Hydrologic/Habitat Modification	Petroleum Activities

Figure 11.2. Five Leading Sources of Water Quality Impairment Related to Human Activities. Source: Based on 1994 Section 305(b) reports submitted by States, Tribes, Territories, Commissions, and the District of Columbia.

Rivers and Streams

Rivers and streams are characterized by flow. Perennial rivers and streams flow continuously, all year round. Non-perennial rivers and streams stop flowing for some period of time, usually due to dry conditions or upstream withdrawals. Many rivers and streams originate in non-perennial headwaters that flow only during snowmelt or heavy showers. Non-perennial streams provide critical habitats for non-fish species, such as amphibians and dragonflies, as well as safe havens for juvenile fish to escape from predation by larger fish.

The health of rivers and streams is directly linked to habitat integrity on shore and in adjacent wetlands. Stream quality will deteriorate if activities damage shoreline (i.e., riparian) vegetation and wetlands, which filter pollutants from runoff and bind soils. Removal of vegetation also eliminates shade that moderates stream temperature as well as the land temperature that can warm runoff entering

127

surface waters. Stream temperature, in turn, affects the availability of dissolved oxygen in the water column for fish and other aquatic organisms.

Overall Water Quality

River Miles Surveyed

- Total rivers = 3.5 million miles
- Total surveyed = 615,806 miles—17 percent Surveyed—83 percent Not Surveyed

Levels of Overall Use Support—Rivers

- Good (Fully Supporting)—57 percent
- Good (Threatened)—7 percent
- Fair (Partially Supporting)—22 percent
- Poor (Not Supporting)—14 percent
- Poor (Not Attainable)—< less than 1 percent

For the 1994 Report, 58 States, Territories, Tribes, Commissions, and the District of Columbia surveyed 615,806 miles (17 percent) of the Nation's total 3.5 million miles of rivers and streams. The surveyed rivers and streams represent 48 percent of the 1.3 million miles of perennial rivers and streams that flow year round in the lower 48 States.

Altogether, the States and Tribes surveyed 27,075 fewer river miles in 1994 than in 1992. Individually, most States reported that they surveyed more river miles in 1994, but their increases were offset by a decline of 85,000 surveyed river miles reported by Montana, Mississippi, and Maryland. For 1994, these States reported use support status for only those river miles that they surveyed in direct monitoring programs or evaluations rather than using inferences for unsurveyed waters. The following discussion applies exclusively to surveyed waters and cannot be extrapolated to describe conditions in the Nation's rivers as a whole because the States, Tribes, and other jurisdictions do not consistently use statistical or probabilistic survey methods to characterize all their waters at this time. EPA is working with the States, Tribes, and other jurisdictions to expand survey coverage of the Nation's waters and expects future survey information to cover a greater portion of the Nation's rivers and streams.

Of the Nation's 615,806 surveyed river miles, the States, Tribes, and other jurisdictions found that 64 percent have good water quality.

Of these waters, 57 percent fully support their designated uses, and an additional 7 percent support uses but are threatened and may become impaired if pollution control actions are not taken.

Some form of pollution or habitat degradation prevents the remaining 36 percent (224,236 miles) of the surveyed river miles from fully supporting a healthy aquatic community or human activities all year round. Twenty-two percent of the surveyed river miles have fair water quality that partially supports designated uses. Most of the time, these waters provide adequate habitat for aquatic organisms and support human activities, but periodic pollution interferes with these activities and/or stresses aquatic life. Fourteen percent of the surveyed river miles have poor water quality that consistently stresses aquatic life and/or prevents people from using the river for activities such as swimming and fishing.

What Is Polluting Our Rivers and Streams?

The States and Tribes report that bacteria pollute 76,397 river miles (which equals 34 percent of the impaired river miles). Bacteria provide evidence of possible fecal contamination that may cause illness if the public ingests the water. Siltation, composed of tiny soil particles, remains one of the most widespread pollutants impacting rivers and streams. The States and Tribes reported that siltation impairs 75,792 river miles (which equals 34 percent of the impaired river miles).

Siltation alters aquatic habitat and suffocates fish eggs and bottom-dwelling organisms. Excessive siltation can also interfere with drinking water treatment processes and recreational use of a river.

In addition to siltation and bacteria, the States and Tribes also reported that nutrients, oxygen-depleting substances, metals, and habitat alterations impact more miles of rivers and streams than other pollutants and processes. Often, several pollutants and processes impact a single river segment. For example, a process, such as removal of shoreline vegetation, may accelerate erosion of sediment and nutrients into a stream.

Where Does this Pollution Come from?

The States and Tribes reported that agriculture is the most widespread source of pollution in the Nation's surveyed rivers. Agriculture generates pollutants that degrade aquatic life or interfere with public use of 134,557 river miles (which equals 60 percent of the impaired river miles) in 49 States and Tribes.

Twenty-one States reported the size of rivers impacted by specific types of agricultural activities:

- **Non-irrigated Crop Production**—crop production that relies on rain as the sole source of water.

- **Irrigated Crop Production**—crop production that uses irrigation systems to supplement rainwater.

- **Rangeland**—land grazed by animals that is seldom enhanced by the application of fertilizers or pesticides, although managers sometimes modify plant species to a limited extent.

- **Pastureland**—land upon which a crop (such as alfalfa) is raised to feed animals, either by grazing the animals among the crops or harvesting the crops.

- **Feedlots**—facilities where animals are fattened and confined at high densities.

- **Animal Holding Areas**—facilities where animals are confined briefly before slaughter.

The States reported that non-irrigated crop production impaired the most river miles, followed by irrigated crop production, rangeland, feedlots, pastureland, and animal holding areas.

Many States reported declines in pollution from sewage treatment plants and industrial discharges as a result of sewage treatment plant construction and upgrades and permit controls on industrial discharges. Despite the improvements, municipal sewage treatment plants remain the second most common source of pollution in rivers (impairing 37,443 miles) because population growth increases the burden on our municipal facilities.

Hydrologic modifications and habitat alterations are a growing concern to the States. Hydrologic modifications include activities that alter the flow of water in a stream, such as channelization, dewatering, and damming of streams. Habitat alterations include removal of streamside vegetation that protects the stream from high temperatures, and scouring of stream bottoms. Additional gains in water quality conditions will be more subtle and require innovative management strategies that go beyond point source controls. The States, Tribes, and other jurisdictions also reported that urban runoff and storm sewers impair 26,862 river miles (12 percent of the impaired rivers), resource extraction impairs 24,059 river miles (11 percent of the impaired rivers), and removal of streamside vegetation impairs 21,706 river miles (10 percent of the impaired rivers). The States, Tribes, and other jurisdictions also report that "natural" sources impair significant stretches of rivers and streams.

"Natural" sources, such as low flow and soils with arsenic deposits, can prevent waters from supporting uses in the absence of human activities.

Lakes, Ponds, and Reservoirs

Lake Acres Surveyed

- Total lakes = 40.8 million acres
- Total surveyed = 17.1 million acres—42 percent Surveyed—58 percent Not Surveyed

Levels of Overall Use Support—Lakes

- Good (Fully Supporting)—50 percent
- Good (Threatened)—13 percent
- Fair (Partially Supporting)—28 percent
- Poor (Not Supporting)—9 percent
- Poor (Not Attainable)—less than 1 percent

Lakes are sensitive to pollution inputs because lakes flush out their contents relatively slowly. Even under natural conditions, lakes undergo eutrophication, an aging process that slowly fills in the lake with sediment and organic matter. The eutrophication process alters basic lake characteristics such as depth, biological productivity, oxygen levels, and water clarity. The eutrophication process is commonly defined by a series of trophic states.

Overall Water Quality

Forty-eight States, Tribes, and other jurisdictions surveyed overall use support in more than 17.1 million lake acres representing 42 percent of the approximately 40.8 million total acres of lakes, ponds, and reservoirs in the Nation. For 1994, the States surveyed about 1 million fewer lake acres than in 1992.

131

The number of surveyed lake acres declined because several States separated fish tissue data from their survey of overall use support. Some of these States, such as Minnesota, have established massive databases of fish tissue contamination information (which is used to establish fish consumption advisories), but lack other types of water quality data for many of their lakes. In 1994, these States chose not to assess overall use support entirely with fish tissue data alone, which is a very narrow indicator of water quality.

The States and Tribes reported that 63 percent of their surveyed 17.1 million lake acres have good water quality. Waters with good quality include 50 percent of the surveyed lake acres fully supporting uses and 13 percent of the surveyed lake acres that are threatened and might deteriorate if we fail to manage potential sources of pollution.

Some form of pollution or habitat degradation impairs the remaining 37 percent of the surveyed lake acres. Twenty-eight percent of the surveyed lake acres have fair water quality that partially supports designated uses. Most of the time, these waters provide adequate habitat for aquatic organisms and support human activities, but periodic pollution interferes with these activities and/or stresses aquatic life. Nine percent of the surveyed lake acres suffer from poor water quality that consistently stresses aquatic life and/or prevents people from using the lake for activities such as swimming and fishing.

What Is Polluting Our Lakes, Ponds, and Reservoirs?

Forty-one States, the District of Columbia, and Puerto Rico reported the number of lake acres impacted by individual pollutants and processes.

Thirty-seven States and Puerto Rico identified more lake acres polluted by nutrients than any other pollutant or process. The States and Puerto Rico reported that extra nutrients pollute 2.8 million lake acres (which equals 43 percent of the impaired lake acres). Healthy lake ecosystems contain nutrients in small quantities, but extra inputs of nutrients from human activities unbalance lake ecosystems.

In addition to nutrients, the States, Puerto Rico, and the District of Columbia report that siltation pollutes 1.8 million lake acres (which equals 28 percent of the impaired lake acres), enrichment by organic wastes that deplete oxygen impacts 1.6 million lake acres (which equals 24 percent of the impaired lake acres), and metals pollute 1.4 million acres (which equals 21 percent of the impaired lake acres).

Metals declined from the most widespread pollutant impairing lakes in the 1992 305(b) reporting cycle to the fourth leading pollutant impairing lakes in 1994. The decline is due to changes in State reporting and assessment methods rather than a measured decrease in metals contamination. In 1994, several States chose to no longer assess overall use support with fish contamination data alone. Much of that data consisted of measurements of metals in fish tissue. As a result of excluding these fish tissue data, the national estimate of lake acres impaired by metals fell by over 2 million acres in 1994.

Where Does this Pollution Come from?

Forty-two States and Puerto Rico reported sources of pollution in some of their impacted lakes, ponds, and reservoirs. These States and Puerto Rico reported that agriculture is the most widespread source of pollution in the Nation's surveyed lakes. Agriculture generates pollutants that degrade aquatic life or interfere with public use of 3.3 million lake acres (which equals 50 percent of the impaired lake acres).

The States and Puerto Rico also reported that municipal sewage treatment plants pollute 1.3 million lake acres (19 percent of the impaired lake acres), urban runoff and storm sewers pollute 1.2 million lake acres (18 percent of the surveyed lake acres), unspecified nonpoint sources impair 989,000 lake acres (15 percent of the impaired lake acres), hydrologic modifications and habitat alterations degrade 832,000 lake acres (12 percent of the impaired lake acres), and industrial point sources pollute 759,000 lake acres (11 percent of the impaired lake acres). Many States prohibit new point source discharges into lakes, but existing municipal sewage treatment plants remain a leading source of pollution entering lakes.

The States and Puerto Rico listed numerous sources that impact several hundred thousand lake acres, including land disposal of wastes, construction, flow regulation, highway maintenance and runoff, contaminated sediments, atmospheric deposition of pollutants, and on-site wastewater systems (including septic tanks).

The Great Lakes

Great Lakes Shore Miles Surveyed

- Total Great Lakes = 5,559 miles
- Total surveyed = 5,224 miles—94 percent Surveyed—6 percent Not Surveyed

Levels of Overall Use Support — Great Lakes

- Good (Fully Supporting)—2 percent
- Good (Threatened)—1 percent
- Fair (Partially Supporting)—34 percent
- Poor (Not Supporting)—63 percent
- Poor (Not Attainable)—0 percent

The Great Lakes contain one-fifth of the world's fresh surface water and are stressed by a wide range of pollution sources, including air pollution. Many of the pollutants that reach the Great Lakes remain in the system indefinitely because the Great Lakes are a relatively closed water system with few natural outlets. Despite dramatic declines in the occurrence of algal blooms, fish kills, and localized "dead" zones depleted of oxygen, less visible problems continue to degrade the Great Lakes. The States surveyed 94 percent of the Great Lakes shoreline miles for 1994 and reported that fish consumption advisories and aquatic life concerns are the dominant water quality problems, overall, in the Great Lakes. The States reported that most of the Great Lakes nearshore waters are safe for swimming and other recreational activities and can be used as a source of drinking water with normal treatment. However, only 2 percent of the surveyed nearshore waters fully support designated uses, overall, and 1 percent support uses but are threatened. About 97 percent of the surveyed waters do not fully support designated uses, overall, because fish consumption advisories are posted throughout the nearshore waters of the Great Lakes and water quality conditions are unfavorable for supporting aquatic life in many cases. Aquatic life impacts result from persistent toxic pollutant burdens in birds, habitat degradation and destruction, and competition and predation by nonnative species such as the zebra mussel and the sea lamprey.

These figures do not address water quality conditions in the deeper, cleaner, central waters of the Lakes.

What Is Polluting the Great Lakes?

The States reported that most of the Great Lakes shoreline is polluted by toxic organic chemicals—primarily PCB—that are often found in fish tissue samples. The Great Lakes States reported that toxic organic chemicals impact 98 percent of the impaired Great Lakes shoreline miles. Other leading causes of impairment include pesticides, affecting 21 percent; non-priority organic chemicals, affecting

20 percent; nutrients, affecting 6 percent; and metals, affecting 6 percent.

Where Does this Pollution Come from?

Only four of the eight Great Lakes States measured the size of their Great Lakes shoreline polluted by specific sources. These States have jurisdiction over one-third of the Great Lakes shoreline, so their findings do not necessarily reflect conditions throughout the Great Lakes Basin.

- Wisconsin identifies air pollution and discontinued discharges as a source of pollutants contaminating all 1,017 of their surveyed shoreline miles. Wisconsin also identified smaller areas impacted by contaminated sediments, non-point sources, industrial and municipal discharges, agriculture, urban runoff and storm sewers, combined sewer overflows, and land disposal of waste.

- Indiana attributes all of the pollution along its entire 43-mile shoreline to air pollution, urban runoff and storm sewers, industrial and municipal discharges, and agriculture.

- Ohio reports that non-point sources pollute 86 miles of its 236 miles of shoreline, in-place contaminants impact 33 miles, and land disposal of waste impacts 24 miles of shoreline.

- New York identifies many sources of pollutants in their Great Lakes waters, but the State attributes the most miles of degradation to contaminated sediments (439 miles) and land disposal of waste (374 miles).

Estuaries

Estuary Square Miles Surveyed

- Total estuaries = 34,388 square miles
- Total surveyed = 26,847 square miles—78 percent Surveyed— 22 percent Not Surveyed

Levels of Overall Use Support — Estuaries

- Good (Fully Supporting)—57 percent

- Good (Threatened)—6 percent
- Fair (Partially Supporting)—27 percent
- Poor (Not Supporting)—9 percent
- Poor (Not Attainable)—less than 1 percent

Estuaries are areas partially surrounded by land where rivers meet the sea. They are characterized by varying degrees of salinity, complex water movements affected by ocean tides and river currents, and high turbidity levels. They are also highly productive ecosystems with a range of habitats for many different species of plants, shellfish, fish, and animals.

Many species permanently inhabit the estuarine ecosystem; others, such as shrimp, use the nutrient-rich estuarine waters as nurseries before traveling to the sea.

Estuaries are stressed by the particularly wide range of activities located within their watersheds. They receive pollutants carried by rivers from agricultural lands and cities; they often support marinas, harbors, and commercial fishing fleets; and their surrounding lands are highly prized for development. These stresses pose a continuing threat to the survival of these bountiful waters.

Overall Water Quality

Twenty-five coastal States and jurisdictions surveyed 78 percent of the Nation's total estuarine waters in 1994. The States and other jurisdictions reported that 63 percent of the surveyed estuarine waters have good water quality that fully supports designated uses. Of these waters, 6 percent are threatened and might deteriorate if we fail to manage potential sources of pollution.

Some form of pollution or habitat degradation impairs the remaining 37 percent of the surveyed estuarine waters. Twenty-seven percent of the surveyed estuarine waters have fair water quality that partially supports designated uses. Most of the time these waters provide adequate habitat for aquatic organisms and support human activities, but periodic pollution interferes with these activities and/or stresses aquatic life. Nine percent of the surveyed estuarine waters suffer from poor water quality that consistently stresses aquatic life and/or prevents people from using the estuarine waters for activities such as swimming and shellfishing.

What Is Polluting Our Estuaries?

The States identified more square miles of estuarine waters polluted by nutrients and bacteria than any other pollutant or process. Fifteen States reported that extra nutrients pollute 4,548 square miles of estuarine waters (which equals 47 percent of the impaired estuarine waters). As in lakes, extra inputs of nutrients from human activities destabilize estuarine ecosystems.

Twenty-five States reported that bacteria pollute 4,479 square miles of estuarine waters (which equals 46 percent of the impaired estuarine waters). Bacteria provide evidence that an estuary is contaminated with sewage that may contain numerous viruses and bacteria that cause illness in people.

The States also report that oxygen depletion from organic wastes impacts 3,127 square miles (which equals 32 percent of the impaired estuarine waters), habitat alterations impact 1,564 square miles (which equals 16 percent of the impaired estuarine waters), and oil and grease pollute 1,344 square miles (which equals 14 percent of the impaired estuarine waters).

Where Does this Pollution Come from?

Twenty-three States reported that urban runoff and storm sewers are the most widespread source of pollution in the Nation's surveyed estuarine waters. Pollutants in urban runoff and storm sewer effluent degrade aquatic life or interfere with public use of 4,508 square miles of estuarine waters (which equals 46 percent of the impaired estuarine waters).

The States also reported that municipal sewage treatment plants pollute 3,827 square miles of estuarine waters (39 percent of the impaired estuarine waters), agriculture pollutes 3,321 square miles of estuarine waters (34 percent of the impaired estuarine waters), and industrial discharges pollute 2,609 square miles (27 percent of the impaired estuarine waters). Urban sources contribute more to the degradation of estuarine waters than agriculture because urban centers are located adjacent to most major estuaries.

Ocean Shoreline Waters

Although the oceans are expansive, they are vulnerable to pollution from numerous sources, including city storm sewers, ocean outfalls from sewage treatment plants, overboard disposal of debris and sewage, oil spills, and bilge discharges that contain oil and grease. Nearshore ocean waters, in particular, suffer from the same pollution problems that degrade our inland waters.

Overall Water Quality

Ocean Shoreline Waters Surveyed

- Total ocean shore = 58,421 miles including Alaska's shoreline
- Total surveyed = 5,208 miles—9 percent Surveyed—91 percent Not Surveyed

Levels of Overall Use Support — Ocean Shoreline Waters

- Good (Fully Supporting)—89 percent
- Good (Threatened)—4 percent
- Fair (Partially Supporting)—5 percent
- Poor (Not Supporting)—2 percent
- Poor (Not Attainable)—0 percent

Thirteen of the 27 coastal States and Territories surveyed only 9 percent of the Nation's estimated 58,421 miles of ocean coastline. Most of the surveyed waters (4,834 miles, or 93 percent) have good quality that supports a healthy aquatic community and public activities. Of these waters, 225 miles (4 percent of the surveyed shoreline) are threatened and may deteriorate in the future.

Some form of pollution or habitat degradation impairs the remaining 7 percent of the surveyed shoreline (374 miles). Five percent of the surveyed estuarine waters have fair water quality that partially supports designated uses. Most of the time, these waters provide adequate habitat for aquatic organisms and support human activities, but periodic pollution interferes with these activities and/or stresses aquatic life. Only 2 percent of the surveyed shoreline suffers from poor water quality that consistently stresses aquatic life and/or prevents people from using the shoreline for activities such as swimming and shellfishing.

Only six of the 27 coastal States identified pollutants and sources of pollutants degrading ocean shoreline waters. General conclusions cannot be drawn from the information supplied by these States because these States border less than 1 percent of the shoreline along the contiguous States. The six States identified impacts in their ocean shoreline waters from bacteria, metals, nutrients, turbidity, siltation, and pesticides. The six States reported that urban runoff and storm sewers, industrial discharges, land disposal of wastes, septic systems, agriculture, unspecified non-point sources, and combined sewer overflows (CSOs) pollute their coastal shoreline waters.

Wetlands

Wetlands are areas that are inundated or saturated by surface water or ground water at a frequency and duration sufficient to support (and that under normal circumstances does support) a prevalence of vegetation typically adapted for life in saturated soil conditions. Wetlands, which are found throughout the United States, generally include swamps, marshes, bogs, and similar areas.

Wetlands are now recognized as some of the most unique and important natural areas on earth. They vary in type according to differences in local and regional hydrology, vegetation, water chemistry, soils, topography, and climate. Coastal wetlands include estuarine marshes; mangrove swamps found in Puerto Rico, Hawaii, Louisiana, and Florida; and Great Lakes coastal wetlands. Inland wetlands, which may be adjacent to a waterbody or isolated, include marshes and wet meadows, bottomland hardwood forests, Great Plains prairie potholes, cypress-gum swamps, and southwestern playa lakes.

In their natural condition, wetlands provide many benefits, including food and habitat for fish and wildlife, water quality improvement, flood protection, shoreline erosion control, ground water exchange, as well as natural products for human use and opportunities for recreation, education, and research.

Wetlands help maintain and improve water quality by intercepting surface water runoff before it reaches open water, removing or retaining nutrients, processing chemical and organic wastes, and reducing sediment loads to receiving waters. As water moves through a wetland, plants slow the water, allowing sediment and pollutants to settle out. Plant roots trap sediment and are then able to metabolize and detoxify pollutants and remove nutrients such as nitrogen and phosphorus.

Wetlands function like natural basins, storing either floodwater that overflows riverbanks or surface water that collects in isolated depressions. By doing so, wetlands help protect adjacent and downstream property from flood damage. Trees and other wetlands vegetation help slow the speed of flood waters. This action, combined with water storage, can lower flood heights and reduce the water's erosive potential. In agricultural areas, wetlands can help reduce the likelihood of flood damage to crops.

Wetlands within and upstream of urban areas are especially valuable for flood protection because urban development increases the rate and volume of surface water runoff, thereby increasing the risk of flood damage.

Wetlands produce a wealth of natural products, including fish and shellfish, timber, wildlife, and wild rice. Much of the Nation's fishing and shellfishing industry harvests wetlands-dependent species. A national survey conducted by the Fish and Wildlife Service (FWS) in 1991 illustrates the economic value of some of the wetlands-dependent products. Over 9 billion pounds of fish and shellfish landed in the United States in 1991 had a direct, dockside value of $3.3 billion. This served as the basis of a seafood processing and sales industry that generated total expenditures of $26.8 billion. In addition, 35.6 million anglers spent $24 billion on freshwater and saltwater fishing. It is estimated that 71 percent of commercially valuable fish and shellfish depend directly or indirectly on coastal wetlands.

Overall Water Quality

The States, Tribes, and other jurisdictions are making progress in developing specific designated uses and water quality standards for wetlands, but many States and Tribes still lack specific water quality criteria and monitoring programs for wetlands. Without criteria and monitoring data, most States and Tribes cannot evaluate use support. To date, only nine States and Tribes reported the designated use support status for some of their wetlands. Only one State used quantitative data as a basis for the use support decisions.

EPA cannot derive national conclusions about water quality conditions in all wetlands because the States used different methodologies to survey only 3 percent of the total wetlands in the Nation. Summarizing State wetlands data would also produce misleading results because two States (North Carolina and Louisiana) contain 91 percent of the surveyed wetlands acreage.

What Is Polluting Our Wetlands and Where Does this Pollution Come from?

The States have even fewer data to quantify the extent of pollutants degrading wetlands and the sources of these pollutants. Although most States cannot quantify wetlands area impacted by individual causes and sources of degradation, 12 States identified causes and 13 States identified sources known to degrade wetlands integrity to some extent. These States listed sediment as the most widespread cause of degradation impacting wetlands, followed by flow alterations, habitat modifications, and draining. Agriculture topped the list of sources degrading wetlands, followed by urban runoff, hydrologic modification, and municipal point sources.

Wetland Loss: A Continuing Problem

It is estimated that over 200 million acres of wetlands existed in the lower 48 States at the time of European settlement. Since then, extensive wetlands acreage has been lost, with many of the original wetlands drained and converted to farmland and urban development. Today, less than half of our original wetlands remain. The losses amount to an area equal to the size of California. According to the U.S. Fish and Wildlife Service's *Wetlands Losses in the United States 1780's to 1980's*, the three States that have sustained the greatest percentage of wetlands loss are California (91 percent), Ohio (90 percent), and Iowa (89 percent).

According to FWS status and trends reports, the average annual loss of wetlands has decreased over the past 40 years. The average annual loss from the mid-1950s to the mid-1970s was 458,000 acres, and from the mid-1970s to the mid-1980s it was 290,000 acres. Agriculture was responsible for 87 percent of the loss from the mid-1950s to the mid-1970s and 54 percent of the loss from the mid-1970s to the mid-1980s.

A more recent estimate of wetlands losses from the National Resources Inventory (NRI), conducted by the Natural Resources Conservation Service (NRCS), indicates that 792,000 acres of wetlands were lost on non-Federal lands between 1982 and 1992 for a yearly loss estimate of 70,000 to 90,000 acres. This net loss is the result of gross losses of 1,561,300 acres of wetlands and gross gains of 768,700 acres of wetlands over the 10-year period. The NRI estimates are consistent with the trend of declining wetlands losses reported by FWS. Although losses have decreased, we still have to make progress toward our interim goal of no overall net loss of the Nation's remaining wetlands and the long-term goal of increasing the quantity and quality of the Nation's wetlands resource base.

The decline in wetlands losses is a result of the combined effect of several trends:

1. the decline in profitability in converting wetlands for agricultural production;

2. passage of Swampbuster provisions in the 1985 and 1990 Farm Bills that denied crop subsidy benefits to farm operators who converted wetlands to cropland after 1985;

3. presence of the CWA Section 404 permit programs as well as development of State management programs;

4. greater public interest and support for wetlands protection; and

5. implementation of wetlands restoration programs at the Federal, State, and local level.

Nineteen States listed sources of recent wetlands losses in their 1994 305(b) reports. Residential development and urban growth were cited as the leading sources of current losses. Other losses were due to commercial development; construction of roads, highways, and bridges; agriculture; and industrial development. In addition to human activities, a few States also reported that natural sources, such as rising lake levels, resulted in wetlands losses and degradation.

Ground Water

Ninety-five percent of all fresh water available on earth (exclusive of icecaps) is ground water. Ground water—water found in natural underground rock formations called aquifers—is a vital natural resource with many uses. The extent of the Nation's ground water resources is enormous. At least 60 percent of the land area in the conterminous United States overlies aquifers that may be susceptible to contamination. Usable ground water exists in every State.

Aquifers can range in size from thin surficial formations that yield small quantities of ground water to large systems such as the High Plains aquifer that underlies eight western States and provides water to millions. Although the Nation's ground water is of good quality, it is recognized that ground water is more vulnerable to contamination than previously reported and that an increasing number of pollution events and contamination sources are threatening the integrity of the resource.

Ground Water Use

Nationally, 51 percent of the population relies to some extent on ground water as a source of drinking water. This percentage is even higher in rural areas where most residents rely on potable or treatable ground water as an economical source of drinking water. Eighty-one percent of community water systems are dependent on ground water. Seventy-four percent of community water systems are small ground water systems serving 3,300 people or less. Ninety-five percent of the approximately 200,000 noncommunity water systems (serving schools, parks, and other small facilities) are ground water systems.

Irrigation accounts for approximately 63 percent of national ground water withdrawals. Public drinking water supplies account for approximately 19 percent of the Nation's total ground water withdrawals. Domestic, commercial, livestock, industrial, mining, and thermoelectric withdrawals together account for approximately 18 percent of national ground water withdrawals.

Ground Water Quality

Although the 1994 Section 305(b) State Water Quality Reports indicate that, overall, the Nation's ground water is of good quality, many local areas have experienced significant ground water contamination. The sources and types of ground water contamination vary depending upon the region of the country. Those most frequently reported by States include:

- Approximately 1.2 million federally regulated underground storage tanks are buried at over 500,000 sites nationwide. An estimated 139,000 tanks have leaked and impacted ground water quality.

- Seventy-seven percent of the 1.1 billion pounds of pesticides produced annually in the United States is applied to land in agricultural production, which usually overlies aquifers.

- More than 85 percent of all Superfund sites have some degree of ground water contamination. Most of these sites impact aquifers that are currently used, or potentially may be used, for drinking water purposes.

- Approximately 23 million domestic septic tanks are in operation in the United States. These tanks impact ground water quality through the discharge of fluids into or above aquifers.

The most common contaminants associated with these sources include petroleum compounds, nitrates, metals, volatile organic compounds (VOCs), and pesticides.

States are reporting that ground water quality is most likely to be adversely affected by contamination in areas of high demand or stress. To combat these problems, States are developing programs designed to evaluate the overall quality and vulnerability of their ground water resources, to identify potential threats to ground water quality, and to identify methods to protect their ground water resources. Thirty-three States indicate that they have implemented statewide ground water monitoring programs.

Ground water monitoring programs vary widely among the States, depending upon the special needs of each of the States. For example, some States choose to monitor ground water quality in specific areas that are especially vulnerable to contamination, whereas other States may choose to monitor ground water quality on a statewide basis. When it comes to selecting chemicals to test for in the ground water, some States monitor for a large suite of chemicals, whereas other States limit monitoring to one or two specific chemicals that are a definite threat to ground water quality. Ground water monitoring provides a great deal of information about the nature and quality of our Nation's ground water resources. Still, there is much we do not know about how human activities influence ground water quality. Our continued quest for information about the status of our ground water will help protect and preserve this vast and vulnerable resource. Through a greater understanding of how human activities influence ground water quality, we can better ensure the long-term availability of high-quality water for future generations.

Chapter 12

Cryptosporidiosis: Diarrhea-Inducing Parasite

What is cryptosporidiosis?

Cryptosporidiosis (krip-to-spo-rid-e-o-sis)

Cryptosporidiosis is a disease caused by the parasite *Cryptosporidium parvum*, which as late as 1976 was not known to cause disease in humans. Until 1993, when over 400,000 people in Milwaukee, Wisconsin, became ill with diarrhea after drinking water contaminated with the parasite, few people had heard of either cryptosporidiosis or the single-celled intestinal protozoan that causes it.

Since the Milwaukee outbreak, concern about the safety of drinking water in the United States has increased, and new attention has been focused on determining and reducing the risk for cryptosporidiosis—from community and municipal water supplies.

How is cryptosporidiosis spread?

Cryptosporidiosis is spread by putting something in the mouth that has been contaminated with the stool of an infected person or animal. In this way, people swallow the *Cryptosporidium* parasite, which is too small to be seen with the naked eye. A person can become infected by drinking contaminated water or eating raw or undercooked food contaminated with *Cryptosporidium* oocysts (an egg-like form of the parasite that is the infectious stage); direct contact with the

Centers for Disease Control Press Release, June 19, 1995.

droppings of infected animals or stool of infected humans; or hand-to-mouth transfer of oocysts from surfaces that may have become contaminated with microscopic amounts of stool from an infected person or animal.

What are the symptoms of cryptosporidiosis?

Two to ten days after infection by the parasite, symptoms may appear. Although some persons may not have symptoms, others have watery diarrhea, headache, abdominal cramps, nausea, vomiting, and low-grade fever. These symptoms may lead to weight loss and dehydration.

In otherwise healthy persons, these symptoms usually last one to two weeks, at which time the immune system is able to stop the infection. In persons with suppressed immune systems, such as persons who have AIDS or recently have had an organ or bone marrow transplant, the infection may continue and become life-threatening.

What should you do if you suspect that you have cryptosporidiosis?

See your physician. Since the routine stool examination used for most parasites usually fails to detect *Cryptosporidium*, a stool specimen should be examined using stains/tests available especially for this parasite. It is important for persons with a poorly functioning immune system to seek medical attention early in the course of their disease.

What is the treatment for cryptosporidiosis?

No safe and effective cure is available for cryptosporidiosis.

People who have normal immune systems improve without taking antibiotic or antiparasitic medications.

The treatment recommended for this diarrheal illness is to drink plenty of fluids and to get extra rest. Physicians may prescribe medication to slow the diarrhea during recovery.

Who is at risk?

Persons at increased risk for cryptosporidiosis include child care workers; diaper-aged children who attend child care centers; persons exposed to human feces by sexual contact; and caregivers who might come in direct contact with feces while caring for a person infected with cryptosporidiosis at home or in a medical facility. Once infected, persons with suppressed immune systems, such as cancer chemotherapy patients, are at risk for severe disease.

How can you prevent cryptosporidiosis?

- Avoid water or food that may be contaminated.

- Wash hands after using the toilet and before handling food.

- If you work in a child care center where you change diapers, be sure to wash your hands thoroughly with plenty of soap and warm water after every diaper change, even if you wear gloves.

- During community-wide outbreaks caused by contaminated drinking water, boil drinking water for one minute to kill the *Cryptosporidium* parasite. Allow water to cool before drinking it.

- HIV-infected persons should avoid drinking water directly from lakes or rivers; avoid unpasteurized milk or milk products; avoid exposure to calves and lambs and places where these animals are raised; wash hands after contact with pets; and wash hands after gardening or other contact with soil. Because any sexual activity that brings a person in contact with the feces of an infected partner greatly increases the risk for cryptosporidiosis, HIV-infected persons and AIDS patients should follow "safer sex" guidelines and avoid sexual practices that may result in contact with feces.

- If you are a caregiver of cryptosporidiosis patients, wash hands after bathing patients, emptying bedpans, changing soiled linen, or otherwise coming in contact with the stools of patients.

- If you have cryptosporidiosis, wash your hands often to prevent spreading the disease to other members of your household. For more information on cryptosporidiosis, see the following sources:

Cordell RL, Addiss DG. Cryptosporidiosis in child care settings: a review of the literature and recommendations for prevention and control. Pediatr Infect Dis J. 1994;1354):310-17.

Dubey JP, Speer CA, Fayer R. Cryptosporidiosis of man and animals. Boston: CRC Press, 1990.

LeChevallier MW, Norton WD, Lee RG. *Giardia* and *Cryptosporidium* spp. in filtered drinking water supplies. Appl Environ Microbiol 1991;57<9):2617-21.

MacKenzie WR, Hoxie NJ, Proctor ME, Gradus MS, Blair KA, Peterson DE, Kazmierczak JJ, Addiss DG, Fox KR, Rose JB, Davis JP. A massive outbreak in Milwaukee of *Cryptosporidium* infection transmitted through the filtered public water supply. N Engl J Med 1994; 331:161-7.

Rose JB, Gerba CP, and Jakubowski W. Survey of potable water supplies for *Cryptosporidium* and *Giardia*. Environmental Science and Technology 1991;25(8):1393-1400.

Smith PD, Quinn TC, Strober W, Janoff EN, Masur H. Gastrointestinal infections in AIDS. Ann Intern Med 1992;116:63-77.

Chapter 13

What's in the Water?: The Disinfectant Dilemma

When 25 high-level representatives from industry and government, as well as environmental, labor, and civil rights organizations, first sat down together in Washington in the fall of 1993, the event might have been compared to the lion sitting down with the lamb. Often, adversaries over the years, these diverse and critical sectors of American society had been assigned the joint challenge of helping to craft realistic U.S. policies that simultaneously encourage economic growth, create jobs, and protect the environment.

But in 1974, scientists discovered that when chlorine is used to disinfect water, it can react with natural organic matter to form chemicals known as disinfection by-products. Chronic exposure to chlorine and chlorine by-products may cause liver, kidney, heart, and neurological damage, as well as effects to unborn children, according to the EPA. In proposed rules for regulating disinfection by-products, the EPA classifies chloroform, bromate, bromoform, dichloroacetic acid, and bromodichloromethane as probable human carcinogens based on carcinogenicity in animals. By-products such as dichloroacetic acid, trichloroacetic acid, chloral hydrate, and bromodichloromethane are classified as possible carcinogens, based on animal data.

In response, in part, to the potential health effects of chlorinated water, researchers have attempted to find other methods of disinfection. Though work continues in this confounding area, scientists are finding that these alternatives may sometimes offer more problems

NIH publication 95-218. *Environmental Health Perspectives* Volume 103, Number Supplement 1, January 1995.

than solutions. Alternatives to chlorine in water treatment include ozone, chlorine dioxide, chloramines, and ultraviolet radiation, all of which can form disinfection by-products. Now EPA is preparing regulations for 12 contaminants that result from drinking water disinfection.

Consumers, however, must still rely on disinfection to prevent waterborne disease. From 1971 to 1990, more than 140,000 people nationwide became ill from microbial contamination of drinking water, according to a study by the Centers for Disease Control and Prevention. Such numbers on waterborne disease are only speculative, though, according to Robert D. Morris, an epidemiologist with the Department of Family and Community Medicine at the Medical College of Wisconsin, Milwaukee: "The surveillance systems for waterborne disease are designed only to address severe outbreaks. They are useless for dealing with diseases where there is no mortality and which are self-limiting." Thus the numbers of people affected by waterborne disease are likely much higher than reported numbers. Now, through three proposed rules, EPA is attempting to balance risks from microbial contaminants against risks from disinfectants and disinfection by-products.

Disinfection Rules

The Information Collection Rule, proposed in the *Federal Register* in February 1994, would require that water systems collect information on the quality of their source water, on treatment processes they use, and on the quality of the water they provide to customers. Furthermore, the rule would require large water systems (serving 100,000 or more people) to monitor for micro-organisms (including cryptosporidia) and for disinfection by-products in treated water, but it would allow them to choose which technology to use. "We want the final rule to be flexible and cost-effective and for systems to determine how they will comply, without overly burdensome regulation," says Stig Regli, an environmental engineer at EPA's Office of Groundwater and Drinking Water.

In June 1994, EPA also proposed the disinfectants/disinfection by-products rule and the enhanced surface water treatment rule. Under these proposals, communities would be required to meet tighter standards for disinfectants and disinfection by-products, and new standards to protect water systems against harmful micro-organisms such as *giardia* and *cryptosporidia*. In short, regulators will aim to control disinfection by-products without increasing risks in drinking water from dangerous micro-organisms. "We're not asking utilities to do a juggling aa between these risks," says Regli. "Through these rules, we would try to establish a balance between the risks, defining how much total treatment, including filtration and disinfection, a system would need, depending on the degree of pathogen concentration in its source water."

Why Not Chlorinate?

Chlorine, a pale-green gas in its elemental form, is a crucial part of industrial processes. In the United States, 212 industries use chlorine and related chemicals, according to the Chemical Manufacturers Association. Most of the 11 million tons of chlorine produced each year in the United States is used in bleaching paper and in the production of solvents and polyvinyl chloride (PVC). Tile floor coverings, automobile components, and medical equipment are only a few of the products derived from PVC, which represents the fastest growing segment of chlorine use.

In recent decades, scientists have shown that chlorinated chemicals are the cause of reproductive abnormalities in many wildlife species. In addition, chlorinated chemicals could be part of the reason for increases in breast and prostate cancers in humans. The most damaging chlorinated substances are organochlorides, which contain chlorine and carbon. Organochlorides include polychlorinated biphenyls (PCBs), dioxins, and the now-banned pesticide DDT, which have entered the environment primarily through industrial emissions and are highly toxic.

Water treatment represents a relatively small percentage of chlorine's use in the United States. Only about 5 percent of the chlorine produced nationally each year is used to treat drinking water and waste-water. Yet chlorinated water touches everyone. "One of the largest exposures to chlorinated compounds is from drinking water," says Erik D. Olson, senior attorney with the Natural Resources Defense Council. "Virtually every person in the country is exposed daily, even hourly, to chlorinated water."

The question is, exactly how dangerous to human health are chlorination by-products? Since the early 1970s, three kinds of epidemiological studies have attempted to assess the relationship between cancer and long-term consumption of water from various sources, particularly surface water.

Ecological studies have investigated cancer mortality rates over broad geographic areas. Cohort studies have investigated groups of people that differ according to the extent of exposure to a potential cause of disease. Most cohort studies on the health effects of chlorinated water have compared illness rates among populations who drink chlorinated water and populations who drink unchlorinated water or groundwater, which tends to be less heavily chlorinated. Case-control studies have investigated the backgrounds of people with specific diseases—bladder cancer, for example—who drink chlorinated water with people having the same disease who did not drink chlorinated water.

Morris and colleagues at the Medical College of Wisconsin reviewed 10 separate epidemiological studies, published between 1966 and 1991, on the relationships between water chlorination and cancer. In their analysis published in the July 1992 *American Journal of Public Health,* Morris estimated that chlorinated by-products are associated with 10,700 bladder and rectal cancers a year. Morris notes, however, "precise cause and effect cannot be determined."

But in an August 1994 *American Journal of Public Health* editorial, Kenneth Cantor, an epidemiologist at the National Cancer Institutes argued that the initial studies used in the Morris meta-analysis were "subject to many types of bias." For example, many of the initial studies assumed that exposures to contaminants were virtually constant over subjects' lifetimes. Despite his criticism of the methods used in the Morris analysis, Cantor agrees that "several thousand excess cases [of rectal and bladder cancer] each year may be linked to consumption of chlorination by-products from surface water sources in the United States."

Since the mid-1980s, Greenpeace has been pushing for a phase-out of industrial chlorine use, following the lead of Germany's Green Party. Greenpeace's campaign gained strength in 1991 when the International Joint Commission, a Canadian-U.S. government agency that oversees the Great Lakes, also called for phasing out the use of chlorine in industry. Then, in 1994, the Clinton Administration proposed a study of chlorine and chlorinated compounds as part of the reauthorization of the Clean Water Act. This proposal would have required the EPA to gather a task force to "assess the use, environmental and health impacts of chlorine and chlorinated compounds, and availability . . . and safety of substitutes for these substances as used in publicly owned treatment works and drinking water systems," among other uses, including pulp and paper manufacturing. However, the reauthorization bill did not pass.

The chlorine industry is strongly opposed to a ban on the use of chlorine. "Sunsetting" chlorine is unnecessary because emissions are already being phased out through existing law, according to chlorine-industry representatives. "The Clean Water Act has worked very well to control and reduce the release of chlorine compounds in water, air, and waste disposal," says Debbie Schwartz of the Chlorine Chemistry Council.

But Rick Hind, legislative director of Greenpeace Toxics Campaign, says that existing reductions in chlorine emissions are too little, too late. "Small reductions in emissions will be erased as the economy continues to grow, as we see additional and larger industrial uses of chlorine. Some of these [chlorine by-products], such as dioxin, are highly persistent and bioaccumulative, so we will continue to see their buildup in the fatty tissues of animals. The levels of dioxin found in most adults and children are already high enough to represent significant health threats."

Disinfection Alternatives

Few people realistically expect to see the use of chlorine in water treatment banned—or even drastically reduced—anytime soon, because the feasible alternatives do not completely replace chlorine. In fact, none of the major alternatives to chlorine—ozone, chlorine dioxide, and chloramine—fulfills the three most important requirements of a disinfectant: effectiveness, relatively low cost, and the ability to provide a residual in the distribution system to prevent regrowth of micro-organisms. As a result, greater numbers of water suppliers are turning to alternatives in combination with chlorination.

Ozonation. Ozonation, a process of passing ozone through water, is an effective disinfectant, though not a complete answer without chlorination. "Ozonation has a flash effect on killing bacteria," according to Billy Tullos, business manager for Elf Atochem North America, a chemical company based in Philadelphia. "It kills what it touches, but it's short-term, and the water picks up bacteria again in the distribution system." So water suppliers generally must use chlorine in combination with ozone, though in lower dosages, to act as a residual disinfectant.

Ozonation is the most commonly used water treatment method in Europe. The first ozonation plant was built in Nice, France, in 1906. "Many Europeans say they dislike chlorinated water," says Susan Richardson, a scientist at the EPA Research Laboratory in Athens,

Georgia. "They generally prefer the taste and smell of ozonated water."

In the United States, the first ozone plant opened in 1978, and the number of plants had increased to 18 by June 1990. A 1992 study prepared for the American Water Works Association showed that, of 166 water utilities in the United States serving about 72 million people, only about 5 percent of the population served consumed ozonated water. However, this percentage will likely increase as the Federal government further regulates disinfection by-products. The study also showed that ozone was the disinfectant most evaluated by utilities for future use, with 81 percent of the utilities considering ozonation.

Like all disinfectants, ozonation forms potentially harmful by-products. Probably the most dangerous by-product of ozonation is bromate, an animal carcinogen and probably human carcinogen according to the International Agency for Research on Cancer. Bromate's effects on humans are unclear. Fred Hauchman, associate director of EPA's Health Effects Research Laboratory in North Carolina, who has studied bromate's effects on animals, says, "it appears that bromate may be one of the more carcinogenic by-products . . . though as with any contaminant studies performed in the laboratory, these results may not be able to be extrapolated to humans."

Alternatives to chlorine are costly because of necessary capital improvements and changes in treatment processes, though it is difficult to estimate exactly how much each alternative would cost because economies of scale vary from large to small water suppliers. Ozonation is the most expensive alternative because utilities must install ozone production facilities. These facilities are costly to operate and maintain, require specially trained technicians to run them, and are large users of electricity, all of which would contribute to increases in water bills.

Chlorine dioxide. Chlorine dioxide is as effective a disinfectant as chlorine, not much more expensive, and does not produce trihalomethanes, a dangerous by-product of chlorine. In 1977, 103 U.S. water systems were using or had used chlorine dioxide. In 1994, an estimated 500 to 900 municipalities were using chlorine dioxide, although some only seasonally. Chlorine dioxide may also create health problems, though this is not well understood. For example, when chlorine dioxide is added to drinking water, some of the chemical can decompose into a by-product called chlorite. Studies have shown that chlorite administered to rats through drinking water resulted in anemia in the animals, according to the EPA's review of disinfectants and disinfection by-products published in the 29 July 1994 *Federal Register*.

Chlorine dioxide is difficult to produce without generating chlorites and other by-products. Nevertheless, a recent study by the EPA's Richardson, published in the April 1994 *Environmental Science of Technology*, showed that chlorine dioxide forms far fewer dangerous by-products than chlorine. Richardson and colleagues found only trace amounts of toxic by-products of chlorine dioxide in water at a pilot drinking water plant in Evansville, Indiana. According to Richardson, "at least a factor of a thousand less than levels you would find for chlorinated water." In general, though, chlorine dioxide has been studied less intensively than some other disinfectants. "We recognize that health risk data are not substantial on chlorine dioxide and chlorites," say Regli.

Chloramine. Another alternative to chlorine is chloramine, a combination of chlorine and ammonia. Chloramine does not produce chlorites and forms far fewer by-products than chlorine alone, specifically trihalomethanes. After 1979, when the EPA passed the first rule regulating disinfectants and their by-products, many utilities began using chloramines, usually as a residual disinfectant. According to the 1992 American Water Works survey, 31 percent of the population was served by chlorinated water. However, chloramine is far less effective than chlorine, and thus may not be safely used as a primary treatment method. It may be used in combination with lesser amounts of chlorine, thereby reducing by-products. Still, chloramine too may have potential adverse health effects. Chloramines have been reported to damage red blood cells. Chloramines can also interfere with the mechanisms used by red blood cells to prevent and repair this damage. Where chloramines are in the water supply, many dialysis centers have installed reverse osmosis units, along with charcoal filtration systems, to prevent anemia in hemodialysis patients.

Preventing the Problems

Water systems can use two basic strategies to reduce the amount of disinfection by-products in their finished water, according to Richard Miltner, chief of the treatment evaluation section at EPA's Drinking Water Research Division in Cincinnati, Ohio. "First, don't use chlorine; use something else," Miltner suggests. "Second, remove a good deal of the organic matter before disinfecting through clarification and filtering."

Water clarification techniques, such as coagulation, sedimentation, and filtration, remove many organic materials from finished water. Granular activated carbon (GAC), a filtering technique used in many European cities, can be especially successful at removing organic matter. Some American systems have been using GAC for many years to improve the taste or smell of drinking water, but now more are installing GAC as a method of reducing disinfection by-products. GAC is feasible for most surface water in the United States, according to Olson.

Water suppliers, however, argue that GAC is expensive and often can be unnecessary. Utility managers complain that the Natural Resources Defense Council and other environmental groups want every water system in the nation to use the most expensive technologies whether the systems really need them or not. "The quality of our water is very good," says Dean Moss, general manager of the Beaufort-Jasper Water and Sewer Authority, which serves Beaufort, South Carolina, and surrounding communities. "We're meeting all standards. We test for all substances we can, for whatever might be in the water, and we're below detection on virtually everything. To add GAC would be an expensive procedure, and I would see only a minuscule improvement in the quality of the water. I couldn't justify the cost." Moss estimates that a GAC facility would cost $3 to $4 million, while the authority already carries a debt of $10 million. "The costs of implementing proposed technologies are pretty substantial," Moss adds. "I want to deliver the highest quality water I can, but I have to balance what my customers can afford."

Cost Overruns?

How much are you willing to spend for clean water? That is a question Americans should be asking themselves, because the cost of treating water is going up. Since 1991, the EPA has been strengthening federal treatment standards to improve the quality of potable water. As communities conform to these new standards, they are forced to spend more to monitor and test for contaminants and to treat drinking water and sewage.

Water utilities are concerned about the costs of complying with increasingly expensive regulations. Congress, under the Safe Drinking Water Act, which requires the EPA to regulate what comes from our tap, has required the EPA to establish regulations for 25 new contaminants every three years beginning in 1991. In 1986, the EPA required water systems nationwide to meet standards for 23 contaminants, including hazardous chemicals from industry and agriculture. This number rose to 62 chemicals by 1991, to 86 by 1994, and could reach nearly 200 by the year 2000. The Clean Water Act, meanwhile, requires the EPA to regulate what municipalities release into rivers and streams after treatment.

Water suppliers say that water regulations are too often rigid, expensive, and sometimes unnecessary. Consequently, water utilities have joined forces with local and state officials to establish a coalition to lobby Congress. This coalition wants the federal government to pay for growing environmental mandates, thereby reducing or eliminating the financial burden on water systems, and it wants water systems to have more latitude in considering the costs and benefits of different clean-up methods and technologies.

Environmentalists say that clean water is worth the cost of increasing regulations, and that too many Americans are drinking inadequately treated water. The nation's supplies still contain dangerous contaminants, including synthetic organic chemicals, lead, arsenic, and fecal wastes, possibly bringing increased risks of cancer, birth defects, and infections. Industrial toxic wastes are discharged into rivers and streams or disposed in landfills, pits, lagoons, and dumps where they can leak into shallow water tables connected to lakes and streams, and eventually into aquifers. Oil and other contaminants run off streets and parking lots into waterways. And pesticides and fertilizers spread on lawns and cropland filter through the soil into the water table or wash directly into lakes and streams, which supply half of the nation's drinking water.

Researchers, though, have an incomplete understanding of how much pollution is in the nation's supply and where the pollution is concentrated. "We're not monitoring effectively for contaminants that could be in our water, so we don't have a good database for what is there," says Paul Schwartz, public policy advocate at Clean Water Action. Part of the problem is poor monitoring by water systems. "Many systems report no data at all," he says. Although systems that fail to monitor are in violation of EPA and state drinking water regulations.

Experts agree that polluted water and inadequate monitoring are far more common occurrences in small systems (serving 10,000 people or less) than in large ones. Even today, some very small systems (serving less than 100 people) lack chlorination, and some are so inefficient that they are on the verge of bankruptcy and cannot keep up with growing monitoring costs. But even efficient small suppliers have difficulty coping with a regulatory framework that favors larger systems.

The problem is that small systems must comply with standards for treatment that were developed to be affordable for large systems; small systems lack the economies of scale to absorb the growing costs of new rules. By the year 2000, small systems will pay nearly $3 billion to comply with all drinking water regulations according to the EPA.

Yet it is clear that federal regulations have forced the great majority of water systems to improve water quality. Mandates have pushed state agencies to do a better job of monitoring and enforcement. "The Federal government's taking control from the states stopped the absolute decline of resources," says Schwartz.

The coalition of utilities and local and state officials, however, finds the rising costs of water treatment hard to swallow. "Environmental advocates want laboratory-quality water, but we do not have the ability to sustain zero contaminants for 200,000 systems," says Kevin McCarty, assistant executive director of the U.S. Conference of Mayors. "We need to reflect what is possible with setting standards. Water is pretty cheap now, but regulations coming up will be very expensive. We could see unthinkable escalations in the cost of water."

Under today's rules, water suppliers often have a choice between one clean-up technology that is very expensive and very effective and a second clean-up technology that is nearly as effective but much less expensive. But courts usually require that the supplier choose the technology that is most effective, regardless of expense, critics say. So utilities cannot choose clean-up methods that are appropriate for local economic conditions. "When there is a minimal difference in health risks between two technologies, communities should be allowed to choose the less expensive one," says Shaun McGrath, aide to Congressman Jim Slattery (D-Kansas), Who introduced Safe Drinking Water Act amendments in 1994 that failed to pass.

Water suppliers want the option of developing watershed-protection and pollution-prevention programs as methods of compliance. Now most water systems are limited to applying technology. "With more pollution prevention, a lot of contamination of drinking water could be prevented before it reaches the systems," says McGrath. "If a community has a good pollution-prevention program, such as measures to prevent nitrate run-off, it should be regarded." Environmentalists agree with the coalition, in principle, that a community's finances should be given more consideration when clean-up technologies are chosen for water supplies. However, they also believe that the anti-regulatory coalition wants to go too far in weakening standards. If the coalition gets what it wants from Congress, they say, there could be no additional drinking-water regulations for the rest of the decade.

In the meantime, chlorine remains the least expensive and one of the most effective disinfectants. In fact, the widespread use of chlorine is still the public's best protection against the dangers of waterborne diseases, particularly in communities served by smaller water systems that cannot afford expensive alternative technologies. However, because it is still not possible to draw definite conclusions about the precise nature and extent of cancer and non-cancer health effects from consumption of chlorinated by-products, it also remains the most controversial. Most of the factions involved, however, seem to agree that the controversy will spur research into newer safer technologies.

Rigid Regulations

Standing on the banks of the North Saluda Reservoir, north of Greenville, South Carolina, you can see the pebbly bottom through the clear, greenish water. Streams run from the Blue Ridge Mountains to the Table Rock and North Saluda reservoirs, providing most of the water for that city and surrounding communities. The Greenville Water System, which owns every inch of the watersheds that drain into the lakes, has a reputation throughout the Southeast for quality and safety.

Yet Greenville residents must pay for a $75 million filtration plant to reduce micro-organisms in local drinking water. The filtration plant, scheduled to start up by the end of 1999, is already costing consumers 13 percent more in their water bills, an expense that Lynn Stovall, general manager of the Greenville Water System, says is a waste of money. Greenville must build a filtration plant because Congress, under the Safe Drinking Water Act amendments passed in 1986, requires that nearly every supply of surface water in the nation be filtered to reduce bacteria and viruses, and Greenville cannot meet the criteria of the EPA's Surface Water Treatment Rule for avoiding filtration.

The regulation could significantly reduce incidents of illness due to microbial contamination. Only about 50 medium-to-large water systems around the nation have met the avoidance criteria set by the EPA, but they must still protect their watersheds from pollution and meet rigorous treatment requirements.

Greenville's supply should also be allowed to avoid filtration, Stovall argues, because disinfection with chlorine and other treatment methods already reduce micro-organisms to safe levels. Ninety percent of Greenville's water is unfiltered from the protected watersheds, and the other 10 percent is pumped from Lake Keowee and filtered by the Greenville Water System.

"Greenville's watershed protection is unprecedented in South Carolina," agrees Clint Shealy, environmental engineer at the South Carolina Department of Health and Environmental Control. But the EPA rules for water quality are "very stringent," he says. "The Greenville Water System missed deadlines and did not meet some water quality and treatment guidelines. We really had no choice but to require filtration. The state has no authority to give variances."

To Stovall, however, the EPA's policy does not allow for local conditions. The EPA's rules are one-size-fits-all standards, applying to nearly every community in the country, whether they are heavily polluted or, like Greenville's water source, as clean as a mountain stream. "It's difficult to get regulators to hear your point of view when their minds are already made up," Stovall says.

Water suppliers also complain about inflexible regulations that require expensive monitoring for contaminants that are not present in their supplies or are present only in the part per billion or lower range. Utilities point to required nationwide monitoring for a pesticide used primarily in the production of pineapples, DBCP—a substance that has been banned for more than a decade. But Schwartz argues that the DBCP example is misleading. This persistent chemical was used on crops nationwide and still shows up in drinking water. Furthermore, people dump chemicals where they shouldn't, and these toxins can leach into water supplies.

Congressional lawmakers are hoping to give states more flexibility on testing requirements, says Shaun McGrath, legislative aide to Congressman Jim Slattery (D Kansas). "If a water system has tested for contaminants and they haven't been found it for some time, water systems shouldn't have to test four times a year. In those cases, we think systems should be able to test far less often, maybe once every four years."

—by John Tibberts

John Tibberts is a freelance journalist in Charleston, South Carolina.

Chapter 14

Fluoridated Water and the Risk of Cancer

Virtually all water contains fluoride. In the 1940s, scientists discovered that the higher the level of natural fluoride in the community water supply, the fewer the dental caries (cavities) among the residents. Currently, more than half of all Americans live in areas where fluoride is added to the water supply to bring it up to the level considered best for dental health.

The possible relationship between fluoridated water and cancer has been debated at length. Although earlier animal studies revealed no evidence that fluoride is carcinogenic, a National Toxicology Program study completed in April 1990 generated considerable interest in this subject. In this study, a small number of male rats (4 of 130) developed bone cancer after drinking water containing fluoride in amounts that were 25 to 100 times greater than the levels found in municipal fluoridated water. No cancers were seen in the female rats or in the male or female mice that were also tested. According to the scientists who conducted the study, the fact that a few male rats developed tumors could not be used as firm evidence to link fluoride ingestion with cancer.

In February 1991, the Public Health Service reported the results of a year-long survey that showed no evidence of an association between fluoride and cancer in humans. The survey, which involved a review of more than 50 human epidemiology studies produced over the past 40 years, led the investigators to conclude that optimal fluoridation of drinking water "does not pose a detectable risk of cancer to humans."

National Cancer Institute. *Cancer Facts*. May 1995.

In one recent study, scientists at the National Cancer Institute evaluated the relationship between fluoridation of drinking water and the cancer mortality (deaths) in the United States during a 36-year period and the relationship between fluoridation and the cancer incidence (rate) during a 15-year period. After examining more than 2.2 million cancer death records and 125,000 cancer case records in counties using fluoridated water, the researchers saw no indication of a cancer risk associated with fluoridated drinking water.

The Cancer Information Service (CIS), a program of the National Cancer Institute, is a nationwide telephone service for cancer patients and their families, the public, and health care professionals. CIS information specialists have extensive training in providing up-to-date and understandable information about cancer. They can answer questions in English and Spanish and can send free printed material. In addition, CIS offices serve specific geographic areas and have information about cancer-related services and resources in their region. The toll-free number of the CIS is 1-800-4-CANCER (1-800-422-6237).

Chapter 15

Lead in Your Drinking Water

Health Threats from Lead

Too much lead in the human body can cause serious damage to the brain, kidneys, nervous system, and red blood cells.

You have the greatest risk, even with short-term exposure, if:

- you are a young child, or
- you are pregnant.

Sources of Lead in Drinking Water

Lead levels in your drinking water are likely to be highest if:

- your home has faucets or fittings made of brass which contains some lead, or

- your home or water system has lead pipes, or

- your home has copper pipes with lead solder, and
    —the home is less than five years old, or
    —you have naturally soft water, or
    —water often sits in the pipes several hours.

EPA Office of Water EPA/810-F-93-001, June 1993.

Actions You Can Take to Reduce Lead in Drinking Water

Flush Your Pipes Before Drinking. Anytime the water in a particular faucet has not been used for six hours or longer, "flush" your cold-water pipes by running the water until it becomes as cold as it will get. (This could take as little as five to thirty seconds if there has been recent heavy water use such as showering or toilet flushing. Otherwise, it could take two minutes or longer.) The more time water has been sitting in your home's pipes, the more lead it may contain.

Only Use Cold Water for Consumption. Use only water from the cold-water tap for drinking, cooking, and especially for making baby formula. Hot water is likely to contain higher levels of lead.

The two actions recommended above are very important to the health of your family. They will probably be effective in reducing lead levels because most of the lead in household water usually comes from the plumbing in your house, not from the local water supply.

Have Your Water Tested. After you have taken the two precautions above for reducing the lead in water used for drinking or cooking, have your water tested. The only way to be sure of the amount of lead in your household water is to have it tested by a competent laboratory. Your water supplier may be able to offer information or assistance with testing. Testing is especially important for apartment dwellers, because flushing may not be effective in high-rise buildings with lead-soldered central piping.

For more details on the problem of lead in drinking water and what you can do about it, read the questions and answers in the remainder of this chapter. Your local or state department of health or environment might be able to provide additional information.

Why is lead a problem? Although it has been used in numerous consumer products, lead is a toxic metal now known to be harmful to human health if inhaled or ingested. Important sources of lead exposure include: ambient air, soil and dust (both inside and outside the home), food (which can be contaminated by lead in the air or in food containers), and water (from the corrosion of plumbing). On average, it is estimated that lead in drinking water contributes between 10 and 20 percent of total lead exposure in young children. In the last few years, federal controls on lead in gasoline have significantly reduced people's exposure to lead.

The degree of harm depends upon the level of exposure (from all sources). Known effects of exposure to lead range from subtle biochemical changes at low levels of exposure, to severe neurological and toxic effects or even death at extremely high levels.

Does lead affect everyone equally? Young children, infants and fetuses appear to be particularly vulnerable to lead poisoning. A dose of lead that would have little effect on an adult can have a big effect on a small body. Also, growing children will more rapidly adsorb any lead they consume. A child's mental and physical development can be irreversibly stunted by over-exposure to lead. In infants, whose diet consists of liquids made with water—such as baby formula—lead in drinking water makes up an even greater proportion of total lead exposure (40 to 60 percent).

How could lead get into my drinking water? Typically, lead gets into your water after the water leaves your local treatment plant or your well. That is, the source of lead in your home's water is most likely pipe or solder in your home's own plumbing.

The most common cause is corrosion, a reaction between the water and the lead pipes or solder. Dissolved oxygen, low ph. (acidity) and low mineral content in water are common causes of corrosion. All kinds of water, however, may have high levels of lead.

One factor that increases corrosion is the practice of grounding electrical equipment (such as telephones) to water pipes. Any electric current traveling through the ground wire will accelerate the corrosion of lead in the pipes. (Nevertheless, wires should not be removed from pipes unless a qualified electrician installs an adequate alternative grounding system.)

Does my home's age make a difference? Lead-contaminated drinking water is most often a problem in houses that are either very old or very new.

Up through the early 1900s, it was common practice, in some areas of the country, to use lead pipes for interior plumbing. Also, lead piping was often used for the service connections that join residences to public water supplies. (This practice ended only recently in some localities.) Plumbing installed before 1930 is most likely to contain lead.

Copper pipes have replaced lead pipes in most residential plumbing. However, the use of lead solder with copper pipes is widespread. Experts regard this lead solder as the major cause of lead contamination of household water in U.S. homes today. New brass faucets and fittings can also leach lead, even though they are "lead-free."

Scientific data indicate that the newer the home, the greater the risk of lead contamination. Lead levels decrease as a building ages. This is because, as time passes, mineral deposits form a coating on the inside of the pipes (if the water is not corrosive). This coating insulates the water from the solder. But, during the first five years (before the coating forms) water is in direct contact with the lead. More likely than not, water in buildings less than five years old has high levels of lead contamination.

How can I tell if my water contains too much lead? You should have your water tested for lead. Testing costs between $20 and $100. Since you cannot see, taste, or smell lead dissolved in water, testing is the only sure way of telling whether or not there are harmful quantities of lead in your drinking water.

You should be particularly suspicious if your home has lead pipes (lead is a dull gray metal that is soft enough to be easily scratched with a house key), if you see signs of corrosion, frequent leaks, rust-colored water, stained dishes or laundry or if your non-plastic plumbing is less than five years old. Your water supplier may have useful information, including whether or not the service connector used in your home or area is made of lead.

Testing is especially important in high-rise buildings where flushing might not work.

How do I have my water tested? Water samples from the tap will have to be collected and sent to a qualified laboratory for analysis. Contact your local water utility or your local health department for information and assistance. In some instances, these authorities will test your tap water for you, or they can refer you to a qualified laboratory. You may find a qualified testing company under "Laboratories" in the yellow pages of your telephone directory.

You should be sure that the lab you use has been approved by your state or by EPA as being able to analyze drinking water samples for lead contamination. To find out which labs are qualified, contact your state or local department of the environment or health.

What are the testing procedures? Arrangements for sample collection will vary. A few laboratories will send a trained technician to take the samples; but in most cases, the lab will provide sample containers along with instructions as to how you should draw your own tap-water samples. If you collect the samples yourself, make sure you follow the lab's instructions exactly. Otherwise, the results might not be reliable.

Make sure that the laboratory is following EPA's water sampling and analysis procedures. Be certain to take a "first draw" and a "fully flushed" sample. (The first-draw sample—taken after at least six hours of no water use from the tap tested—will have the highest level of lead, while the fully flushed sample will indicate the effectiveness of flushing the tap before using the water.)

How much lead is too much? Federal standards initially limited the amount of lead in water to 50 parts per billion (ppb). In light of new health and exposure data, EPA has set an action level of 15 ppb. If tests show that the level of lead in your household water is in the area of 15 ppb or higher, it is advisable especially if there are young children in the home—to reduce the lead level in your tap water as much as possible. (EPA estimates that more than 40 million U.S. residents use water that can contain lead in excess of 15 ppb.)

Note: One ppb is equal to 1.0 microgram per liter (μg/l) or 0.001 milligram per liter (mg/l).

How can I reduce my exposure? If your drinking water is contaminated with lead, or until you find out for sure, there are several things you can do to minimize your exposure. Two of these actions should be taken right away by everyone who has, or suspects, a problem. The advisability of other actions listed here will depend upon your particular circumstances.

Immediate Steps

- The first step is to refrain from consuming water that has been in contact with your home's plumbing for more than six hours, such as overnight or during your work day. Before using water for drinking or cooking, "flush" the cold water faucet by allowing the water to run until you can feel that the water has become as cold as it will get. You must do this for each drinking water faucet—taking a shower will not flush your kitchen tap. Buildings built prior to about 1930 may have service connectors made of lead. Letting the water run for an extra 15 seconds after it cools should also flush this service connector. Flushing is important because the longer water is exposed to lead pipes or lead solder, the greater the possible lead contamination. (The water that comes out after flushing will not have been in extended contact with lead pipes or solder.)

- Once you have flushed a tap, you might fill one or more bottles with water and put them in the refrigerator for later use that day. (The water that was flushed—usually one to two gallons— can be used for non-consumption purposes such as washing dishes or clothes; it needn't be wasted.)

  Note: Flushing may prove ineffective in high-rise buildings that have large-diameter supply pipes joined with lead solder.

- The second step is to never cook with or consume water from the hot-water tap. Hot water dissolves more lead more quickly than cold water. So, do not use water taken from the hot tap for cooking or drinking, and especially not for making baby formula (If you need hot water, draw water from the cold tap and heat it on the stove.) Use only thoroughly flushed water from the cold tap for any consumption.

Other Actions

- If you are served by a public water system (more than 219 million people are) contact your supplier and ask whether or not the supply system contains lead piping, and whether your water is corrosive. If either answer is yes, ask what steps the supplier is taking to deal with the problem of lead contamination.

  Drinking water can be treated at the plant to make it less corrosive. Cities such as Boston and Seattle have successfully done this for an annual cost of less than one dollar per person. (Treatment to reduce corrosion will also save you and the water supplier money by reducing damage to plumbing.)

  Water mains containing lead pipes can be replaced, as well as those portions of lead service connections that are under the jurisdiction of the supplier.

- If you own a well or another water source, you can treat the water to make it less corrosive. Corrosion control devices for individual households include calcite filters and other devices. Calcite filters should be installed in the line between the water source and any lead service connections or lead-soldered pipe. You might ask your health or water department for assistance in finding these commercially, available products.

Recently a number of cartridge type filtering devices became available on the market. These devices use various types of filtering media, including carbon, ion exchange resins, activated alumina and other privately marketed products. Unless they have been certified as described below, the effectiveness of these devices to reduce lead exposure at the tap can vary greatly.

It is highly recommended that before purchasing a filter, you verify the claims made by the vendor. If you have bought a filter, you should replace the filter periodically as specified by the manufacturer. Failure to do so may result in exposure to high lead levels.

Two organizations can help you decide which type of filter is best for you. The National Sanitation Foundation, International (NSF), and independent testing agency, evaluates and certifies the performance of filtering devices to remove lead from drinking water. Generally, their seal of approval appears on the device and product packaging. The Water Quality Association (WQA) is an independent, not-for-profit organization that represents firms and individuals who produce and sell equipment and services which improves the quality of drinking water. WQA's water quality specialists can provide advice on treatment units for specific uses at home or business.

For additional information regarding the certification program, contact NSF at (313) 769-8010, or WQA at (708) 505-0161, ext. 270.

- You can purchase bottled water for home and office consumption. (Bottled water sold in interstate commerce is regulated by the Food and Drug Administration. Water that is bottled and sold within a state is under state regulation. EPA does not regulate bottled water.)

- When repairing or installing new plumbing in old homes, instruct, in writing, any plumber you hire to use only lead-free materials. See the definition of "lead free" below.

- When building a new home, be sure lead-free materials are used. Before you move into a newly built home, remove all strainers from faucets and flush the water for at least 15 minutes to remove loose solder or flux debris from the plumbing. Occasionally, check the strainers and remove any later accumulation of loose material.

What about lead in sources other that drinking water? As mentioned above, drinking water is estimated to contribute only 10 to 20 percent of the total lead exposure in young children. Ask your local health department or call EPA for more information on other sources of exposure to lead. A few general precautions can help prevent contact with lead in and around your home:

- Avoid removing paint in the home unless you are sure it contains no lead. Lead paint should only be removed by someone who knows how to protect you from lead paint dust. However, by washing floors, window sills, carpets, upholstery and any objects children put in their mouths, you can get rid of this source of lead.

- Make sure children wash their hands after playing outside in the dirt or snow.

- Never store food in open cans. Keep it in glass plastic or stainless steel containers. Use glazed pottery only for display if you don't know whether it contains lead.

- If you work around lead, don't bring it home. Shower and change clothes at work and wash your work clothes separately.

Aren't there a lot of types of treatment devices that would work? There are many devices which are certified for effective lead reduction, but devices that are not designed to remove lead will not work.

It is suggested that you follow the recommendations below before purchasing any device:

- Avoid being misled by false claims and scare tactics. Be wary of "free" water testing that is provided by the salesperson to determine your water quality; many tests are inaccurate or misleading. Research the reputation and legitimacy of the company or sales representative.

- Avoid signing contracts or binding agreements for "onetime offers" or for those that place a lien on your home. Be very careful about giving credit card information over the phone. Check into any offers that involve prizes or sweepstakes winnings.

- As suggested above, verify the claims of manufacturers by contacting the National Sanitation Foundation International or the Water Quality Association.

What is the government doing about the problem of lead in household water? There are two major governmental actions to reduce your exposure to lead:

- Under the authority of the Safe Drinking Water Act, EPA set the action level for lead in drinking water at 15 ppb. This means utilities must ensure that water from the customer's tap does not exceed this level in at least 90 percent of the homes sampled. If water from the tap does exceed this limit, then the utility must take certain steps to correct the problem. Utilities must also notify citizens of all violations of the standard.

- In June 1986, President Reagan signed amendments to the Safe Drinking Water Act. These amendments require the use of "lead-free" pipe, solder, and flux in the installation or repair of any public water system, or any plumbing in a residential or non-residential facility connected to a public water system.

  Under the provisions of these amendments, solders and flux will be considered "lead-free" when they contain not more than 0.2 percent lead. (In the past, solder normally contained about 50 percent lead.) Pipes and fittings will be considered "lead-free" when they contain not more than 8.0 percent lead.

  These requirements went into effect in June 1986. The law gave state governments until June 1988 to implement and enforce these new limitations. Although the states have banned all use of lead materials in drinking water systems, such bans do not eliminate lead contamination within existing plumbing. Also, in enforcing the ban, some states have continued to find illegally used lead solder in new plumbing installations. While responsible plumbers always observe the ban, this suggests that some plumbing installations or repairs using lead solder may be escaping detection by the limited number of enforcement personnel.

Where can I get more information? First contact your county or state department of health or environment for information on local water quality. For more general information on lead, there are now two toll-free telephone services:

EPA Safe Drinking Water Hotline 1-800-426 4791
National Lead Information Center 1-800-LEAD-FYI

Chapter 16

Mercury: The Problem of Quicksilver

Probably best known as the silvery substance in thermometers, mercury has been refined from cinnabar since the 15th or 16th Century B.C. Cinnabar was used as a red paint by primitive peoples long before the process of mercury refining was discovered.

History also chronicles the health hazards of occupational exposure to mercury dating to the time of the Roman conquest of Spain when criminals sentenced to work in the Spanish quicksilver mines had a life expectancy of only three years. However, it was the widespread poisoning of Japanese fisherman and their families from consumption of methyl mercury-contaminated fish in Minamata, Japan, in the fifties, and the recent discovery that most other mercury compounds can be transformed into highly toxic methyl mercury in the environment that generated widespread concern about the health implications of the continued release of mercury into the environment.

This chapter discusses the hazards of mercury and what the U.S. Environmental Protection Agency (EPA) and others are doing to protect public health from the risk of mercury exposure.

Mercury: What Is it?

Mercury is a heavy metal. At room temperature, in its pure form, it is a silvery liquid which vaporizes easily. Mercury is an important industrial metal because of its particular properties: uniform volume

E.P.A. Office of Pesticides and Toxic Substances. Toxics Information Series: Mercury. TS-793.

expansion, liquidity at room temperature, electrical conductivity, high density, low vapor pressure, ability to alloy with almost all common metals (except iron and platinum), and ease of vaporizing and freezing.

Over 3,000 industries utilize mercury in manufacturing and processing. In 1973, U.S. consumption of mercury was approximately 1,900 metric tons. Battery manufacturing (29.9 percent) and chlorine-alkali production (24 percent) accounted for over half; other major uses included paints and industrial instruments. Because of the inherent toxicity of mercury, it was, until recently, widely used in pesticides. Its use in medicines was for its diuretic properties as well as being used as an antiseptic and preservative. Because other more effective diuretics were found the mercurial use in medicine has declined.

Why Is Mercury a Problem?

Mercury is a problem because of its high toxicity and the potential for human exposure. Although all mercury compounds are toxic, methyl mercury is by far the most toxic, and recent discoveries concerning its production have increased concern about its potential exposure to the public. Scientific evidence points to the existence of a mercury cycle, where, in part, elemental mercury and various mercury compounds are transformed in the environment by natural biological and chemical action into methyl mercury. This conversion process, known as methylation, can occur in bacteria found in waterways and in the intestines of mammals. Since mercury is an element and therefore cannot be broken down into harmless components, once released into the environment, it remains available for methylation for many years.

Approximately 80 percent of the mercury used is eventually released back into the environment. Because it is easily vaporized, air emissions are a major source of human exposure, especially near sewage treatment facilities. The largest contributors to air emissions are chlorine-alkali plants, followed by fossil fuels, municipal incinerators, and mercury mines and smelters. Waterways also receive mercury through waste water discharges from industrial plants and municipal sewage. Landfill disposal of wastes contribute to the soil buildup of mercury. There is growing concern that the use of municipal sewage sludge as fertilizer may be compounding the problem of mercury contamination of the soils.

Mercury taken into the body through air, water and food is absorbed in varying amounts depending on its chemical form and the route of intake. Absorption of mercury present in water and food varies the most, from about 0.01 percent for elemental mercury to nearly 100 percent for methyl mercury. The major food sources of mercury are fish and shellfish.

Health Effects

In the human body, mercury accumulates in the liver, kidney, brain and blood and causes both acute and chronic health effects depending on the form of mercury. Acute poisoning, although seldom seen today, can cause severe gastrointestinal damage, cardiovascular collapse, and acute kidney failure, all of which can result in death.

Chronic symptoms of inorganic and organo-mercury compounds which are most often seen in industrial workers and in cases of contaminated food consumption may include birth defects, and central nervous system and kidney damage. Genetic damage is also suspected. Loss of appetite and weight loss are often the first signs of chronic mercury poisoning.

Nervous system damage: The most universal effects of mercury are damage to the nervous system. Increased excitability, mental instability, apathy and a tendency to weep which are often followed by fine tremors in the hands and feet can occur after exposure to mercury vapor. Personality changes such as timidity, nervousness and dizziness or insomnia may also occur. Symptoms of methyl mercury poisoning include tunnel vision, loss of muscle coordination, hearing impairment and impairment of gait.

Kidney damage: Inorganic mercury causes a transient kidney condition evidenced by excessive protein in the urine. The condition does not occur in all persons exposed to toxic doses of mercury. Although we do not know what level causes kidney failure, "high" levels almost always do.

Birth defects: Infants prenatally exposed to methyl mercury compounds ingested by their mothers have been born with primarily neurological defects. Symptoms include mental disturbance, poor muscle coordination, gait impairment, speech difficulties, and difficulties in chewing and swallowing.

Genetic effects: In laboratory tests with insects and plants mercury has been shown to cause chromosomal damage similar to that which causes Down Syndrome (mongolism) in humans. Scientists are concerned that mercury may cause similar damage in humans, resulting in congenital disorders and possibly cancer, although it has yet to be documented.

What Is the Government Doing about this Hazard?

Recognizing the toxic effects of mercury, the Federal government has taken steps to reduce the public's exposure to the chemical and its compounds. EPA has issued effluent guidelines for industry to reduce the release of mercury into water, and is preparing final water quality criteria for mercury. Based on the latest scientific information, the criteria can be used for further regulation of mercury by the Agency or individual states. Both effluent guidelines and water quality criteria are authorized by the Clean Water Act, administered by EPA.

Under the authority of the Clean Air Act, EPA is reviewing the current national air emission standards for mercury together with several other hazardous substances, in order to reduce the risk of mercury exposure through the ambient air. More importantly, under the Clean Air Act, EPA has limited emissions of mercury from certain industries. As hazardous waste, under the provisions of the Resource Conservation and Recovery Act, certain mercury wastes are regulated by EPA from point of origin to final disposal.

In February 1976, EPA ordered an immediate halt to the production, sale and use of most mercurial pesticides. Subsequent to resulting litigation, the original cancellation order was modified to allow registration under the Federal Insecticide, Fungicide and Rodenticide Act of mercurial pesticides only. This was for a few fungicidal uses, such as in-can preservatives in latex paints, mildew inhibitors on outdoor fabrics and in outdoor paints, control of brown mold on lumber, control of winter turf diseases, and control of Dutch Elm Disease (currently being reconsidered).

Because of the risk to workers in industries utilizing mercury, the Occupational Safety and Health Administration is reviewing the current occupational exposure standard of 0.1 milligrams of mercury per cubic meter of air (0.1 mg/m^3) to determine whether or not that standard should be reduced to 0.05 mg/m^3 to assure protection of the workers. The Food and Drug Administration (FDA) is developing methods to determine the concentration of methyl mercury in fish and other foods. In order to protect the public from contaminated fish, the FDA has issued an action level of 1.0 part mercury per million parts fish (1 ppm) in fish and shellfish as the maximum amount of mercury it will allow in those foods.

Research is continuing to define more clearly the tolerable levels of exposure to mercury, the health effects of increased burning of coal and the effects of chronic exposure to low levels of mercury compounds on unborn children. Results of this research will enable regulatory agencies to better assess the threat to public health and to institute appropriate control measures.

In summary, the toxic effects of mercury, although not completely defined, are of grave concern, as is the continued release of mercury to the environment where it can remain and affect future generations. The Federal government has taken several steps to reduce the public's exposure to mercury, and is investigating means to further reduce the mercury risk in this country.

Children at Risk

As in the case with other toxic chemicals such as lead, children are especially susceptible to the adverse effects of methyl mercury. Methyl mercury easily crosses the placental barrier and concentrates in the fetus more readily than in the mother. Thus, a woman exposed to toxic levels of mercury may not exhibit any signs of mercury poisoning, but her child may be born with brain damage quite similar to cerebral palsy.

Children may also react adversely to mercury exposure after they are born. Mercury can be transmitted through breast milk, as well as through the environmental media of air, water and food. Neurological symptoms are very similar to those seen in adults. In addition, children may develop dermatitis, eczema and mucous membrane irritation. Acrodynia, or "pink disease" affects only children from four months to four years of age. Characterized by a distinctive rash, coldness, swelling and irritation of the hands, feet, cheeks and nose, usually followed by peeling and ulceration; typical neurological and psychological symptoms, and profuse perspiration, acrodynia has been almost totally eradicated by withdrawal of mercury from common medications used in children (cough medicines, ointments, antiseptics, etc.).

Mercury in Fish: Cause for Concern?

FDA Consumer, September 1994.

Swordfish and shark taste great, especially grilled or broiled. But reports that these and some other large predatory fish may contain methyl mercury levels in excess of the Food and Drug Administration's 1 part per million (ppm) limit has dampened some fish lovers' appetites.

FDA scientists responsible for seafood safety are also concerned about the safety of eating these types of fish, but they agree that the fish are safe, provided they are eaten infrequently (no more than once a week) as part of a balanced diet.

Mercury Is Everywhere

Mercury occurs naturally in the environment. According to FDA toxicologist Mike Bolger, Ph.D., approximately 2,700 to 6,000 tons of mercury are released annually into the atmosphere naturally by degassing from the Earth's crust and oceans. Another 2,000 to 3,000 tons are released annually into the atmosphere by human activities, primarily from burning household and industrial wastes, and especially from fossil fuels such as coal.

Mercury vapor is easily transported in the atmosphere, deposited on land and water, and then, in part, released again to the atmosphere. Trace amounts of mercury are soluble in bodies of water, where bacteria can cause chemical changes that transform mercury to methyl mercury, a more toxic form.

Fish absorb methyl mercury from water as it passes over their gills and as they feed on aquatic organisms. Larger predator fish are exposed to higher levels of methyl mercury from their prey.

Methyl mercury binds tightly to the proteins in fish tissue, including muscle. Cooking does not appreciably reduce the methyl mercury content of the fish.

Nearly all fish contain trace amounts of methyl mercury, some more than others. In areas where there is industrial mercury pollution, the levels in the fish can be quite elevated. In general, however, methyl mercury levels for most fish range from less than 0.01 ppm to 0.5 ppm. It's only in a few species of fish that methyl mercury levels reach the FDA limit for human consumption of 1 ppm. This most frequently occurs in some large predator fish, such as shark and swordfish. Certain species of very large tuna, typically sold as fresh steaks or sushi, can have levels over 1 ppm. (Canned tuna, composed of smaller species of tuna such as skipjack and albacore, has much lower levels of methyl mercury, averaging only about 0.17 ppm.) The average concentration of methyl mercury for commercially important species (mostly marine in origin) is less than 0.3 ppm. (See the Table 16.1.)

FDA works with state regulators when commercial fish, caught and sold locally, are found to contain methyl mercury levels exceeding 1 ppm. The agency also checks imported fish at ports and refuses entry if methyl mercury levels exceed the FDA limit.

Sport-caught predator fresh-water species like pike and walleye sometimes have methyl mercury levels in the 1 ppm range. Other fresh-water species also have elevated levels, particularly in areas where mercury levels in the local environment are elevated.

FDA suggests sports fishers check with state or local governments for advisories about water bodies or fish species. These advisories provide up-to-date public health information on local areas and warn of areas or species where mercury (or other contamination) is of concern.

Safety Studies

Eating commercially available fish should not be a problem, say FDA toxicologists. The 1 ppm limit FDA has set for commercial fish is considerably lower than levels of methyl mercury in fish that have caused illness.

For information about the likely outcome of eating fish with low levels of methyl mercury, scientists look to studies of persons exposed to high levels: in particular, studies of two poisoning episodes from highly contaminated fish in Japan in the 1960s, and another poisoning incident in Iraq in the 1970s involving contaminated grain.

In the first episode, which occurred in Minamata, Japan, 111 people died or became very ill (mostly from nervous system damage) from eating fish (often daily over extended periods) from waters that were severely polluted with mercury from local industrial discharge.

Following a similar incident in Nigata, Japan, where 120 persons were poisoned, studies showed that the harm caused by methyl mercury poisoning, particularly the neurological symptoms, can progress over a period of years after exposure has ended. The average mercury content of fish samples from both areas ranged from 9 to 24 ppm, though in Minamata, some fish were found to have levels as high as 40 ppm. Fortunately, no similar incidents have occurred in the United States.

Table 16.1. Mercury Levels by Fish Species. Results of FDA sampling for methyl mercury by species for October 1990 to October 1991 (the action level is 1 ppm).

Fish Species	Range (ppm)
Bass, fresh water	0.15-0.34
Catfish, fresh and salt water	<0.10-0.31
Cod	Trace
Crabs	0.10-0.15
Croaker	0.13-0.32
Flounder	ND-0.08
Grouper	0.35-0.48
Haddock	Trace
Lobster	0.10-0.14
Mackerel	0.10-0.23
Mahi mahi (dolphin)	0.11-0.21
Marlin	0.10-0.92
Orange roughy	0.42-0.71
Oysters	< 0.10
Perch, fresh water	ND 0.31
Perch, ocean(rosefish, red rockfish)	Trace-0.03
Pike	Trace-0.16
Pollock	ND-0.10
Salmon	ND-0.11
Shrimp	< 0.10
Shark	0.23-2.95
Snapper, red	0.07-0.26
Swordfish	0.26-3.22
Trout	Trace-0.13
Tuna, canned	ND-0.75

ND means none detected

The best indexes of exposure to methyl mercury are concentrations in hair and blood. The average concentration of total mercury in non-exposed people is about 8 parts per billion (ppb) in blood and 2 ppm in hair. From the Japanese studies, toxicologists learned that the lowest mercury in adults associated with toxic effects (paresthesia) was 200 ppb in blood and 50 ppm in hair, accumulated over months to years of eating contaminated food.

The Japanese studies did not, however, provide information on what levels of methyl mercury might adversely affect the fetus and infant.

"There is no doubt that when humans are exposed to high levels of methyl mercury, poisoning and problems in the nervous system can occur," Bolger says.

The types of symptoms reflect the degree of exposure. Paresthesia (numbness and tingling sensations around the lips, fingers and toes) usually is the first symptom. A stumbling gait and difficulty in articulating words is the next progressive symptom, along with a constriction of the visual fields, ultimately leading to tunnel vision and impaired hearing. Generalized muscle weakness, fatigue, headache, irritability, and inability to concentrate often occur. In severe cases, tremors or jerks are present. These neurological problems frequently lead to coma and death.

"During prenatal life, humans are susceptible to the toxic effects of high methyl mercury exposure levels because of the sensitivity of the developing nervous system," Bolger explains. Methyl mercury easily crosses the placenta, and the mercury concentration rises to 30 percent higher in fetal red blood cells than in those of the mother.

"But none of the studies of methyl mercury poisoning victims have clearly shown the level at which newborns can tolerate exposure," Bolger says. "It is clear that at exposure levels that affect the fetus, adults are also susceptible to adverse effects. What is not clear is the effect, if any, on fetuses at much lower levels—those that approach current exposure levels through normal fish consumption."

Studies of the poisoning incident in Iraq have provided limited data about what effects low levels of methyl mercury exposures to the fetus have on the infant. One possible effect, for example, is lateness in walking. In the fall and winter of 1971-72, wheat seed intended for planting—and which had therefore been treated with an alkyl mercury fungicide—was mistakenly used to prepare bread; more that 6,500 Iraqis were hospitalized with neurological symptoms and 459 died. The vast majority of the mothers experienced exposures that resulted in hair levels greater than the lowest levels associated with effects in adults. But there was no clear evidence that the fetus was more sensitive than the adult to methyl mercury.

Another study on methyl mercury toxicity was published by the World Health Organization in 1990. It concluded, "the general population does not face a significant health risk from methyl mercury." Bolger says there is a consensus among scientists on all the results of this study except for the findings related to the relationship between low exposure levels and fetal toxicity.

Searching for More Information

FDA and the National Institute of Environmental Health Sciences are supporting a study by the University of Rochester to gather conclusive data on the effects of long-term exposure to low levels of methyl mercury in the fetus and infant. The study is being conducted in the Seychelles Islands, off the coast of East Africa in the Indian Ocean.

Fish is the major source of protein for people in the Seychelles Islands. Begun about 10 years ago, the study focuses on the approximately 700 pregnancies that occur on the islands each year.

"That's a much more significant database than we had in the Iraqi study," says Bolger. "Also, the population is mostly Muslim," he says, a religion that prohibits smoking and drinking, behaviors that could affect the prenatal health of fetuses (and interfere with efforts to understand the subtle effects of methyl mercury).

The study tracks women from pregnancy to childbirth, and monitors the babies' consumption of breast milk. As children grow older, they are followed for any signs of nervous system disorders. Reports from the Seychelles study are not ready for publication, but Bolger expects the results to make a significant contribution to the consideration of whether further regulatory controls or other actions may be needed.

Advice for Consumers on Fish Consumption

Fish is an important source of high-quality protein, vitamins and minerals. FDA seafood specialists say that eating a variety of types of fish, the normal pattern of consumption, does not put anyone in danger of mercury poisoning. It is when people eat fad diets—frequently eating only one type of food or a particular species of fish—that they put themselves at risk.

Pregnant women and women of childbearing age who may become pregnant, however, are advised by FDA experts to limit their consumption of shark and swordfish to no more than once a month. These fish have much higher levels of methyl mercury than other commonly consumed fish. Since the fetus may be more susceptible than the mother to the adverse effects of methyl mercury, FDA experts say that it is prudent to minimize the consumption of fish that have higher levels of methyl mercury, like shark and swordfish. This advice covers both pregnant women and women of childbearing age who might become pregnant, since the first trimester of pregnancy appears to be the critical period of exposure for the fetus. Dietary practices immediately before pregnancy would have a direct bearing on fetal exposure during the first trimester, the period of greatest concern.

FDA toxicologists have determined that for persons other than pregnant women and women of childbearing age who may become pregnant, regular consumption of fish species with methyl mercury levels around 1 part per million (ppm)—such as shark and swordfish—should be limited to about 7 ounces per week (about one serving) to stay below the acceptable daily intake for methyl mercury. For fish with levels averaging 0.5 ppm, regular consumption should be limited to about 14 ounces per week. Current evidence indicates that nursing women who follow this advice do not expose their infants to increased risk from methyl mercury.

Consumption advice is unnecessary for the top 10 seafood species, making up about 80 percent of the seafood market: canned tuna, shrimp, pollock, salmon, cod, catfish, clams, flatfish, crabs, and scallops. This is because the methyl mercury levels in these species are all less than 0.2 ppm and few people eat more than the suggested weekly limit of fish (2.2 pounds) for this level of methyl mercury contamination.

FDA's action level of 1 ppm for methyl mercury in fish was established to limit consumers' methyl mercury exposure to levels 10 times lower than the lowest levels associated with adverse effects (paresthesia) observed in the poisoning incidents. FDA based its action level on the lowest level at which adverse effects were found to occur in adults. This is because that level of exposure was actually lower than the lowest level found to affect fetuses, affording them greater protection.

FDA toxicologists are developing a more complete database for addressing low-level methyl mercury exposures from fish; however, they consider the 1-ppm limit to provide an adequate margin of safety.

This doesn't mean that it is safe to regularly and frequently eat fish that contain 1 ppm methyl mercury. The limit was established taking into consideration the types of fish people eat, the levels of methyl mercury present in each species, and the amounts of fish that are normally consumed.

Not everyone agrees, however, about what advice to provide to consumers. This is particularly evident in sport fish advisories provided by states around the country. Because states often use different criteria for their fish advisories, adjoining states may provide different advice about fish from the same bodies of water. Some states have adopted a zero risk approach and have advised consumers not to eat certain species, while others have advocated a limit on intake that is more consistent with the FDA approach.

Despite these differences, efforts by the states remain a valuable guide for alerting people to possible mercury contamination in certain fish species in particular bodies of water. Federal efforts are being made to increase uniformity in fishing advisories.

Questions?

FDA invites consumers who have questions about methyl mercury in fish or other seafood concerns to telephone the 24-hour FDA Seafood Hotline at (1-800) FDA-4010 or (202) 205-4314 (in the Washington, D.C., area). The automated hot line and Flash Fax service are available 24 hours a day. Public affairs specialists can be reached at the same numbers from noon to 4 p.m. Eastern time, Monday through Friday.

— by Judith E. Foulke

Judith E. Foulke is a member of FDA's public affairs staff.

Part Four

Indoor Pollution

Chapter 17

The Inside Story: A Guide to Indoor Air Quality

Indoor Air Quality Concerns

All of us face a variety of risks to our health as we go about our day-to-day lives. Driving in cars, flying in planes, engaging in recreational activities, and being exposed to environmental pollutants all pose varying degrees of risk. Some risks are simply unavoidable. Some we choose to accept because to do otherwise would restrict our ability to lead our lives the way we want. And some are risks we might decide to avoid if we had the opportunity to make informed choices. Indoor air pollution is one risk that you can do something about.

In the last several years, a growing body of scientific evidence has indicated that the air within homes and other buildings can be more seriously polluted than the outdoor air in even the largest and most industrialized cities. Other research indicates that people spend approximately 90 percent of their time indoors. Thus, for many people, the risks to health may be greater due to exposure to air pollution indoors than outdoors.

In addition, people who may be exposed to indoor air pollutants for the longest periods of time are often those most susceptible to the effects of indoor air pollution. Such groups include the young, the elderly, and the chronically ill, especially those suffering from respiratory or cardiovascular disease.

Environmental Protection Agency. EPA 402-K-93-007. *The Inside Story: A Guide to Indoor Air Quality*. September 1993.

What Causes Indoor Air Problems?

Indoor pollution sources that release gases or particles into the air are the primary cause of indoor air quality problems in homes. Inadequate ventilation can increase indoor pollutant levels by not bringing in enough outdoor air to dilute emissions from indoor sources and by not carrying indoor air pollutants out of the home. High temperature and humidity levels can also increase concentrations of some pollutants.

Pollutant Sources

There are many sources of indoor air pollution in any home. These include combustion sources such as oil, gas, kerosene, coal, wood, and tobacco products; building materials and furnishings as diverse as deteriorated, asbestos-containing insulation, wet or damp carpet, and cabinetry or furniture made of certain pressed wood products; products for household cleaning and maintenance, personal care, or hobbies; central heating and cooling systems and humidification devices; and outdoor sources such as radon, pesticides, and outdoor air pollution.

The relative importance of any single source depends on how much of a given pollutant it emits and how hazardous those emissions are. In some cases, factors such as how old the source is and whether it is properly maintained are significant. For example, an improperly adjusted gas stove can emit significantly more carbon monoxide than one that is properly adjusted.

Some sources, such as building materials, furnishings, and household products like air fresheners, release pollutants more or less continuously. Other sources, related to activities carried out in the home, release pollutants intermittently. These include smoking, the use of unvented or malfunctioning stoves, furnaces, or space heaters, the use of solvents in cleaning and hobby activities, the use of paint strippers in re-decorating activities, and the use of cleaning products and pesticides in housekeeping. High pollutant concentrations can remain in the air for long periods after some of these activities.

Amount of Ventilation

If too little outdoor air enters a home, pollutants can accumulate to levels that can pose health and comfort problems. Unless they are built with special mechanical means of ventilation, homes that are designed and constructed to minimize the amount of outdoor air that can "leak" into and out of the home may have higher pollutant levels than other homes. However, because some weather conditions can drastically reduce the amount of outdoor air that enters a home, pollutants can build up even in homes that are normally considered "leaky."

How Does Outdoor Air Enter a House?

Outdoor air enters and leaves a house by: infiltration, natural ventilation, and mechanical ventilation. In a process known as infiltration, outdoor air flows into the house through openings, joints, and cracks in walls, floors, and ceilings, and around windows and doors. In natural ventilation, air moves through opened windows and doors. Air movement associated with infiltration and natural ventilation is caused by air temperature differences between indoors and outdoors and by wind. Finally, there are a number of mechanical ventilation devices, from outdoor-vented fans that intermittently remove air from a single room, such as bathrooms and kitchen, to air handling systems that use fans and duct work to continuously remove indoor air and distribute filtered and conditioned outdoor air to strategic points throughout the house. The rate at which outdoor air replaces indoor air is described as the air exchange rate. When there is little infiltration, natural ventilation, or mechanical ventilation, the air exchange rate is low and pollutant levels can increase.

What If You Live in an Apartment?

Apartments can have the same indoor air problems as single-family homes because many of the pollution sources, such as the interior building materials, furnishings, and household products, are similar. Indoor air problems similar to those in offices are caused by such sources as contaminated ventilation systems, improperly placed outdoor air intakes, or maintenance activities.

Solutions to air quality problems in apartments, as in homes and offices, involve such actions as: eliminating or controlling the sources of pollution, increasing ventilation, and installing air cleaning devices. Often a resident can take the appropriate action to improve the indoor air quality by removing a source, altering an activity, unblocking an air supply vent, or opening a window to temporarily increase

1. Moisture
2. Pressed Wood Furniture
3. Humidifier
4. Moth Repellents
5. Dry-Cleaned Goods
6. House Dust Mites
7. Personal Care Products
8. Air Freshener
9. Stored Fuels
10. Car Exhaust
11. Paint Supplies
12. Paneling
13. Woodstove
14. Tobacco Smoke
15. Carpets
16. Pressed Wood Subflooring
17. Drapes
18. Fireplace
19. Household Chemicals
20. Asbestos Floor Tiles
21. Pressed Wood Cabinets
22. Unvented Gas Stove
23. Asbestos Pipe Wrap
24. Radon
25. Unvented Clothes Dryer
26. Pesticides
27. Stored Hobby Products
28. Lead-Based Paint

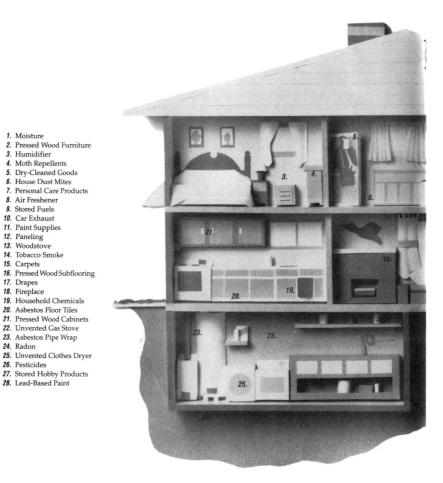

Figure 17.1. *Air Pollution Sources in the Home*

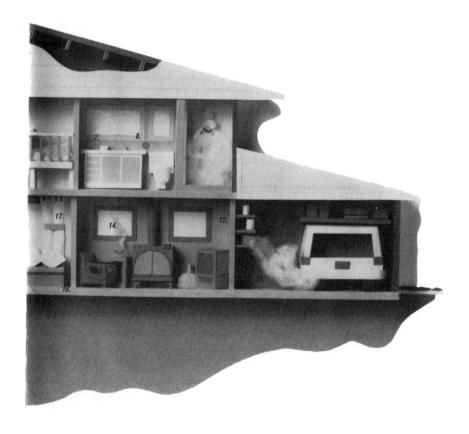

the ventilation; in other cases, however, only the building owner or manager is in a position to remedy the problem. You can encourage building management to follow guidance in EPA and NIOSH's *Building Air Quality: A Guide for Building Owners and Facility Managers.* It is available from the Superintendent of Documents, P.O. Box 371954, Pittsburgh, PA 15250-7954; stock # 055-000-00390-4.

Indoor Air and Your Health

Health effects from indoor air pollutants may be experienced soon after exposure or, possibly, years later.

Immediate effects may show up after a single exposure or repeated exposures. These include irritation of the eyes, nose, and throat, headaches, dizziness, and fatigue. Such immediate effects are usually short-term and treatable. Sometimes the treatment is simply eliminating the person's exposure to the source of the pollution, if it can be identified. Symptoms of some diseases, including asthma, hypersensitivity pneumonitis, and humidifier fever, may also show up soon after exposure to some indoor air pollutants.

The likelihood of immediate reactions to indoor air pollutants depends on several factors. Age and preexisting medical conditions are two important influences. In other cases, whether a person reacts to a pollutant depends on individual sensitivity, which varies tremendously from person to person. Some people can become sensitized to biological pollutants after repeated exposures, and it appears that some people can become sensitized to chemical pollutants as well.

Certain immediate effects are similar to those from colds or other viral diseases, so it is often difficult to determine if the symptoms are a result of exposure to indoor air pollution. For this reason, it is important to pay attention to the time and place the symptoms occur. If the symptoms fade or go away when a person is away from the home and return when the person returns, an effort should be made to identify indoor air sources that may be possible causes. Some effects may be made worse by an inadequate supply of outdoor air or from the heating, cooling, or humidity conditions prevalent in the home.

Other health effects may show up either years after exposure has occurred or only after long or repeated periods of exposure. These effects, which include some respiratory diseases, heart disease, and cancer, can be severely debilitating or fatal. It is prudent to try to improve the indoor air quality in your home even if symptoms are not noticeable.

While pollutants commonly found in indoor air are responsible for many harmful effects, there is considerable uncertainty about what concentrations or periods of exposure are necessary to produce specific health problems. People also react very differently to exposure to indoor air pollutants. Further research is needed to better understand which health effects occur after exposure to the average pollutant concentrations found in homes and which occur from the higher concentrations that occur for short periods of time.

Identifying Air Quality Problems

Some health effects can be useful indicators of an indoor air quality problem, especially if they appear after a person moves to a new residence, remodels or refurnishes a home, or treats a home with pesticides. If you think that you have symptoms that may be related to your home environment, discuss them with your doctor or your local health department to see if they could be caused by indoor air pollution. You may also want to consult a board-certified allergist or an occupational medicine specialist for answers to your questions.

Another way to judge whether your home has or could develop indoor air problems is to identify potential sources of indoor air pollution. Although the presence of such sources (see illustration at the beginning of this chapter) does not necessarily mean that you have an indoor air quality problem, being aware of the type and number of potential sources is an important step toward assessing the air quality in your home.

A third way to decide whether your home may have poor indoor air quality is to look at your lifestyle and activities. Human activities can be significant sources of indoor air pollution. Finally, look for signs of problems with the ventilation in your home. Signs that can indicate your home may not have enough ventilation include moisture condensation on windows or walls, smelly or stuffy air, dirty central heating and air cooling equipment, and areas where books, shoes, or other items become moldy. To detect odors in your home, step outside for a few minutes, and then upon reentering your home, note whether odors are noticeable.

Measuring Pollutant Levels

The federal government recommends that you measure the level of radon in your home. Without measurements there is no way to tell whether radon is present because it is a colorless, odorless, radioactive gas. Inexpensive devices are available for measuring radon. EPA provides guidance as to risks associated with different levels of exposure and when the public should consider corrective action. There are specific mitigation techniques that have proven effective in reducing levels of radon in the home.

For pollutants other than radon, measurements are most appropriate when there are either health symptoms or signs of poor ventilation and specific sources or pollutants have been identified as possible causes of indoor air quality problems. Testing for many pollutants can be expensive. Before monitoring your home for pollutants besides radon, consult your state or local health department or professionals who have experience in solving indoor air quality problems in nonindustrial buildings.

Weatherizing Your Home

The federal government recommends that homes be weatherized in order to reduce the amount of energy needed for heating and cooling. While weatherization is underway, however, steps should also be taken to minimize pollution from sources inside the home. In addition, residents should be alert to the emergence of signs of inadequate ventilation, such as stuffy air, moisture condensation on cold surfaces, or mold and mildew growth. Additional weatherization measures should not be undertaken until these problems have been corrected.

Weatherization generally does not cause indoor air problems by adding new pollutants to the air. (There are a few exceptions, such as caulking, that can sometimes emit pollutants.) However, measures such as installing storm windows, weather stripping, caulking, and blown-in wall insulation can reduce the amount of outdoor air infiltrating into a home. Consequently, after weatherization, concentrations of indoor air pollutants from sources inside the home can increase.

Three Basic Strategies to Improve Air Quality in Your Home

Source Control

Usually the most effective way to improve indoor air quality is to eliminate individual sources of pollution or to reduce their emissions.

Some sources, like those that contain asbestos, can be sealed or enclosed; others, like gas stoves, can be adjusted to decrease the amount of emissions. In many cases, source control is also a more cost-efficient approach to protecting indoor air quality than increasing ventilation because increasing ventilation can increase energy costs. Specific sources of indoor air pollution in your home are listed later in this section.

Ventilation Improvements

Another approach to lowering the concentrations of indoor air pollutants in your home is to increase the amount of outdoor air coming indoors. Most home heating and cooling systems, including forced air heating systems, do not mechanically bring fresh air into the house. Opening windows and doors, operating window or attic fans, when the weather permits, or running a window air conditioner with the vent control open increases the outdoor ventilation rate. Local bathroom or kitchen fans that exhaust outdoors remove contaminants directly from the room where the fan is located and also increase the outdoor air ventilation rate.

It is particularly important to take as many of these steps as possible while you are involved in short-term activities that can generate high levels of pollutants—for example, painting, paint stripping, heating with kerosene heaters, cooking, or engaging in maintenance and hobby activities such as welding, soldering, or sanding. You might also choose to do some of these activities outdoors, if you can and if weather permits.

Advanced designs of new homes are starting to feature mechanical systems that bring outdoor air into the home. Some of these designs include energy-efficient heat recovery ventilators (also known as air-to-air heat exchangers). For more information about air-to-air heat exchangers, contact the Conservation and Renewable Energy Inquiry and Referral Service (CAREIRS), PO Box 3048, Merrifield, VA 22116; (800) 523-2929.

Air Cleaners

There are many types and sizes of air cleaners on the market, ranging from relatively inexpensive tabletop models to sophisticated and expensive whole-house systems. Some air cleaners are highly effective at particle removal, while others, including most table-top models, are much less so. Air cleaners are generally not designed to remove gaseous pollutants.

The effectiveness of an air cleaner depends on how well it collects pollutants from indoor air (expressed as a percentage efficiency rate) and how much air it draws through the cleaning or filtering element (expressed in cubic feet per minute). A very efficient collector with a low air-circulation rate will not be effective, nor will a cleaner with a high air-circulation rate but a less efficient collector. The long-term performance of any air cleaner depends on maintaining it according to the manufacturer's directions.

Another important factor in determining the effectiveness of an air cleaner is the strength of the pollutant source. Table-top air cleaners, in particular, may not remove satisfactory amounts of pollutants from strong nearby sources. People with a sensitivity to particular sources may find that air cleaners are helpful only in conjunction with concerted efforts to remove the source.

Over the past few years, there has been some publicity suggesting that houseplants have been shown to reduce levels of some chemicals in laboratory experiments. There is currently no evidence, however, that a reasonable number of houseplants remove significant quantities of pollutants in homes and offices. Indoor houseplants should not be over-watered because overly damp soil may promote the growth of micro-organisms which can affect allergic individuals.

At present, EPA does not recommend using air cleaners to reduce levels of radon and its decay products. The effectiveness of these devices is uncertain because they only partially remove the radon decay products and do not diminish the amount of radon entering the home. EPA plans to do additional research on whether air cleaners are, or could become, a reliable means of reducing the health risk from radon. EPA's booklet, *Residential Air-Cleaning Devices*, provides further information on air-cleaning devices to reduce indoor air pollutants.

For most indoor air-quality problems in the home, source control is the most effective solution.

Indoor Air Pollution: Questions That May Be Asked

American Lung Association, 1996.

The subject of indoor air pollution is not without some controversy. Indoor air quality is an evolving issue; it is important to keep informed about continuing developments in this area. The following questions may be asked of physicians and other health professionals.

What is "multiple chemical sensitivity" or "total allergy"?

The diagnostic label of multiple chemical sensitivity (MCS) also referred to as "chemical hypersensitivity" or "environmental illness" is being applied increasingly, although definition of the phenomenon is elusive and its pathogenesis as a distinct entity is not confirmed. Multiple chemical sensitivity has become more widely known and increasingly controversial as more patients received the label.

Persons with the diagnostic label of multiple chemical sensitivity are said to suffer multi-system illness as a result of contact with, or proximity to, a spectrum of substances, including airborne agents. These may include both recognized pollutants discussed earlier (such as tobacco smoke, formaldehyde, et al.) and other pollutants ordinarily considered innocuous. Some who espouse the concept of MCS believe that it may explain such chronic conditions as some forms of arthritis and colitis, in addition to generally recognized types of hypersensitivity reactions.

Some practitioners believe that the condition has a purely psychological basis. One study reported a 65 percent incidence of current or past clinical depression, anxiety disorders, or somatoform disorders in subjects with this diagnosis compared with 28 percent in controls. Others, however, counter that the disorder itself may cause such problems, since those affected are no longer able to lead a normal life, or that these conditions stem from effects on the nervous system.

The current consensus is that in cases of claimed or suspected MCS, complaints should not be dismissed as psychogenic, and a thorough workup is essential. Primary care givers should determine that the individual does not have an underlying physiological problem and should consider the value of consultation with allergists and other specialists.

Who are "clinical ecologists"?

"Clinical ecology", while not a recognized conventional medical specialty, has drawn the attention of health care professionals as well as laypersons. The organization of clinical ecologists physicians who treat individuals believed to be suffering from "total allergy" or "multiple chemical sensitivity" was founded as the Society for Clinical Ecology and is now known as the American Academy of Environmental Medicine. Its ranks have attracted allergists and physicians from other traditional medical specialties.

What are ionizers and other ozone generating air cleaners?

Ion generators act by charging the particles in a room so that they are attracted to walls, floors, tabletops, draperies, occupants, etc. Abrasion can result in these particles being re-suspended into the air. In some cases these devices contain a collector to attract the charged particles back to the unit. While ion generators may remove small particles (e.g., those in tobacco smoke) from the indoor air, they do not remove gases or odors, and may be relatively ineffective in removing large particles such as pollen and house dust allergens. Although some have suggested that these devices provide a benefit by rectifying a hypothesized ion imbalance, no controlled studies have confirmed this effect.

Ozone, a lung irritant, is produced indirectly by ion generators and some other electronic air cleaners and directly by ozone generators. While indirect ozone production is of concern, there is even greater concern with the direct, and purposeful introduction of a lung irritant into indoor air. There is no difference, despite some marketers' claims, between ozone in smog outdoors and ozone produced by these devices. Under certain use conditions ion generators and other ozone generating air cleaners can produce levels of this lung irritant significantly above levels thought harmful to human health. A small percentage of air cleaners that claim a health benefit may be regulated by FDA as a medical device. The Food and Drug Administration has set a limit of 0.05 parts per million of ozone for medical devices. Although ozone can be useful in reducing odors and pollutants in unoccupied spaces (such as removing smoke odors from homes involved in fires) the levels needed to achieve this are above those generally thought to be safe for humans.

Can other air cleaners help?

Ion generators and ozone generators are types of air cleaners; others include mechanical filter air cleaners, electronic air cleaners (e.g., electrostatic precipitators), and hybrid air cleaners utilizing two or more techniques. Generally speaking, existing air cleaners are not appropriate single solutions to indoor air quality problems, but can be useful as an adjunct to effective source control and adequate ventilation. Air cleaning alone cannot adequately remove all pollutants typically found in indoor air.

The value of any air cleaner depends upon a number of factors, including its basic efficiency, proper selection for the type of pollutant to be removed, proper installation in relation to the space, and faithful maintenance. Drawbacks, varying with type, may include inadequate pollutant removal, re-dispersement of pollutants, deceptive masking rather than removal, generation of ozone, and unacceptable noise levels.

The EPA and CPSC have not taken a position either for or against the use of these devices in the home.

Should I have my ducts cleaned?

As awareness of the importance of indoor air quality grows, more people are looking at duct cleaning as a way to solve indoor air quality problems. Individuals considering having ducts cleaned should determine that contaminated ducts are the cause of their health problems. Even when contaminants are found in ducts, the source may lie elsewhere, and cleaning ducts may not permanently solve the problem. The duct cleaning industry is expanding to meet demand, using extensive advertising to encourage people to use their services. Individuals who employ such services should verify that the service provider takes steps to protect individuals from exposure to dislodged pollutants and chemicals used during the cleaning process. Such steps may range from using HEPA filtration on cleaning equipment, providing respirators for workers, and occupants vacating the premises during cleaning.

Can carpet make people sick?

Like many other household products and furnishings, new carpet can be a source of chemical emissions. Carpet emits volatile organic compounds, as do products that accompany carpet installation such as adhesives and padding. Some people report symptoms such as eye, nose and throat irritation; headaches; skin irritations; shortness of breath or cough; and fatigue, which they may associate with new carpet installation. Carpet can also act as a "sink" for chemical and biological pollutants including pesticides, dust mites, and fungi.

Individuals purchasing new carpet should ask retailers for information to help them select lower emitting carpet, cushion, and adhesives. Before new carpet is installed, they should ask the retailer to unroll and air out the carpet in a clean, well-ventilated area. They should consider leaving the premises during and immediately after carpet installation or schedule the installation when the space is unoccupied. Opening doors and windows and increasing the amount of fresh air indoors will reduce exposure to most chemicals released from newly installed carpet. During and after installation in a home, use of window fans and room air conditioners to exhaust fumes to the outdoors is recommended. Ventilation systems should be in proper working order, and should be operated during installation, and for 48 to 72 hours after the new carpet is installed.

Individuals should request that the installer follow the Carpet and Rug Institute's installation guidelines. If new carpet has an objectionable odor, they should contact their carpet retailer. Finally, carpet owners should follow the manufacturer's instructions for proper carpet maintenance.

Can plants control indoor air pollution?

Recent reports in the media and promotions by the decorative houseplant industry characterize plants as "nature's clean air machine," claiming that National Aeronautics and Space Administration (NASA) research shows plants remove indoor air pollutants. While it is true that plants remove carbon dioxide from the air, and the ability of plants to remove certain other pollutants from water is the basis for some pollution control methods, the ability of plants to control indoor air pollution is less well established. Most research to date used small chambers without any air exchange which makes extrapolation to real world environments extremely uncertain. The only available study of the use of plants to control indoor air pollutants in an actual building could not determine any benefit from the use of plants. As a practical means of pollution control, the plant removal mechanisms appear to be inconsequential compared to common ventilation and air exchange rates. In other words, the ability of plants to actually improve indoor air quality is limited in comparison with provision of adequate ventilation.

While decorative foliage plants may be aesthetically pleasing, it should be noted that over-damp planter soil conditions may actually promote growth of unhealthy micro-organisms.

Chapter 18

Environmental Tobacco Smoke

Environmental tobacco smoke (ETS) is the mixture of smoke that comes from the burning end of a cigarette, pipe, or cigar, and smoke exhaled by the smoker. It is a complex mixture of over 4,000 compounds, more than 40 of which are known to cause cancer in humans or animals and many of which are strong irritants. ETS is often referred to as "secondhand smoke" and exposure to ETS is often called "passive smoking."

Health Problems Related to Environmental Tobacco Smoke

Key Signs/Symptoms in Adults:

- rhinitis/pharyngitis, nasal congestion, persistent cough
- conjunctival irritation
- headache
- wheezing (bronchial constriction)
- exacerbation of chronic respiratory conditions

Key Signs/Symptoms in Infants and Children

- asthma onset

Extracted from EPA publication #EPA402-K-93-007, *The Inside Story: A Guide to Indoor Air Quality* and from *Indoor Air Pollution: An Introduction for Health Professionals*

- increased severity of, or difficulty in controlling, asthma
- frequent upper respiratory infections and/or episodes of otitis media
- persistent middle-ear effusion
- snoring
- repeated pneumonia, bronchitis

Health Effects of Environmental Tobacco Smoke

In 1992, EPA completed a major assessment of the respiratory health risks of ETS (Respiratory Health Effects of Passive Smoking: Lung Cancer and Other Disorders EPA/600/6-90/ 006F). The report concludes that exposure to ETS is responsible for approximately 3,000 lung cancer deaths each year in nonsmoking adults and impairs the respiratory health of hundreds of thousands of children.

Infants and young children whose parents smoke in their presence are at increased risk of lower respiratory tract infections (pneumonia and bronchitis) and are more likely to have symptoms of respiratory irritation like cough, excess phlegm, and wheeze. EPA estimates that passive smoking annually causes between 150,000 and 300,000 lower respiratory tract infections in infants and children under 18 months of age, resulting in between 7,500 and 15,000 hospitalizations each year. These children may also have a build-up of fluid in the middle ear, which can lead to ear infections. Older children who have been exposed to secondhand smoke may have slightly reduced lung function.

Asthmatic children are especially at risk. EPA estimates that exposure to secondhand smoke increases the number of episodes and severity of symptoms in hundreds of thousands of asthmatic children, and may cause thousands of non-asthmatic children to develop the disease each year. EPA estimates that between 200,000 and 1,000,000 asthmatic children have their condition made worse by exposure to secondhand smoke each year.

Exposure to secondhand smoke causes eye, nose, and throat irritation. It may affect the cardiovascular system and some studies have linked exposure to secondhand smoke with the onset of chest pain. For publications about ETS, contact EPA's Indoor Air Quality Information Clearinghouse (IAQ INFO), 800-438-4318.

Reducing Exposure to Environmental Tobacco Smoke

- Don't smoke at home or permit others to do so. Ask smokers to smoke outdoors.

The 1986 Surgeon General's report concluded that physical separation of smokers and nonsmokers in a common air space, such as different rooms within the same house, may reduce—but will not eliminate nonsmokers' exposure to environmental tobacco smoke.

- If smoking indoors cannot be avoided, increase ventilation in the area where smoking takes place.

Open windows or use exhaust fans. Ventilation, a common method of reducing exposure to indoor air pollutants, also will reduce but not eliminate exposure to environmental tobacco smoke. Because smoking produces such large amounts of pollutants, natural or mechanical ventilation techniques do not remove them from the air in your home as quickly as they build up. In addition, the large increases in ventilation it takes to significantly reduce exposure to environmental tobacco smoke can also increase energy costs substantially. Consequently, the most effective way to reduce exposure to environmental tobacco smoke in the home is to eliminate smoking there.

- Do not smoke if children are present, particularly infants and toddlers.

Children are particularly susceptible to the effects of passive smoking. Do not allow baby-sitters or others who work in your home to smoke indoors. Discourage others from smoking around children. Find out about the smoking policies of the day care center providers, schools, and other care givers for your children. The policy should protect children from exposure to ETS.

- Expectant mothers should not smoke or allow smoking around them.

The impact of maternal smoking on fetal development has been well documented. Maternal smoking is also associated with increased incidence of Sudden Infant Death Syndrome, although it has not been determined to what extent this increase is due to in utero versus post-natal (lactational and ETS) exposure.

Chapter 19

Formaldehyde: An Irritating Volatile Organic Compound

What is formaldehyde?

Formaldehyde is an important industrial chemical used to make other chemicals, building materials, and household products. It is one of the large family of chemical compounds called volatile organic compounds or "VOCs." The term volatile means that the compounds vaporize, that is, become a gas, at normal room temperatures. Formaldehyde serves many purposes in products. It is used as a part of:

- the glue or adhesive in pressed wood products (particle board, hardwood plywood, and fiberboard);
- preservatives in some paints, coatings, and cosmetics;
- the coating that provides permanent press quality to fabrics and draperies;
- the finish used to coat paper products; and
- certain insulation materials (urea-formaldehyde foam insulation).

Formaldehyde is released into the air by burning wood, kerosene or natural gas, by automobiles, and by cigarettes. Formaldehyde can off-gas from materials made with it. It is also a naturally occurring substance.

U.S. Consumer Products Safety Commission. *An Update on Formaldehyde.* October 1990.

Why should you be concerned?

Formaldehyde is a colorless, strong-smelling gas. When present in the air at levels above 0.1 ppm (parts in a million parts of air), it can cause watery eyes, burning sensations in the eyes, nose and throat, nausea, coughing, chest tightness, wheezing, skin rashes, and allergic reactions. It also causes cancer in laboratory animals and may cause cancer in humans.

Formaldehyde can affect people differently. Some people are very sensitive to formaldehyde while others may not have any noticeable reaction to the same level.

Persons have developed allergic reactions (allergic skin disease and hives) to formaldehyde through skin contact with solutions of formaldehyde or durable-press clothing containing formaldehyde. Others have developed asthmatic reactions and skin rashes from exposure to formaldehyde.

You should understand that formaldehyde is just one of several gases present indoors that may cause illnesses. Many of these gases, as well as colds and flu, cause similar symptoms.

What levels of formaldehyde are normal?

Formaldehyde is normally present at low levels, usually less than 0.03 ppm, in both outdoor and indoor air. The outdoor air in rural areas has lower concentrations while urban areas have higher concentrations. Residences or offices that contain products that release formaldehyde to the air can have formaldehyde levels of greater than 0.03 ppm. Products that may add formaldehyde to the air include particle board used as sub-flooring or shelving, fiberboard in cabinets and furniture, plywood wall panels, and urea-formaldehyde as insulation. As formaldehyde levels increase, illness or discomfort is more likely to occur and may be more serious.

Efforts have been made by both the government and industry to reduce exposure to formaldehyde. The Consumer Products Safety Commission (CPSC) voted to ban urea-formaldehyde foam insulation. That ban was overturned in the courts, but these actions greatly reduced the residential use of the product. CPSC, the Department of Housing and Urban Development, and other federal agencies are working with the pressed wood industry to further reduce the release of the chemical from their products. However, it would be unrealistic to expect to completely remove formaldehyde from the air. Some persons who are extremely sensitive to formaldehyde may need to reduce or stop using these products.

What affects formaldehyde levels?

Formaldehyde levels in the indoor air depend mainly on what is releasing the formaldehyde (the source), the temperature, the humidity, and the air exchange rate (the amount of outdoor air entering or leaving the indoor area). Increasing the flow of outdoor air to the inside decreases the formaldehyde levels. Decreasing this flow of outdoor air by sealing the residence or office increases the formaldehyde level in the indoor air.

As the temperature rises, more formaldehyde comes off from the product. The reverse is also true; less formaldehyde comes off at lower temperature. Humidity also affects the release of formaldehyde from the product. As humidity rises more formaldehyde is released.

The formaldehyde levels in a residence change with the season and from day-to-day and day-to-night. Levels may be high on a hot and humid day and low on a cool, dry day. Understanding these factors is important when you consider measuring the levels of formaldehyde.

Some sources—such as pressed wood products containing urea-formaldehyde glues, urea-formaldehyde foam insulation, durable-press fabrics, and draperies—release more formaldehyde when new. As they age, the formaldehyde release decreases.

What are the major sources?

1. Urea-formaldehyde foam insulation: During the 1970s, many owners installed this insulation to save energy. Many of these homes had high levels of formaldehyde soon afterwards. Sale of urea formaldehyde foam insulation has largely stopped. Formaldehyde release from this product decreases rapidly after the first few months and reaches background levels in a few years. Therefore, urea-formaldehyde foam insulation installed 5 to 10 years ago is unlikely to still release formaldehyde.

2. Durable-press fabrics, draperies, and coated paper products: In the early 1960s, there were several reports of allergic reactions to formaldehyde from durable-press fabrics and coated paper products. Such reports have declined in recent years as

industry has taken steps to reduce formaldehyde levels. Draperies made of formaldehyde treated durable press fabrics may add slightly to indoor formaldehyde levels

3. Cosmetics, paints, coatings, and some wet-strength paper products: The amount of formaldehyde present in these products is small and is of slight concern. However, persons sensitive to formaldehyde may have allergic reactions.

4. Pressed Wood Products: Pressed wood products, especially those containing urea-formaldehyde glues, are a source of formaldehyde. These products include particle board used in subfloors, shelves, cabinets, and furniture; plywood wall panels, and medium-density fiberboard used in drawers, cabinets, and furniture. Medium-density fiberboard, which contains a higher glue content, has the potential to release the most formaldehyde.

5. Combustion Sources: Burning materials such as wood, kerosene, cigarettes, and natural gas, and operating internal combustion engines (e.g., automobiles), produces small quantities of formaldehyde. Combustion sources add small amounts of formaldehyde to indoor air.

6. Products such as carpets or gypsum board do not contain formaldehyde when new. They may trap formaldehyde emitted from other sources and later release the formaldehyde into the indoor air when the temperature and humidity change.

Do you have formaldehyde-related symptoms?

There are several formaldehyde-related symptoms, such as watery eyes, runny nose, burning sensation in eyes, nose, and throat, headaches, and fatigue. These symptoms may also occur because of the common cold, the flu or other pollutants that may be present in the indoor air. If these symptoms lessen when you are away from home or office but reappear upon your return, they may be caused by indoor pollutants, including formaldehyde. Examine your environment. Have you recently moved into a new or different home or office? Have you recently remodeled or installed new cabinets, or furniture?

Symptoms may be due to formaldehyde exposure. You should contact your physician and/or state or local health department for help. Your physician can help to determine if the cause of your symptoms is formaldehyde or other pollutants.

Should you measure formaldehyde?

Only trained professionals should measure formaldehyde because they know how to interpret the results. If you become ill, and the illness persists following the purchase of furniture or remodeling with pressed wood products, you might not need to measure formaldehyde. Since these are likely sources, you can take action. You may become ill after painting, sealing, making repairs, and/or applying pest control treatment in your home or office. In such cases, indoor air pollutants other than formaldehyde may be the cause. If the source is not obvious, you should consult an physician to determine whether or not your symptoms might relate to indoor air quality problems. If your physician believes that you may be sensitive to formaldehyde, you may want to make some measurements. As discussed earlier, many factors can affect the level of formaldehyde on a given day in an office or residence. This is why a professional is best suited to make an accurate measurement of the levels.

Do-it-yourself formaldehyde measuring devices are available. These devices can only provide a "ball park" figure for the formaldehyde level in the area. If you use such a device, you must carefully follow the instructions.

How do you reduce formaldehyde exposure?

Every day you probably use many products that contain formaldehyde. You may not be able to avoid coming in contact with some formaldehyde in your normal daily routine. If you are sensitive to formaldehyde, you will need to avoid many everyday items to reduce symptoms. For most people, a low-level exposure to formaldehyde (up to 0.1 ppm) does not produce symptoms. People who suspect they are sensitive to formaldehyde should work closely with a knowledgeable physician to make sure that formaldehyde is causing their symptoms.

You can avoid exposure to higher levels by:

- Purchasing low formaldehyde-releasing pressed wood products for use in construction or remodeling of homes, and for furniture, cabinets etc. These could include oriented strand board and softwood plywood for construction, low-formaldehyde-emitting pressed wood products or solid wood for furniture and cabinets. Some products are labeled as low-emitting, or ask for help in identifying low-emitting products.

• Using alternative products such as lumber or metal.

• Avoiding the use of foamed-in-place insulation containing formaldehyde, especially urea-formaldehyde foam insulation.

• Washing durable-press fabrics before use.

How do you reduce existing formaldehyde levels?

The choice of methods to reduce formaldehyde is unique to your situation. People who can help you select appropriate methods are your state or local health department, physician, or professional expert in indoor air problems. Here are some of the methods to reduce indoor levels of formaldehyde.

1. Bring large amounts of fresh air into the home. Increase ventilation by opening doors and windows and installing an exhaust fan(s).

2. Reduce the humidity level in your home.

3. Seal the surfaces of the formaldehyde-containing product. You may use a vapor barrier such as some paints, varnishes, or a layer of vinyl or polyurethane-like materials. Be sure to seal completely, with a material that does not itself contain formaldehyde.

4. Remove from your home the product that is releasing formaldehyde in the indoor air. When other materials in the area such as carpets, gypsum boards, etc., have absorbed formaldehyde, these products may also start releasing it into the air. Overall levels of formaldehyde can be lower if you increase the ventilation over an extended period.

One method NOT recommended by CPSC is a chemical treatment with strong ammonia (28-29 percent ammonia in water) which results in a temporary decrease in formaldehyde levels. We strongly discourage such treatment since ammonia in this strength is extremely dangerous to handle. Ammonia may damage the brass fittings of a natural gas system, adding a fire and explosion danger.

Where do I go for more information:

The Formaldehyde Institute Inc.
1330 Connecticut Ave., N.W.
Washington, D.C. 20036

Local and State Health Departments

Formaldehyde and Cancer

National Cancer Institute. *Cancer Facts*. May 1995.

In 1980, laboratory findings showed that exposure to formaldehyde could cause nasal cancer in rats. Since then, the question of whether exposure to formaldehyde increases a person's risk of cancer has been the subject of considerable controversy.

Early concerns focused on the use of formaldehyde in the manufacture of mobile homes. Soon, however, questions were raised about workers routinely exposed to the substance: anatomists, embalmers, pathologists, other medical workers, and industrial workers who produce formaldehyde (and formaldehyde resins and plastics), plywood, photographic film, and permanent press fabrics.

During the 1980s, many studies, including major ones by the National Cancer Institute (NCI), were conducted to determine whether these workers had a greater risk for developing cancer than people in the general population. Much of this research was intended to help two regulatory agencies, the Environmental Protection Agency (EPA) and the Occupational Safety and Health Administration (OSHA), develop regulations, if necessary, to protect the public and workers from unnecessary risks of cancer because of formaldehyde exposure. Investigations at NCI have focused on professionals (anatomists and embalmers) as well as industrial workers. Anatomists and embalmers were at greater risk for leukemia and brain cancer than the general population, but industrial workers were not. Industrial workers employed in the chemical, plastics, plywood, and photographic film industries developed nasopharyngeal cancer more often than the general population. The risk increased seven-fold for workers with heavy exposure to formaldehyde. Studies in the Netherlands and Denmark have shown elevated rates of nasal cancer in many persons exposed to formaldehyde.

An NCI study that revealed a 30-percent increase in lung cancer mortality among industrial workers generated the most controversy. The rate of lung cancer did not increase with the level of exposure, and an excess rate of lung cancer among workers was not evident at all industrial plants. The increased incidence of lung cancer was confined to workers in resin and molding compound production, which led NCI investigators to conclude that factors other than formaldehyde might have been involved. Other scientists believe formaldehyde exposure may be the cause of the lung cancer excess.

By 1987, enough evidence had been gathered to prompt EPA to classify formaldehyde as a "probable human carcinogen" under conditions of unusually high or prolonged exposure. The International Agency for Research on Cancer also concluded that formaldehyde is a probable human carcinogen. OSHA and EPA concluded that new rules governing exposure limits were necessary. In November 1987, OSHA proposed that the occupational standard for formaldehyde exposure be reduced from 3 parts per million (ppm) to 1 ppm, averaged over an 8-hour workday; this proposal became law the following month. In May 1992, the law was amended, and the formaldehyde exposure limit was reduced to 0.75 ppm. (Information is available from the Occupational Safety and Health Administration, 200 Constitution Avenue NW, Room N3647, Washington, D.C. 20210.)

Formaldehyde use also has been studied in non-industrial settings. In February 1982, the Consumer Product Safety Commission (CPSC) ordered a ban on all sales of urea-formaldehyde foam insulation (UFFI) for homes and schools. The CPSC ruled that because formaldehyde gas often is released from foam after installation, UFFI presents an "unreasonable health risk." In April 1983, however, a Federal appellate court struck down this ban. The court ruled that there was not sufficient scientific evidence to justify the ban. The CPSC still believes that the evidence shows that risks are associated with UFFI. However, CPSC officials advise consumers to leave insulation alone if they have not experienced any health problems.

For information about health risks posed by home products, you may write to the Consumer Product Safety Commission Public Affairs

Office, 4330 East-West Highway, Bethesda, MD 20816. The CPSC also operates a toll-free hotline; the telephone number is 1-800-638-CPSC (1-800-638-2772). When you dial this number, you will be able to get information from CPSC's pamphlet "UFFI: Urea-Formaldehyde Foam Insulation." When you are instructed to press the three-digit code, press 300. An information operator can read to you from the publication. You cannot order the publication by phone but instead must write to the above address. The teletypewriter number for the hearing impaired is 1-800-638-8270.

Formaldehyde also is used in cosmetics, drug products, paper, textiles, and a variety of other products for the home. Information about drugs and cosmetics may be obtained from the U.S. Food and Drug Administration, 5600 Fishers Lane, Rockville, MD 20857. The telephone number is 301-443-4190.

The Cancer Information Service (CIS), a program of the National Cancer Institute, provides a nationwide telephone service for cancer patients and their families, the public, and health care professionals. CIS information specialists have extensive training in providing up-to-date and understandable information about cancer and cancer research. They can answer questions in English and Spanish and can send free printed material. In addition, CIS offices serve specific geographic areas and have information about cancer-related services and resources in their region. The toll-free number of the CIS is 1-800-4-CANCER (1-800-422-6237).

Chapter 20

Citizen's Guide to Radon

Introduction

EPA Recommends:

- Test your home for radon—it's easy and inexpensive.
- Fix your home if your radon level is 4 picocuries per liter (pCi/L) or higher.
- Radon levels less than 4 pCi/L still pose a risk, and in many cases may be reduced.

Radon is a cancer-causing, radioactive gas. You can't see radon. And you can't smell it or taste it. But it may be a problem in your home.

Radon is estimated to cause many thousands of deaths each year. That's because when you breathe air containing radon, you can get lung cancer. In fact, the Surgeon General has warned that radon is the second leading cause of lung cancer in the United States today. Only smoking causes more lung cancer deaths. If you smoke and your home has high radon levels, your risk of lung cancer is especially high.

Radon can be found all over the U.S.. Radon comes from the natural (radioactive) breakdown of uranium in soil, rock and water and gets into the air you breathe. Radon can be found all over the U.S. It can get into any type of building (homes, offices, and schools) and build up to high levels. But you and your family are most likely to get your greatest exposure at home. That's where you spend most of your time.

EPA publication number 402-K92-001. September 1994.

217

You should test for radon. Testing is the only way to know if you and your family are at risk from radon. EPA and the Surgeon General recommend testing all homes below the third floor for radon. EPA also recommends testing in schools.

Testing is inexpensive and easy. It should only take a few minutes of your time. Millions of Americans have already tested their homes for radon.

You can fix a radon problem. There are simple ways to fix a radon problem that aren't too costly. Even very high levels can be reduced to acceptable levels.

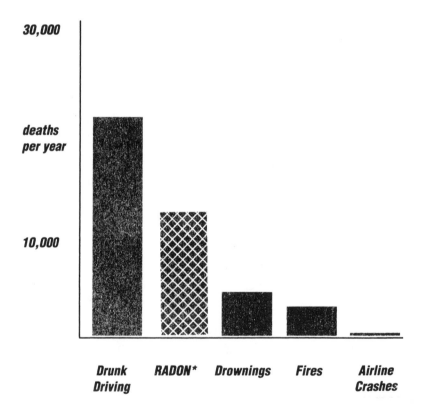

Figure 20.1. *Radon Deaths. Radon is estimated to cause about 14,000 deaths per year—however, this number could range from 7,000 to 30,000 deaths per year. The numbers of deaths from other causes are taken from 1990 National Safety Council reports.*

How Does Radon Get into Your Home?

Radon is a radioactive gas. It comes from the natural decay of uranium that is found in nearly all soils. It typically moves up through the ground to the air above and into your home through cracks and other holes in the foundation. Your home traps radon inside, where it can build up. Any home may have radon problem. This means new and old homes, well-sealed and drafty homes, and homes with or without basements.

Radon from soil gas is the main cause of radon problems. Sometimes radon enters the home through well water. In a small number of homes, the building materials can give off radon, too. However, building materials rarely cause radon problems by themselves.

Radon gets in through:

1. Cracks in solid floors
2. Construction joints
3. Cracks in walls
4. Gaps in suspended floors
5. Gaps around service pipes
6. Cavities inside walls
7. The water supply.

Nearly 1 out of every 15 homes in the U.S. is estimated to have elevated radon levels. Elevated levels of radon gas have been found in homes in your state. Contact your state radon office for general information about radon in your area. While radon problems may be more common in some areas, any home may have a problem. The only way to know about your home is to test.

Radon can be a problem in schools and workplaces, too. Ask your state radon office about radon problems in schools and workplaces in your area.

How to Test Your Home

You can't see radon, but it's not hard to find out if you have a radon problem in your home. All you need to do is test for radon. Testing is easy and should only take a few minutes of your time.

The amount of radon in the air is measured in "picocuries per liter of air," or "pCi/L." Sometimes test results are expressed in Working

219

Levels (WL) rather than picocuries per liter (pCi/L). There are many kinds of low-cost "do it yourself" radon test kits you can get through the mail and in hardware stores and other retail outlets. Make sure you buy a test kit that has passed EPA's testing program or is state-certified. These kits will usually display the phrase "Meets EPA Requirements." If you prefer, or if you are buying or selling a home, you can hire a trained contractor to do the testing for you. Make certain you hire an EPA-qualified or state-certified radon tester. Call your state radon office for a list of these testers.

General Ways to Test for Radon

Short-term Testing: The quickest way to test is with short-term tests. Short-term tests remain in your home for two days to 90 days, depending on the device. "Charcoal canisters," "alpha track," "electret ion chamber," "continuous monitors, " and "charcoal liquid scintillation" detectors are most commonly used for short-term testing. Because radon levels tend to vary from day to day and season to season, a short-term test is less likely than a long-term test to tell you your year-round average radon level. If you need results quickly, however, a short-term test followed by a second short-term test may be used to decide whether to fix your home.

Long-term Testing: Long-term tests remain in your home for more than 90 days. "Alpha track" and "electret" detectors are commonly used for this type of testing. A long-term test will give you a reading that is more likely to tell you your home's year-round average radon level than a short-term test

How to Use a Test Kit

Follow the instructions that come with your test kit. If you are doing a short-term test, close your windows and outside doors and keep them closed as much as possible during the test. (If you are doing a short-term test lasting just two or three days, be sure to close your windows and outside doors at least 12 hours before beginning the test, too. You should not conduct short-term tests lasting just two or three days during unusually severe storms or periods of unusually high winds.) The test kit should be placed in the lowest lived-in level of the home (for example, the basement if it is frequently used, otherwise the first floor). It should be put in a room that is used regularly (like a living room, playroom, den or bedroom) but *not* your kitchen or bathroom. Place the kit at least 20 inches above the floor in a location where it won't be disturbed—away from drafts, high heat, high humidity, and exterior walls. Leave the kit in place for as long as the package says. Once you've finished the test, reseal the package and send it to the lab specified on the package right away for study. You should receive your test results within a few weeks.

EPA Recommends the Following Testing Steps:

1. Take a short-term test. If your result is 4 pCi/L or higher* take a follow-up test (Step 2) to be sure.

2. Follow up with either a long-term test or a second short-term test:

    *   For a better understanding of your year-round average radon level, take a long-term test.
    *   If you need results quickly, take a second short-term test.

    The higher your initial short-term test result, the more certain you can be that you should take a short-term rather than a long-term follow-up test. If your first short-term test result is several times the action level—for example, about 10 pCi/L or higher—you should take a second short-term test immediately

3. If you followed up with a long-term test: Fix your home if your long-term test result is 4 pCi/L or more*

    *   If you followed up with a second short-term test: The higher your short-term results, the more certain you can be that you should fix your home. Consider fixing your home if the average of your first and second test is 4 pCi/L or higher *

* 0.02 Working Levels (WL) or higher.

What Your Test Results Mean

The average indoor radon level is estimated to be about 1.3 pCi/L, and about 0.4 pCi/L of radon is normally found in the outside air. The

U.S. Congress has set a long-term goal that indoor radon levels be no more than outdoor levels. While this goal is not yet technologically achievable in all cases, most homes today can be reduced to 2 pCi/L or below.

Sometimes short-term tests are less definitive about whether or not your home is above 4 pCi/L. This can happen when your results are close to 4 pCi/L. For example, if the average of your two short-term test results is 4.1 pCi/L, there is about a 50 percent chance that your year-round average is somewhat below 4 pCi/L. However, EPA believes that any radon exposure carries some risk, no level of radon is safe. Even radon levels below 4 pCi/L pose some risk, and you can reduce your risk of lung cancer by lowering your radon level.

If your living patterns change and you begin occupying a lower level of your home (such as a basement) you should retest your home on that level. Even if your test result is below 4 pCi/L, you may want to test again sometime in the future.

Radon and Home Sales

More and more, home buyers and renters are asking about radon levels before they buy or rent a home. Because real estate sales happen quickly, there is often little time to deal with radon and other issues. The best thing to do is to test for radon NOW and save the results in case the buyer is interested in them. Fix a problem if it exists so it won 't complicate your home sale. If you are planning to move, call your state radon office for EPA's pamphlet "Home Buyer's and Seller's Guide to Radon," which addresses some common questions. During home sales:

- Buyers often ask if a home has been tested, and if elevated levels were reduced.

- Buyers frequently want tests made by someone who is not involved in the home sale. Your state office has a list of qualified testers.

- Buyers might want to know the radon levels in areas of the home (like a basement they plan to finish) that the seller might not otherwise test.

Today many homes are built to prevent radon from coming in. Your state or local area may require these radon-resistant construction features. Radon-resistant construction features usually keep radon levels in new homes below 2 pCi/L. If you are buying or renting a new home, ask the owner or builder if it has radon-resistant features.

Radon in Water

Compared to radon entering the home through soil, radon entering the home through water will in most cases be a small source of risk. Radon gas can enter the home through well water. It can be released into the air you breathe when water is used for showering and other household uses. Research suggests that swallowing water with high radon levels may pose risks, too, although risks from swallowing water containing radon are believed to be much lower than those from breathing air containing radon.

While radon in water is not a problem in homes served by most public water supplies, it has been found in well water. If you've tested the air in your home and found a radon problem, and your water comes from a well, contact a lab certified to measure radiation in water to have your water tested. If you're on a public water supply and are concerned that radon may be entering your home through the water, call your public water supplier.

Radon problems in water can be readily fixed. The most effective treatment is to remove radon from the water before it enters the home. This is called point-of-entry treatment. Treatment at your water tap is called point-of-use treatment. Unfortunately, point-of-use treatment will not reduce most of the inhalation risk from radon.

Call your state office or the EPA Drinking Water Hotline (800-426-4791) for more information on radon in water.

How to Lower the Radon Level in Your Home

Since there is no known safe level of radon, there can always be some risk. But the risk can be reduced by lowering the radon level in your home.

A variety of methods are used to reduce radon in your home. In some cases, sealing cracks in floors and walls may help to reduce radon. In other cases, simple systems using pipes and fans may be used to reduce radon. Such systems are called "sub-slab depressurization," and do not require major changes to your home. These systems remove radon gas from below the concrete floor and the foundation before it can enter the home. Similar systems can also be installed in houses with crawl spaces. Radon contractors use other methods that may also work in your home. The right system depends on the design of your home and other factors.

Ways to reduce radon in your home are discussed in EPA's "Consumer's Guide to Radon Reduction." You can get a copy from your state radon office.

The cost of making repairs to reduce radon depends on how your home was built and the extent of the radon problem. Most homes can be fixed for about the same cost as other common home repairs like painting or having a new hot water heater installed. The average house costs about $1,200 for a contractor to fix, although this can range from about $500 to about $2,500.

Lowering high radon levels requires technical knowledge and special skills. You should use a contractor who is trained to fix radon problems. The EPA Radon Contractor Proficiency (RCP) Program tests these contractors. EPA provides a list of RCP contractors to state radon offices. A contractor who has passed the EPA test will carry a special RCP identification card. A trained RCP contractor can study the radon problem in your home and help you pick the right treatment method.

Check with your state radon office for names of qualified or state certified radon contractors in your area. Picking someone to fix your radon problem is much like choosing a contractor for other home repairs, you may want to get references and more than one estimate.

If you plan to fix the problem in your home yourself, you should first contact your state radon office for EPA's technical guide, "Radon Reduction Techniques for Detached Houses."

You should also test your home again after it is fixed to be sure that radon levels have been reduced. Most radon reduction systems include a monitor that will alert you if the system needs servicing. In addition, it's a good idea to retest your home sometime in the future to be sure radon levels remain low.

Radon and Home Renovations

If you are planning any major structural renovation, such as converting an unfinished basement area into living space, it is especially important to test the area for radon before you begin the renovation. If your test results indicate a radon problem, radon-resistant techniques can be inexpensively included as part of the renovation. Because major renovations can change the level of radon in any home, always test again after work is completed.

The Risk of Living with Radon

Radon gas decays into radioactive particles that can get trapped in your lungs when you breathe. As they break down further, these particles release small bursts of energy. This can damage lung tissue and lead to lung cancer over the course of your lifetime. Not everyone exposed to elevated levels of radon will develop lung cancer. And the amount of time between exposure and the onset of the disease may be many years.

Like other environmental pollutants, there is some uncertainty about the magnitude of radon health risks. However, we know more about radon risks than risks from most other cancer-causing substances. This is because estimates of radon risks are based on studies of cancer in humans (underground miners). Additional studies on more typical populations are under way.

Smoking combined with radon is an especially serious health risk. Stop smoking and lower your radon level to reduce your lung cancer risk.

Children have been reported to have greater risk than adults of certain types of cancer from radiation, but there are currently no conclusive data on whether children are at greater risk than adults from radon.

Your chances of getting lung cancer from radon depend mostly on:

* How much radon is in your home

* The amount of time you spend in your home

* Whether you are a smoker or have ever smoked.

Radon Myths

MYTH: Scientists aren't sure radon really is a problem.

FACT: Although some scientists dispute the precise number of deaths due to radon, all major health organizations (like the Centers for Disease Control, the American Lung Association and the American Medical Association) agree with estimates that radon causes thousands of preventable lung cancer deaths every year. This is especially true among smokers, since the risk to smokers is much greater than to non-smokers.

MYTH: Radon testing is difficult, time consuming and expensive.

FACT: Radon testing is inexpensive and easy—it should take only a little of your time.

MYTH: Radon test kits are not reliable and are difficult to find.

FACT: Reliable test kits are available through the mail, in hardware stores and other retail outlets. Call your state radon office for a list of test kit companies that have met EPA requirements for reliability or are state certified.

MYTH: Homes with radon problems can't be fixed.

FACT: There are simple solutions to radon problems in homes. Thousands of homeowners have already fixed radon problems in their homes. Radon levels can be readily lowered for about $500 to $2,500. Call your state radon office for a list of contractors that have met EPA requirements or are state certified.

MYTH: Radon only affects certain kinds of homes.

FACT: House construction can affect radon levels. However, radon can be a problem in homes of all types: old homes, new homes, drafty homes, insulated homes, homes with basements and homes without basements.

MYTH: Radon is only a problem in certain parts of the country.

FACT: High radon levels have been found in every state. Radon problems do vary from area to area, but the only way to know your radon level is to test.

MYTH: A neighbor's test result is a good indication of whether your home has a problem.

FACT: It's not. Radon levels vary from home to home. The only way to know if your home has a radon problem is to test it.

MYTH: Everyone should test their water for radon.

FACT: While radon gets into some homes through the water, you should first test the air in your home for radon. If you find high levels and your water comes from a well, contact a lab certified to measure radiation in water to have your water tested.

MYTH: It's difficult to sell homes where radon problems have been discovered.

FACT: Where radon problems have been fixed, home sales have not been blocked or frustrated. The added protection is sometimes a good selling point.

MYTH: I've lived in my home for so long, it doesn't make sense to take action now.

FACT: You will reduce your risk of lung cancer when you reduce radon levels, even if you've lived with a radon problem for a long time.

MYTH: Short-term tests can't be used for making a decision about whether to fix your home.

FACT: A short-term test followed by a second short-term test may be used to decide whether to fix your home. However, the closer the average of your two short-term tests is to 4 pCi/L, the less certain you can be about whether your year-round average is above or below that level. Keep in mind that radon levels below 4 pCi/l still pose some risk. Radon levels can be reduced in most homes to 2 pCi/L or below.

For Further Information

For more information on how to reduce your radon health risk, ask your state radon office to send you these guides:

- *Home Buyer's and Seller's Guide to Radon*
- *Radon in Schools*
- *Radon: A Physician's Guide*
- *Consumer's Guide to Radon Reduction*
- *Technical Support Document*

If you plan to make repairs yourself, be sure to contact your state radon office for a current copy of EPA's technical guidance on radon mitigation, "Application of Radon Reduction Techniques for Detached Houses."

Surgeon General Health Advisory

"Indoor radon gas is a national health problem. Radon causes thousands of deaths each year. Millions of homes have elevated radon levels. Homes should be tested for radon. When elevated levels are confirmed, the problem should be corrected."

Alabama	**800/582-1866**	Montana	**406/444-3671**
Alaska	**800/478-8324**	Nebraska	**800/334-9491**
Arizona	**602/255-4845**	Nevada	**702/687-5394**
Arkansas	**501/661-2301**	New Hampshire	**800/852-3345 x4674**
California	**800/745-7236**	New Jersey	**800/648-0394**
Colorado	**800/846-3986**	New Mexico	**505/827-4300**
Connecticut	**203/566-3122**	New York	**800/458-1158**
Delaware	**800/554-4636**	North Carolina	**919/571-4141**
District of Columbia	**202/727-5728**	North Dakota	**701/221-5188**
Florida	**800/543-8279**	Ohio	**800/523-4439**
Georgia	**800/745-0037**	Oklahoma	**405/271-1902**
Hawaii	**808/586-4700**	Oregon	**503/731-4014**
Idaho	**800/445-8647**	Pennsylvania	**800/237-2366**
Illinois	**800/325-1245**	Puerto Rico	**809/767-3563**
Indiana	**800/272-9723**	Rhode Island	**401/277-2438**
Iowa	**800/383-5992**	South Carolina	**800/768-0362**
Kansas	**913/296-6183**	South Dakota	**800/438-3367**
Kentucky	**502/564-3700**	Tennessee	**800/232-1139**
Louisiana	**800/256-2494**	Texas	**512/834-6688**
Maine	**800/232-0842**	Utah	**800/536-4250**
Maryland	**800/872-3666**	Vermont	**800/640-0601**
Massachusetts	**413/586-7525**	Virginia	**800/468-0138**
Michigan	**800/723-6642**	West Virginia	**800/922-1255**
Minnesota	**800/798-9050**	Wisconsin	**608/267-4795**
Mississippi	**800/626-7739**	Wyoming	**800/458-5847**
Missouri	**800/669-7236**		

INDIAN NATIONS			
All Indian Pueblo Council	**505-881-2254**	Oneida Indian Nation	**315-361-6300**
Cherokee Nation	**918-458-5496**	Seneca Nation	**716-532-0024**
Chickasaw Nation	**405-436-2603**	St. Regis Mohawk Tribe	**518-358-3141**
Hopi Tribe	**602-734-2441**	For Indian Nations in the	
Inner Tribal Council	**602-248-0071**	States of MN,WI,IL,	
Jicarilla Apache Tribe	**505-759-3242**	MI, IN,and OH,call	**312-886-6063**
Navajo Nation	**602-871-7754**		

Table 20.1. State Radon Contacts

Chapter 21

Burning Up Your Air: Combustion Appliances and Indoor Air Pollution

What You Should Know about Combustion Appliances and Indoor Air Pollution

Hazards may be associated with almost all types of appliances. The purpose of this chapter is to answer some common questions you may have about the potential for one specific type of hazard—indoor air pollution—associated with one class of appliances—combustion appliances.

Combustion appliances are those which burn fuels for warmth, cooking, or decorative purposes. Typical fuels are gas, both natural and liquefied petroleum (LP); kerosene; oil; coal; and wood. Examples of the appliances are space heaters, ranges, ovens, stoves, furnaces, fireplaces, water heaters, and clothes dryers. These appliances are usually safe. However, under certain conditions, these appliances can produce combustion pollutants that can damage your health, or even kill you.

POSSIBLE HEALTH EFFECTS range from headaches, dizziness, sleepiness, and watery eyes to breathing difficulties or even death. Similar effects may also occur because of common medical problems or other indoor air pollutants.

©1991 American Lung Association®, U.S. Consumer Product Safety Commission, and U.S. Environmental Protection Agency. Reprinted with permission.

This chapter was written:

1. to encourage the proper use, maintenance, and installation of combustion appliances;

2. to discuss the pollutants produced by these appliances;

3. to describe how these pollutants can affect your health; and

4. to tell you how you can reduce your exposure to them.

Should I be concerned about indoor air pollution?

Yes. Studies have shown that the air in our homes can be even more polluted than the outdoor air in big cities. Because people spend a lot of time indoors, the quality of the air indoors can affect their health. Infants, young children and the elderly are a group shown to be more susceptible to pollutants. People with chronic respiratory or cardio-vascular illness or immune system diseases are also more susceptible than others to pollutants.

Many factors determine whether pollutants in your home will affect your health. They include the presence, use, and condition of pollutant sources, the level of pollutants both indoors and out, the amount of ventilation in your home, and your overall health.

Most homes have more than one source of indoor air pollution. For example, pollutants come from tobacco smoke, building materials, decorating products, home furnishings, and activities such as cooking, heating, cooling, and cleaning. Living in areas with high outdoor levels of pollutants usually results in high indoor levels. Combustion pollutants are one category of indoor air pollutants.

What are combustion pollutants?

Combustion pollutants are gases or particles that come from burning materials. The combustion pollutants discussed in this chapter come from burning fuels in appliances. The common fuels burned in these appliances are natural or LP gas, fuel oil, kerosene, wood, or coal. The types and amounts of pollutants produced depend upon the type of appliance, how well the appliance is installed, maintained, and vented, and the kind of fuel it uses. Some of the common pollutants produced from burning these fuels are carbon monoxide, nitrogen dioxide, particles, and sulfur dioxide. Particles can have hazardous chemicals attached to them. Other pollutants that can be produced by some appliances are unburned hydrocarbons and aldehydes. Combustion always produces water vapor. Water vapor is not usually considered a pollutant, but it can act as one. It can result in high humidity and wet surfaces. These conditions encourage the growth of biological pollutants such as house dust mites, molds, and bacteria.

Where do combustion pollutants come from?

Combustion pollutants found indoors include: outdoor air, tobacco smoke, exhaust from car and lawn mower internal combustion engines, and some hobby activities such as welding, woodburning, and soldering. Combustion pollutants can also come from vented or unvented combustion appliances. These appliances include space heaters, gas ranges and ovens, furnaces, gas water heaters, gas clothes dryers, wood or coal-burning stoves, and fireplaces. As a group these are called "combustion appliances."

What is a vented appliance? What is an unvented appliance?

Vented appliances are appliances designed to be used with a duct, chimney, pipe, or other device that carry the combustion pollutants outside the home. These appliances can release large amounts of pollutants directly into your home if a vent is not properly installed or is blocked or leaking.

Unvented appliances do not vent to the outside, so they release combustion pollutants directly into the home.

Look at Table 21.1 below for typical appliance problems that cause the release of pollutants in your home. Many of these problems are hard for a homeowner to identify. A professional is needed.

Can I use charcoal grills or charcoal hibachis indoors?

No. Never use these appliances inside homes, trailers, truck-caps, or tents. Carbon monoxide from burning and smoldering charcoal can kill you if you use it indoors for cooking or heating. There are about 25 deaths each year from the use of charcoal grills and hibachis indoors.

NEVER burn charcoal inside homes, trailers, tents, or other enclosures. The carbon monoxide can kill you.

Appliances	Fuel	Typical Potential Problems
Central Furnaces Room Heaters Gas Fireplaces	Natural or Liquified Petroleum Gas	Cracked heat exchanger Not enough air to burn fuel properly Defective/blocked flue Maladjusted burner
Central Furnaces	Oil	Cracked heat exchanger Not enough air to burn fuel properly Defective/blocked flue Maladjusted burner
Central Heaters Room Heaters	Wood	Cracked heat exchanger Not enough air to burn fuel properly Defective/blocked flue Green or treated wood
Central Furnaces Stoves	Coal	Cracked heat exchanger Not enough air to burn fuel properly Defective/blocked flue Defective grate
Room Heaters Central Heaters	Kerosene	Improper adjustment Wrong fuel (not K-1) Wrong wick or wick height Not enough air to burn fuel properly
Water Heaters	Natural or Liquefied Petroleum Gas	Not enough air to burn fuel properly Defective/blocked flue Maladjusted burner
Ranges Ovens	Natural or Liquefied Petroleum Gas	Not enough air to burn fuel properly Maladjusted burner Misuse as a room heater
Stoves Fireplaces	Wood Coal	Not enough air to burn fuel properly Defective/blocked flue Green or treated wood Cracked heat exchanger or firebox

Table 21.1. Combustion Appliances and Potential Problems

What are the health effects of combustion pollutants?

The health effects of combustion pollutants range from headaches and breathing difficulties to death. The health effects may show up immediately after exposure or occur after being exposed to the pollutants for a long time. The effects depend upon the type and amount of pollutants and the length of time of exposure to them. They also depend upon several factors related to the exposed person. These include the age and any existing health problems. There are still some questions about the level of pollutants or the period of exposure needed to produce specific health effects. Further studies to better define the release of pollutants from combustion appliances and their health effects are needed.

The sections below discuss health problems associated with some common combustion pollutants. These pollutants include carbon monoxide, nitrogen dioxide, particles, and sulfur dioxide. Even if you are healthy, high levels of carbon monoxide can kill you within a short time. The health effects of the other pollutants are generally more subtle and are more likely to affect susceptible people. It is always a good idea to reduce exposure to combustion pollutants by using and maintaining combustion appliances properly.

Carbon Monoxide

Each year, according to CPSC, there are more than 200 carbon monoxide deaths related to the use of all types of combustion appliances in the home. Exposure to carbon monoxide reduces the blood's ability to carry oxygen. Often a person or an entire family may not recognize that carbon monoxide is poisoning them. The chemical is odorless and some of the symptoms are similar to common illnesses. This is particularly dangerous because carbon monoxide's deadly effects will not be recognized until it is too late to take action against them.

Carbon monoxide exposures especially affect unborn babies, infants, and people with anemia or a history of heart disease. Breathing low levels of the chemical can cause fatigue and increase chest pain in people with chronic heart disease. Breathing higher levels of carbon monoxide causes symptoms such as headaches, dizziness, and weakness in healthy people. Carbon monoxide also causes sleepiness, nausea, vomiting, confusion, and disorientation. At very high levels it causes loss of consciousness and death.

233

Nitrogen Dioxide (NO_2)

Breathing high levels of nitrogen dioxide causes irritation of the respiratory tract and causes shortness of breath. Compared to healthy people, children, and individuals with respiratory illnesses such as asthma, may be more susceptible to the effects of nitrogen dioxide.

Some studies have shown that children may have more colds and flu when exposed to low levels of nitrogen dioxide. When people with asthma inhale low levels of nitrogen dioxide while exercising, their lung airways can narrow and react more to inhaled materials.

Particles

Particles suspended in the air can cause eye, nose, throat, and lung irritation. They can increase respiratory symptoms, especially in people with chronic lung disease or heart problems. Certain chemicals attached to particles may cause lung cancer, if they are inhaled. The risk of lung cancer increases with the amount and length of exposure. The health effects from inhaling particles depend upon many factors, including the size of the particle and its chemical make-up.

Sulfur Dioxide (SO_2)

Sulfur dioxide at low levels of exposure can cause eye, nose, and respiratory tract irritation. At high exposure levels, it causes the lung airways to narrow. This causes wheezing, chest tightness, or breathing problems. People with asthma are particularly susceptible to the effects of sulfur dioxide. They may have symptoms at levels that are much lower than the rest of the population.

Other Pollutants

Combustion may release other pollutants. They include unburned hydrocarbons and aldehydes. Little is known about the levels of these pollutants in indoor air and the resulting health effects.

What do I do if I suspect that combustion pollutants are affecting my health?

If you suspect you are being subjected to carbon monoxide poisoning get fresh air immediately. Open windows and doors for more ventilation, turn off any combustion appliances, and leave the house. You could lose consciousness and die of carbon monoxide poisoning if you do nothing. It is also important to contact a doctor **IMMEDIATELY** for a proper diagnosis. Remember to tell your doctor that you suspect carbon monoxide poisoning is causing your problems. Prompt medical attention is important.

Remember that some symptoms from combustion pollutants— headaches, dizziness, sleepiness, coughing, and watery eyes—may also occur because of common medical problems. These medical problems include colds, the flu, or allergies. Similar symptoms may also occur because of other indoor air pollutants. Contact your doctor for a proper diagnosis.

To help your doctor make the correct diagnosis, try to have answers to the following questions:

- Do your symptoms occur only in the home? Do they disappear or decrease when you leave home, and reappear when you return?

- Is anyone else in your household complaining of similar symptoms, such as headaches, dizziness, or sleepiness? Are they complaining of nausea, watery eyes, coughing, or nose and throat irritation?

- Do you always have symptoms?

- Are your symptoms getting worse?

- Do you often catch colds or get the flu?

- Are you using any combustion appliances in your home?

- Has anyone inspected your appliances lately? Are you certain they are working properly?

Your doctor may take a blood sample to measure the level of carbon monoxide in your blood if he or she suspects carbon monoxide poisoning. This sample will help determine whether carbon monoxide is affecting your health.

Contact qualified appliance service people to have your appliances inspected and adjusted if needed. You should be able to find a qualified person by asking your appliance distributor or your fuel supplier. In some areas, the local fuel company may be able to inspect and adjust the appliance.

How can I reduce my exposure to combustion pollutants?

Proper selection, installation, inspection and maintenance of your appliances are extremely important in reducing your exposure to these pollutants. Providing good ventilation in your home and correctly using your appliance can also reduce your exposure to these pollutants.

Additionally, there are several different residential carbon monoxide detectors for sale. The CPSC is encouraging the development of detectors that will provide maximum protection. These detectors would warn consumers of harmful carbon monoxide levels in the home. They may soon be widely available to reduce deaths from carbon monoxide poisoning.

Appliance Selection

- Choose vented appliances whenever possible.

- Only buy combustion appliances that have been tested and certified to meet current safety standards. Examples of certifying organizations are Underwriters Laboratories (UL) and the American Gas Association (AGA) Laboratories. Look for a label that clearly shows the certification.

- All currently manufactured vented gas heaters are required by industry safety standards to have a safety shut-off device. This device helps protect you from carbon monoxide poisoning by shutting off an improperly vented heater.

- Check your local and state building codes and fire ordinances to see if you can use an unvented space heater, if you consider purchasing one. They are not allowed to be used in some communities, dwellings, or certain rooms in the house.

- If you must replace an unvented gas space heater with another, make it a new one. Heaters made after 1982 have a pilot light safety system called an oxygen depletion sensor (ODS). This system shuts off the heater when there is not enough fresh air, before the heater begins producing large amounts of carbon monoxide. Look for the label that tells you that the appliance has this safety system. Older heaters will not have this protection system.

- Consider buying gas appliances that have electronic ignitions rather than pilot lights. These appliances are usually more energy efficient and eliminate the continuous low-level pollutants from pilot lights.

- Buy appliances that are the correct size for the area you want to heat. Using the wrong size heater may produce more pollutants in your home and is not an efficient use of energy.

- Talk to your dealer to determine the type and size of appliance you will need. You may wish to write to the appliance manufacturer or association for more information on the appliance. Some addresses are in the back of this chapter.

- All new woodstoves are EPA-certified to limit the amounts of pollutants released into the outdoor air. For more information on selecting, installing, operating, and maintaining woodburning stoves, write to the EPA Wood Heater Program. Their address is in the back of this chapter. Before buying a woodstove check your local laws about the installation and use of woodstoves.

Proper Installation

- You should have your appliances professionally installed. Professionals should follow the installation directions and applicable building codes. Improperly installed appliances can release dangerous pollutants in your home and may create a fire hazard. Be sure that the installer checks for backdrafting on all vented appliances. A qualified installer knows how to do this.

Ventilation

- To reduce indoor air pollution, a good supply of fresh outdoor air is needed. The movement of air into and out of your home is very important. Normally, air comes through cracks around doors and windows. This air helps reduce the level of pollutants indoors. This supply of fresh air is also important to help carry pollutants up the chimney, stovepipe, or flue to the outside.

- Keep doors open to the rest of the house from the room where you are using an unvented gas space heater or kerosene heater, and crack open a window. This allows enough air for proper combustion and reduces the level of pollutants, especially carbon monoxide.

- Use a hood fan, if you are using a range. They reduce the level of pollutants you breath, if they exhaust to the outside. Make sure that enough air is coming into the house when you use an exhaust fan. If needed, slightly open a door or window, especially if other appliances are in use. For proper operation of most combustion appliances and their venting system, the air pressure in the house should be greater than that outside. If not, the vented appliances could release combustion pollutants into the house rather than outdoors. If you suspect that you have this problem you may need the help of a qualified person to solve it.

- Make sure that your vented appliance has the vent connected and that nothing is blocking it. Make sure there are no holes or cracks in the vent. Do not vent gas clothes dryers or water heaters into the house for heating. This is unsafe.

- Open the stove's damper when adding wood. This allows more air into the stove. More air helps the wood burn properly and prevents pollutants from being drawn back into the house instead of going up the chimney. Visible smoke or a constant smoky odor inside the home when using a woodburning stove is a sign that the stove is not working properly. Soot on furniture in the rooms where you are using the stove also tells this. Smoke and soot are signs that the stove is releasing pollutants into the indoor air.

Correct Use

- Read and follow the instructions for all appliances so you understand how they work. Keep the owner's manual in a convenient place to refer to when needed. Also, read and follow the warning labels because they tell you important safety information that you need to know. Reading and following the instructions and warning labels could save your life.

- Always use the correct fuel for the appliance.

- Only use water-clear ASTM 1-K kerosene for kerosene heaters. The use of kerosene other than 1-K could lead to a release of more pollutants in your home. Never use gasoline in a kerosene heater because it can cause a fire or an explosion. Using even small amounts of gasoline could cause a fire.

- Use seasoned hardwoods (elm, maple, oak) instead of softwoods (cedar, fir, pine) in woodburning stoves and fireplaces. Hardwoods are better because they burn hotter and form less creosote, an oily, black tar that sticks to chimneys and stove pipes. Do not use green or wet woods as the primary wood because they make more creosote and smoke. Never burn painted scrap wood or wood treated with preservatives, because they could release highly toxic pollutants, such as arsenic or lead. Plastics, charcoal, and colored paper such as comics, also produce pollutants. Never burn anything that the stove or fireplace manufacturer does not recommend.

- Never use a range, oven, or dryer to heat your home. When you misuse gas appliances in this way, they can produce fatal amounts of carbon monoxide. They can produce high levels of nitrogen dioxide, too.

- Never use an unvented combustion heater overnight or in a room where you are sleeping. Carbon monoxide from combustion heaters can reach dangerous levels.

- Never ignore a safety device when it shuts off an appliance. It means that something is wrong. Read your appliance instructions to find out what you should do or have a professional check out the problem.

- Never ignore the smell of fuel. This usually indicates that the appliance is not operating properly or is leaking fuel. Leaking fuel will not always be detectible by smell. If you suspect that you have a fuel leak have it fixed as soon as possible. In most cases you should shut off the appliance, extinguish any other flames or pilot lights, shut off other appliances in the area, open windows and doors, call for help, and leave the area.

Inspection and Maintenance

- Have your combustion appliance regularly inspected and maintained to reduce your exposure to pollutants. Appliances that are not working properly can release harmful and even fatal amounts of pollutants, especially carbon monoxide.

- Have chimneys and vents inspected when installing or changing vented heating appliances. Some modifications may be required. For example, if a change was made in your heating system from oil to natural gas, the flue gas produced by the gas system could be hot enough to melt accumulated oil combustion debris in the chimney or vent. This debris could block the vent forcing pollutants into the house. It is important to clean your chimney and vents especially when changing heating systems.

What are the inspection and maintenance procedures?

The best advice is to follow the recommendations of the manufacturer. The same combustion appliance may have different inspection and maintenance requirements, depending upon where you live.

In general, check the flame in the furnace combustion chamber at the beginning of the heating season. Natural gas furnaces should have a blue flame with perhaps only a slight yellow tip. Call your appliance service representative to adjust the burner if there is a lot of yellow in the flame, or call your local utility company for this service. LP units should have a flame with a bright blue center that may have a light yellow tip. Pilot lights on gas water heaters and gas cooking appliances should also have a blue flame. Have a trained service representative adjust the pilot light if it is yellow or orange.

Before each heating season, have flues and chimneys inspected and cleaned for leakage and for blockage by creosote or debris. Creosote buildup or leakage could cause black stains on the outside of the chimney or flue. These stains can mean that pollutants are leaking into the house.

The chart below, Table 21.2, shows how and when to take care of your appliance.

This chapter discussed the types of pollutants that may be produced by combustion appliances, described how they might affect your health, and suggested ways you could reduce your exposure to them. It also explained that proper appliance selection, installation, operation,

Applicance	Inspection/ Frequency	Maintenance/ Frequency
Gas Hot Air Heating System	Air Filters – Monthly	Clean/change filter – As needed
	Look at flues for rust and soot – Yearly	Qualified person check/ clean chimney, clean combustion chamber, adjust burners, check heat exchanger and operation Yearly (at start of heating season)
Gas/Oil Water/Steam Heating Systems and Water Heaters	Look at flues for rust and soot – Yearly	Qualified person check/ clean chimney, clean combustion chamber, adjust burners, check operation Yearly (at start of heating season)
Kerosene Space Heaters	Look to see that mantle is properly seated – Daily when in use	Check and replace wick Yearly (at start of heating season)
	Look to see that fuel tank is free of water or other contaminants – Daily or before refueling	Clean combustion chamber Yearly (at start of heating season) Drain fuel tank Yearly (at end of heating season)
Wood/Coal Stoves	Look at flues for rust and soot – Yearly	Qualified person check/clean chimney, check seams and gaskets, check operation Yearly (at start of heating season)

Table 21.2. Inspection and Maintenance Schedules

inspection, and maintenance are very important in reducing exposure to combustion pollutants.

For more information:

For a copy of CPSC's booklets *What You Should Know About Space Heaters* and *What You Should Know About Kerosene Heaters,* and for information on asbestos, biological pollutants, lead, methylene chloride, humidifiers, and formaldehyde in your home, write to:

U.S. Consumer Product Safety Commission
Washington, D.C. 20207

For a copy of *The Inside Story: A Guide to Indoor Air Quality,* (extracted in this sourcebook) and additional information on indoor air quality write:

Public Information Center (PM-211B)
U.S. Environmental Protection Agency
401 M Street, SW
Washington, D.C. 20460

Information on indoor air quality is also available from local American Lung Association (ALA) offices. They are listed in the white pages of the phone book.

For information on woodstoves write:

Wood Heater Program (EN-341W)
U.S. Environmental Protection Agency
401 M Street, SW
Washington, DC 20460

For information on kerosene heaters, write or call:

National Kerosene Heater Association
3100 West End Avenue, Suite 250
Nashville, TN 37203
(Telephone: 615-269-9015)

For information on gas heating appliances, write:

Gas Appliance Manufacturers Association, Inc.
1901 North Moore Street, Suite 1100
Arlington, VA 22209
American Gas Association
1515 Wilson Blvd.
Arlington, VA 22209

For a copy of *Straight Answers to Burning Questions* or other woodburning information, write:

Wood Heating Alliance
1101 Connecticut Ave N.W., Suite 700
Washington, DC 20036

Chapter 22

Asbestos in Your Home

This chapter will help you understand asbestos: what it is, its health effects, where it is in your home, and what to do about it.

Even if asbestos is in your home, this is usually NOT a serious problem. The mere presence of asbestos in a home or a building is not hazardous. The danger is that asbestos materials may become damaged over time. Damaged asbestos may release asbestos fibers and become a health hazard. THE BEST THING TO DO WITH ASBESTOS MATERIAL IN GOOD CONDITION IS TO LEAVE IT ALONE! Disturbing it may create a health hazard where none existed before. Read this chapter before you have any asbestos material inspected, removed, or repaired.

What is asbestos?

Asbestos is a mineral fiber. It can be positively identified only with a special type of microscope. There are several types of asbestos fibers. In the past, asbestos was added to a variety of products to strengthen them and to provide heat insulation and fire resistance.

How can asbestos affect my health?

From studies of people who were exposed to asbestos in factories and shipyards, we know that breathing high levels of asbestos fibers can lead to an increased risk of:

American Lung Association. September 1990.

- lung cancer;
- mesothelioma, a cancer of the lining of the chest and the abdominal cavity; and
- asbestosis, in which the lungs become scarred with fibrous tissue.

The risk of lung cancer and mesothelioma increases with the number of fibers inhaled. The risk of lung cancer from inhaling asbestos fibers is also greater if you smoke. People who get asbestosis have usually been exposed to high levels of asbestos for a long time. The symptoms of these diseases do not usually appear until about 20 to 30 years after the first exposure to asbestos.

Most people exposed to small amounts of asbestos, as we all are in our daily lives, do not develop these health problems. However, if disturbed, asbestos material may release asbestos fibers, which can be inhaled into the lungs. The fibers can remain there for a long time, increasing the risk of disease. Asbestos material that would crumble easily if handled, or that has been sawed, scraped, or sanded into a powder, is more likely to create a health hazard.

Where can I find asbestos and when can it be a problem?

Most products made today do not contain asbestos. Those few products made which still contain asbestos that could be inhaled are required to be labeled as such. However, until the 1970s, many types of building products and insulation materials used in homes contained asbestos. Common products that might have contained asbestos in the past, and conditions which may release fibers, include:

- **Steam Pipes, Boilers, and Furnace Ducts** insulated with an asbestos blanket or asbestos paper tape. These materials may release asbestos fibers if damaged, repaired, or removed improperly.

- **Resilient Floor Tiles (vinyl asbestos, asphalt, and rubber), the backing on Vinyl Sheet Flooring, and Adhesives** used for installing floor tile. Sanding tiles can release fibers. So may scraping or sanding the backing of sheet flooring during removal.

- **Cement sheet, millboard, and paper** used as insulation around furnaces and wood-burning stoves. Repairing or removing appliances may release asbestos fibers. So may cutting, tearing, sanding, drilling, or sawing insulation.

- **Door gaskets** in furnaces, wood stoves, and coal stoves. Worn seals can release asbestos fibers during use.

- **Soundproofing or decorative material** sprayed on walls and ceilings. Loose, crumbly, or water-damaged material may release fibers. So will sanding, drilling, or scraping the material.

- **Patching and joint compounds** for walls and ceilings, and **textured paints**. Sanding, scraping, or drilling these surfaces may release asbestos.

- **Asbestos cement roofing, shingles, and siding.** These products are not likely to release asbestos fibers unless sawed, drilled, or cut.

- **Artificial ashes and embers** sold for use in gas-fired fireplaces. Also, other older household products such as fireproof gloves, stove-top pads, ironing board covers, and certain hairdryers.

- **Automobile brake pads and linings, clutch facings, and gaskets.**

What should be done about asbestos in the home?

If you think asbestos may be in your home, don't panic! Usually, the best thing is to LEAVE asbestos material that is in good condition ALONE. Generally, material in good condition will not release asbestos fibers. THERE IS NO DANGER unless fibers are released and inhaled into the lungs.

Check material regularly if you suspect it may contain asbestos. Don't touch it, but look for signs of wear or damage such as tears, abrasions, or water damage. Damaged material may release asbestos fibers. This is particularly true if you often disturb it by hitting, rubbing, or handling it, or if it is exposed to extreme vibration or air flow.

Sometimes, the best way to deal with slightly damaged material is to limit access to the area and not touch or disturb it. Discard damaged

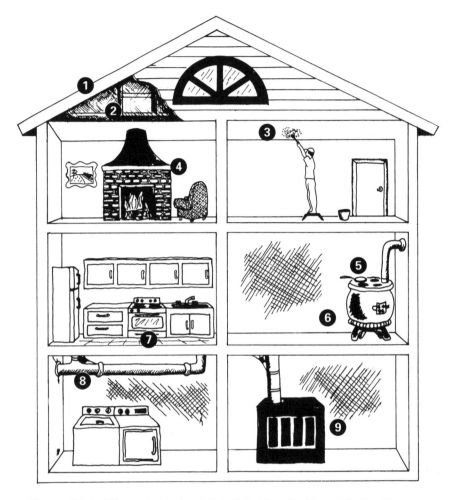

Figure 22.1. Where Asbestos Materials May Be Found in the Home

1. Some roofing and siding shingles are made of asbestos cement.
2. Houses built between 1930 and 1950 may have asbestos as insulation.
3. Asbestos may be present in textured paint and in patching compounds used on wall and ceiling joints. Their use was banned in 1977.
4. Artificial ashes and embers sold for use in gas-fired fireplaces may contain asbestos.
5. Older products such as stove-top pads may have some asbestos compounds.
6. Walls and floors around wood-burning stoves may be protected with asbestos paper, millboard, or cement sheets.
7. Asbestos is found in some vinyl floor tiles and the backing on vinyl sheet flooring and adhesives.
8. Hot water and steam pipes in older houses may be coated with an asbestos material or covered with an asbestos blanket or tape.
9. Oil and coal furnaces and door gaskets may have asbestos insulation

or worn asbestos gloves, stove-top pads, or ironing board covers. Check with local health, environmental, or other appropriate officials to find out proper handling and disposal procedures.

If asbestos material is more than slightly damaged, or if you are going to make changes in your home that might disturb it, repair or removal by a professional is needed. Before you have your house remodeled, find out whether asbestos materials are present.

How to identify materials that contain asbestos?

You can't tell whether a material contains asbestos simply by looking at it, unless it is labeled. If in doubt, treat the material as if it contains asbestos or have it sampled and analyzed by a qualified professional. A professional should take samples for analysis, since a professional knows what to look for, and because there may be an increased health risk if fibers are released. In fact, if done incorrectly, sampling can be more hazardous than leaving the material alone. Taking samples yourself is not recommended. If you nevertheless choose to take the samples yourself, take care not to release asbestos fibers into the air or onto yourself. Material that is in good condition and will not be disturbed (by remodeling, for example) should be left alone. Only material that is damaged or will be disturbed should be sampled. Anyone who samples asbestos-containing materials should have as much information as possible on the handling of asbestos before sampling, and at a minimum, should observe the following procedures:

- Make sure no one else is in the room when sampling is done.

- Wear disposable gloves or wash hands after sampling.

- Shut down any heating or cooling systems to minimize the spread of any released fibers.

- Do not disturb the material any more than is needed to take a small sample.

- Place a plastic sheet on the floor below the area to be sampled.

- Wet the material using a fine mist of water containing a few drops of detergent before taking the sample. The water/detergent mist will reduce the release of asbestos fibers.

- Carefully cut a piece from the entire depth of the material using, for example, a small knife, corer, or other sharp object. Place the small piece into a clean container (for example, a 35-mm film canister, small glass or plastic vial, or high quality resealable plastic bag).

- Tightly seal the container after the sample is in it.

- Carefully dispose of the plastic sheet. Use a damp paper towel to clean up any material on the outside of the container or around the area sampled. Dispose of asbestos materials according to state and local procedures.

- Label the container with an identification number and clearly state when and where the sample was taken.

- Patch the sampled area with the smallest possible piece of duct tape to prevent fiber release.

- Send the sample to an EPA-approved laboratory for analysis. The National Institute for Standards and Technology (NIST) has a list of these laboratories. You can get this list from the Laboratory Accreditation Administration, NIST, Gaithersburg, MD 20899 (telephone 301-975-4016). Your state or local health department may also be able to help.

How to manage an asbestos problem

If the asbestos material is in good shape and will not be disturbed, do nothing! If it is a problem, there are two types of corrections: repair and removal.

REPAIR usually involves either sealing or covering asbestos material.

Sealing. Sealing (encapsulation) involves treating the material with a sealant that either binds the asbestos fibers together or coats the material so fibers are not released. Pipe, furnace, and boiler insulation can sometimes be repaired this way. This should be done only by a professional trained to handle asbestos safely.

Covering. Covering(enclosure)involves placing something over or around the material that contains asbestos to prevent release of fibers.

Exposed insulated piping may be covered with a protective wrap or jacket.

With any type of repair, the asbestos remains in place. Repair is usually cheaper than removal, but it may make later removal of asbestos, if necessary, more difficult and costly. Repairs can either be major or minor.

Major repairs must be done only by a professional trained in methods for safely handling asbestos.

Minor repairs should also be done by professionals since there is always a risk of exposure to fibers when asbestos is disturbed.

Doing minor repairs yourself is not recommended since improper handling of asbestos materials can create a hazard where none existed. If you nevertheless choose to do minor repairs, you should have as much information as possible on the handling of asbestos before doing anything. Contact your state or local health department or regional EPA office for information about asbestos training programs in your area. Your local school district may also have information about asbestos professionals and training programs for school buildings. Even if you have completed a training program, do not try anything more than minor repairs. Before undertaking minor repairs, carefully examine the area around the damage to make sure it is stable. As a general matter, any damaged area which is bigger than the size of your hand is not a minor repair.

Before undertaking minor repairs, be sure to follow all the precautions described earlier for sampling asbestos material. Always wet the asbestos material using a fine mist of water containing a few drops of detergent. Commercial products designed to fill holes and seal damaged areas are available. Small areas of material such as pipe insulation can be covered by wrapping a special fabric, such as re-wettable glass cloth, around it. These products are available from stores (listed in the telephone directory under "Safety Equipment and Clothing") which specialize in asbestos materials and safety items.

Removal. Removal is usually the most expensive method and, unless required by state or local regulations, should be the last option considered in most situations. This is because removal poses the greatest risk of fiber release. However, removal may be required when remodeling or making major changes to your home that will disturb asbestos material. Also, removal may be called for if asbestos material is damaged extensively and cannot be otherwise repaired. Removal is complex and must be done only by a contractor with special training. Improper removal may actually increase the health risks to you and your family.

Asbestos Do's and Don'ts for the Homeowner

- Do keep activities to a minimum in any areas having damaged material that may contain asbestos.

- Do take every precaution to avoid damaging asbestos material.

- Do have removal and major repair done by people trained and qualified in handling asbestos. It is highly recommended that sampling and minor repair also be done by asbestos professionals.

- Don't dust, sweep, or vacuum debris that may contain asbestos.

- Don't saw, sand, scrape, or drill holes in asbestos materials.

- Don't use abrasive pads or brushes on power strippers to strip wax from asbestos flooring. Never use a power stripper on a dry floor.

- Don't sand or try to level asbestos flooring or its backing. When asbestos flooring needs replacing, install new floor covering over it, if possible.

- Don't track material that could contain asbestos through the house. If you cannot avoid walking through the area, have it cleaned with a wet mop. If the material is from a damaged area, or if a large area must be cleaned, call an asbestos professional.

Asbestos Professionals: Who Are They and What Can They Do?

Asbestos professionals are trained in handling asbestos material. The type of professional will depend on the type of product and what needs to be done to correct the problem. You may hire a general asbestos contractor or, in some cases, a professional trained to handle specific products containing asbestos.

Asbestos professionals can conduct home inspections, take samples of suspected material, assess its condition, and advise about what corrections are needed and who is qualified to make these corrections. Once again, material in good condition need not be sampled unless it is likely to be disturbed. Professional correction or abatement contractors repair or remove asbestos materials.

Some firms offer combinations of testing, assessment, and correction. A professional hired to assess the need for corrective action should not be connected with an asbestos-correction firm. It is better to use two different firms so there is no conflict of interest. Services vary from one area to another around the country.

The federal government has training courses for asbestos professionals around the country. Some state and local governments also have or require training or certification courses. Ask asbestos professionals to document their completion of federal or state approved training. Each person performing work in your home should provide proof of training and licensing in asbestos work, such as completion of EPA-approved training. State and local health departments or EPA regional offices may have listings of licensed professionals in your area.

If you have a problem that requires the services of asbestos professionals, check their credentials carefully. Hire professionals who are trained, experienced, reputable, and accredited—especially if accreditation is required by state or local laws. Before hiring a professional, ask for references from previous clients. Find out if they were satisfied. Ask whether the professional has handled similar situations. Get cost estimates from several professionals, as the charges for these services can vary.

Though private homes are usually not covered by the asbestos regulations that apply to schools and public buildings, professionals should still use procedures described during federal or state—approved training. Homeowners should be alert to the chance of misleading claims by asbestos consultants and contractors. There have been reports of firms incorrectly claiming that asbestos materials in homes must be replaced. In other cases, firms have encouraged unnecessary removals or performed them improperly. Unnecessary removals are a waste of money. Improper removals may actually increase the health risks to you and your family. To guard against this, know what services are available and what procedures and precautions are needed to do the job properly.

In addition to general asbestos contractors, you may select a roofing, flooring, or plumbing contractor trained to handle asbestos when it is necessary to remove and replace roofing, flooring, siding, or asbestos-cement pipe that is part of a water system. Normally, roofing and flooring contractors are exempt from state and local licensing requirements because they do not perform any other asbestos-correction work. Call 1-800-USA-ROOF for names of qualified roofing contractors in your area. (Illinois residents call 708-318-6722.) For information on asbestos in floors, read "Recommended Work Procedures for Resilient Floor Covers." You can write for a copy from the Resilient Floor Covering Institute, 966 Hungerford Drive, Suite 12-B, Rockville, MD 20850. Enclose a stamped, business-size, self-addressed envelope.

Asbestos containing automobile brake pads and linings, clutch facings, and gaskets should be repaired and replaced only by a professional using special protective equipment. Many of these products are now available without asbestos. For more information, read "Guidance for Preventing Asbestos Disease Among Auto Mechanics," available from regional EPA offices.

If you hire a professional asbestos inspector

- Make sure that the inspection will include a complete visual examination and the careful collection and lab analysis of samples. If asbestos is present, the inspector should provide a written evaluation describing its location and extent of damage, and give recommendations for correction or prevention.

- Make sure an inspecting firm makes frequent site visits if it is hired to assure that a contractor follows proper procedures and requirements. The inspector may recommend and perform checks after the correction to assure the area has been properly cleaned.

If you hire a corrective-action contractor

- Check with your local air pollution control board, the local agency responsible for worker safety, and the Better Business Bureau. Ask if the firm has had any safety violations. Find out if there are legal actions filed against it.

- Insist that the contractor use the proper equipment to do the job. The workers must wear approved respirators, gloves, and other protective clothing.

- Before work begins, get a written contract specifying the work plan, cleanup, and the applicable federal, state, and local regulations which the contractor must follow (such as notification requirements and asbestos disposal procedures). Contact your state and local health departments, EPA's regional office, and the Occupational Safety and Health Administration's regional office to find out what the regulations are. Be sure the contractor follows local asbestos removal and disposal laws. At the end of the job, get written assurance from the contractor that all procedures have been followed.

- Assure that the contractor avoids spreading or tracking asbestos dust into other areas of your home. They should seal the work area from the rest of the house using plastic sheeting and duct tape, and also turn off the heating and air-conditioning system. For some repairs, such as pipe insulation removal, plastic glove bags may be adequate. They must be sealed with tape and properly disposed of when the job is complete.

- Make sure the work site is clearly marked as a hazard area. Do not allow household members and pets into the area until work is completed.

- Insist that the contractor apply a wetting agent to the asbestos material with a hand sprayer that creates a fine mist before removal. Wet fibers do not float in the air as easily as dry fibers and will be easier to clean up.

- Make sure the contractor does not break removed material into small pieces. This could release asbestos fibers into the air. Pipe insulation was usually installed in preformed blocks and should be removed in complete pieces.

- Upon completion, assure that the contractor cleans the area well with wet mops, wet rags, sponges, or HEPA (high efficiency particulate air) vacuum cleaners. A regular vacuum cleaner must never be used. Wetting helps reduce the chance of spreading asbestos fibers in the air. All asbestos materials and disposable equipment and clothing used in the job must be placed in sealed, leak-proof, and labeled plastic bags. The work site should be visually free of dust and debris. Air monitoring (to make sure there is no increase of asbestos fibers in the air) may be necessary to assure that the contractor's job is done properly. This should be done by someone not connected with the contractor.

Caution! Do not dust, sweep, or vacuum debris that may contain asbestos. These steps will disturb tiny asbestos fibers and may release them into the air. Remove dust by wet mopping or with a special HEPA vacuum cleaner used by trained asbestos contractors.

For More Information

For more information, contact your local American Lung Association for copies of:

Indoor Air Pollution Fact Sheet-Asbestos

Air Pollution in Your Home?

Other publications on indoor pollution

For more information on asbestos in other consumer products, call the CPSC Hotline or write to the U.S. Consumer Product Safety Commission, Washington, D.C. 20207. The CPSC Hotline has information on certain appliances and products, such as the brands and models of hairdryers that contain asbestos. Call CPSC at 1-800-638-CPSC. A teletypewriter (TTY) for the hearing impaired is available at 1-800-638-8270. The Maryland TTY number is 1-800-492-8104.

To find out whether your state has a training and certification program for asbestos removal contractors, and for information on EPA's asbestos programs, call the EPA at 202-554-1404.

For more information on asbestos identification and control activities, contact the Asbestos Coordinator in the EPA Regional Office for your region, or your state or local health department.

Chapter 23

Health Threats from Under the Sink: Household Products

What are they?

The household cleaning agents, personal care products, pesticides, paints, hobby products, and solvents that make our lives so easy are also sources of hundreds of potentially harmful chemicals. The range of household products that contain potentially harmful substances that contribute to indoor air pollution is wide-reaching and diverse. Some of these products release contaminants into the air right away; others do so gradually, over a period of time. The harmful components in many household and personal care products can cause dizziness, nausea, allergic reactions, and eye, skin, and respiratory tract irritation; some can cause cancer.

What are the problems?

Contamination from household products, if limited to low levels for short periods of time, does not pose a serious health threat. However, contamination can occur over a long period of time from a variety of sources, and harmful effects can occur. Where there is prolonged exposure and where there is a possible multiplying effect from the presence of contamination from many different products, the effects can be serious, even fatal.

©1987 American Lung Association. Reprinted with Permission.

Pesticides present a particular problem over and above other household products because many designed for home use are sold without adequate safety testing for cancer, potential for causing birth defects, and other possible health effects. Overuse of pesticides in the home or in closed spaces is dangerous. The best way to avoid indoor air pollution from pesticides is not to use them or to use them very sparingly, with proper ventilation. Avoid using highly toxic pesticides; in many cases, a less toxic product will suffice.

There are four basic rules to follow when using hazardous household products:

1. Whenever possible, avoid using hazardous household products. Use nontoxic alternatives instead.

2. When purchasing household products, buy only as much as you need; do not buy bulk quantities. Store hazardous products and materials carefully.

3. Dispose of hazardous products carefully.

4. Always read the product label and follow manufacturer instructions.

5. Minimize exposure when using hazardous products.

The following lists the health effects and presents some possible solutions to the problems posed by various household products.

Aerosol spray products, including health, beauty, and cleaning products.

Some aerosol products release particles in the air that can be inhaled into the lungs and then absorbed into the bloodstream. Unusually large quantities of these particles can cause headaches, nausea, shortness of breath, eye, throat and lung irritation, skin rashes, burns, and liver damage. Aerosol containers will explode if exposed to heat, causing burns and very serious injury.

Buy products in a non-aerosol form. Most products also come in creams, liquids, and pump sprays. If you use aerosol products, do not inhale them. Do not expose aerosol containers to heat.

Phosphate detergents.

These products are highly alkaline and can cause skin and eye irritations. They are very dangerous if swallowed.

Use soap. Phosphates are not biodegradable, and accumulation pollutes water systems.

Chlorine bleach.

Chlorine bleaches can irritate and burn skin and eyes. Even the fumes from chlorine bleach are irritating to eyes and nose. Never mix chlorine bleach with other substances to make a cleaning solution. These mixtures produce very dangerous gases that can be deadly.

If you use chlorine bleach, handle it carefully. Instead of using chlorine bleach as a cleaning agent, make your own cleaning solution by mixing baking soda in water.

Spot removers and dry cleaning fluids.

Inhalation of toxic vapors from these products can cause depression of the central nervous system. Symptoms include nausea, disorientation, and loss of appetite.

Remove spots as soon as they happen. Use club soda; lemon juice and hot water; borax and cold water. Use bleach-type removers rather than solvent-types.

Oven cleaners.

Oven cleaners contain lye and other strong chemicals that can irritate and burn skin and eyes.

Wipe your oven out after using; this reduces the need to use strong cleaners. Clean your oven with a homemade solution of ammonia or baking soda dissolved in water. Apply this solution to the oven (**Be careful with ammonia**), wait, and wipe with a damp cloth.

Furniture and floor polish.

These products may contain chemicals, such as mineral spirits and petroleum distillates, that can irritate skin, eyes, and nose. Some of these chemicals can cause photosensitization (sensitivity to light).

These products are often very flammable. Use soapy water to clean, and a soft cloth to shine some items. Make your own polish by mixing one part lemon juice to two parts olive or vegetable oil.

Rug and upholstery cleaners.

These products may contain some chemicals which, when inhaled excessively, can cause anemia, liver damage, convulsions, and possible coma.

Use soap or non-aerosol shampoo. Wear gloves and work in a well-ventilated area.

Paints.

Chemical components in paints can irritate eyes, skin, and lungs. Inhaling paint fumes can cause headaches and nausea. Other chemicals in paints can cause respiratory problems, muscle weakness, and liver and kidney damage. Some paints are flammable.

If you can, paint items outside. When you paint indoors, make certain you have adequate ventilation. Using water-soluble paints eliminates the need to use paint thinners, which contain additional toxic chemicals.

Air fresheners.

These products may contain chemicals that can irritate and burn skin and may cause cancer in animals. They also interfere with the natural sense of smell.

Open a window to ventilate unpleasant odors. A dish of hot vinegar removes room odor. Put a box of baking soda in the refrigerator to remove strong odors that start there.

Moth repellents.

Moth crystals, moth flakes, and moth balls contain chemicals that can cause cancer in animals.

Use cedar chips.

Hobby materials: photography and metal work.

Many of the chemicals used to develop photographs and in metalwork are very dangerous. They are flammable and can cause skin, eye, and lung irritations. Some acidic chemicals can burn and cause blindness. Some are poisonous and cause cancer in laboratory animals.

Work with these materials only in a well-ventilated area. Wear goggles and gloves. Store in unbreakable containers away from heat. Store acids in nonmetal containers. Never mix water with acids. Avoid products.

Hobby materials: clay and stone papier-mache glues and epoxy.

These substances can irritate skin and lungs. Some supplies used in paper mache materials contain asbestos. If inhaled, asbestos can cause cancer. Excessive inhalation of fumes from certain glues can be fatal.

Work in well-ventilated areas. Wear gloves and a dust mask. Avoid using products containing asbestos. Use white or yellow glue.

Chapter 24

Protect Your Family from Lead in Your Home

Are You Planning to Buy, Rent, or Renovate a Home Built Before 1978?

Many houses and apartments built before 1978 have paint that contains lead (called lead-based paint). Lead from paint, chips, and dust can pose serious health hazards if not taken care of properly.

By 1996, federal law will require that individuals receive certain information before renting, buying, or renovating pre-1978 housing:

- **Landlords** will have to disclose known information on lead-based paint hazards before leases take effect. Leases will include a federal form about lead-based paint.

- **Sellers** will have to disclose known information on lead-based paint hazards before selling a house. Sales contracts will include a federal form about lead-based paint in the building. Buyers will have up to 10 days to check for lead hazards.

- **Renovators** will have to give you the pamphlet form of this chapter before starting work.

If you want more information on these requirements, call the National Lead Information Clearinghouse at 1-800-424-LEAD.

EPA publication EPA747-K-94-001. May 1995.

Lead From Paint, Dust, and Soil Can Be Dangerous If Not Managed Properly

Fact: Lead exposure can harm young children and babies even before they are born.

Fact: Even children that seem healthy can have high levels of lead in their bodies.

Fact: People can get lead in their bodies by breathing or swallowing lead dust, or by eating soil or paint chips with lead in them.

Fact: People have many options for reducing lead hazards. In most cases, lead-based paint that is in good condition is not a hazard.

Fact: Removing lead-based paint improperly can increase the danger to your family.

If you think your home might have lead hazards, read this chapter to learn some simple steps to protect your family.

Lead Gets in the Body in Many Ways

One out of every eleven children in the United States has dangerous levels of lead in the bloodstream.

Even children who appear healthy can have dangerous levels of lead.

People can get lead in their body if they:

- Put their hands or other objects covered with lead dust in their mouths.
- Eat paint chips or soil that contains lead.
- Breathe in lead dust (especially during renovations that disturb painted surfaces).

Lead is even more dangerous to children than adults because:

- Babies and young children often put their hands and other objects in their mouths. These objects can have lead dust on them.
- Children's growing bodies absorb more lead.
- Children's brains and nervous systems are more sensitive to the damaging effects of lead.

264

Lead's Effects

If not detected early, children with high levels of lead in their bodies can suffer from:

- Damage to the brain and nervous system
- Behavior and learning problems (such as hyperactivity)
- Slowed growth
- Hearing problems
- Headaches

Lead is also harmful to adults. Adults can suffer from:

- Difficulties during pregnancy
- Other reproductive problems (in both men and women)
- High blood pressure
- Digestive problems
- Nerve disorders
- Reproductive problems
- Memory and concentration (Adults) problems
- Muscle and joint pain

Checking Your Family for Lead

Get your children tested if you think your home has high levels of lead.

A simple blood test can detect high levels of lead. Blood tests are important for:

- Children who are six months to one year old (six months if you live in an older home with cracking or peeling paint).
- Family members that you think might have high levels of lead.

If your child is older than one year, talk to your doctor about whether your child needs testing.

Your doctor or health center can do blood tests. They are inexpensive and sometimes free. Your doctor will explain what the test results mean. Treatment can range from changes in your diet to medication or a hospital stay.

Where Lead-based Paint Is Found

In general, the older your home, the more likely it has lead-based paint.

Many homes built before 1978 have lead-based paint. The federal government banned lead-based paint from housing in 1978. Some states stopped its use even earlier. Lead can be found:

- In homes in the city, country, or suburbs.

- In apartments, single-family homes, and both private and public housing.

- Inside and outside of the house.

- In soil around a home. (Soil can pick up lead from exterior paint, or other sources such as past use of leaded gas in cars.)

Where Lead Is Likely to Be a Hazard

Lead-based paint that is in good condition is usually not a hazard.

Peeling, chipping, chalking, or cracking lead-based paint is a hazard and needs immediate attention.

Lead-based paint may also be a hazard when found on surfaces that children can chew or that get a lot of wear-and-tear. These areas include:

- Windows and window sills.
- Doors and door frames.
- Stairs, railings, and banisters.
- Porches and fences.

Lead dust can form when lead-based paint is dry scraped, dry sanded, or heated. Dust also forms when painted surfaces bump or rub together. Lead chips and dust can get on surfaces and objects that people touch. Settled lead dust can reenter the air when people vacuum, sweep, or walk through it.

Lead in soil can be a hazard when children play in bare soil or when people bring soil into the house on their shoes. Call your state agency to find out about soil testing for lead.

Lead from paint chips, which you can see, and lead dust, which you can't always see, can both be serious hazards.

Checking Your Home for Lead Hazards

Just knowing that a home has lead-based paint may not tell you if there is a hazard.

You can get your home checked for lead hazards in one of two ways, or both:

- A paint inspection tells you the lead content of every painted surface in your home. It won't tell you whether the paint is a hazard or how you should deal with it.

- A risk assessment tells you if there are any sources of serious lead exposure (such as peeling paint and lead dust). It also tells you what actions to take to address these hazards.

Have qualified professionals do the work. The federal government is writing standards for inspectors and risk assessors. Some states might already have standards in place. Call your state agency for help with locating qualified professionals in your area.

Trained professionals use a range of methods when checking your home, including:

- Visual inspection of paint condition and location.
- Lab tests of paint samples.
- Surface dust tests.
- A portable x-ray fluorescence machine.

Home test kits for lead are available, but recent studies suggest that they are not always accurate. Consumers should not rely on these tests before doing renovations or to assure safety.

What You Can Do Now to Protect Your Family

If you suspect that your house has lead hazards, you can take some immediate steps to reduce your family's risk:

- If you rent, notify your landlord of peeling or chipping paint.

- Clean up paint chips immediately.

- Clean floors, window frames, window sills, and other surfaces weekly. Use a mop or sponge with warm water and a general all-purpose cleaner or a cleaner made specifically for lead. **REMEMBER: NEVER MIX AMMONIA AND BLEACH PRODUCTS TOGETHER SINCE THEY CAN FORM A DANGEROUS GAS.**

- Thoroughly rinse sponges and mop heads after cleaning dirty or dusty areas.

- Wash children's hands often, especially before they eat and before nap time and bed time.

- Keep play areas clean. Wash bottles, pacifiers, toys, and stuffed animals regularly.

- Keep children from chewing window sills or other painted surfaces.

- Clean or remove shoes before entering your home to avoid tracking in lead from soil.

- Make sure children eat nutritious, low-fat meals high in iron and calcium, such as spinach and low-fat dairy products. Children with good diets absorb less lead.

How to Significantly Reduce Lead Hazards

Removing lead improperly can increase the hazard to your family by spreading even more lead dust around the house.

Always use a professional who is trained to remove lead hazards safely.

In addition to day-to-day cleaning and good nutrition:

- You can temporarily reduce lead hazards by taking actions such as repairing damaged painted surfaces and planting grass to cover soil with high lead levels. These actions (called "interim controls") are not permanent solutions and will need ongoing attention.

- To permanently remove lead hazards, you must hire a lead "abatement" contractor. Abatement (or permanent hazard elimination) methods include removing, sealing, or enclosing lead-based paint with special materials. Just painting over the hazard with regular paint is not enough.

Always hire a person with special training for correcting lead problems—someone who knows how to do this work safely and has the proper equipment to clean up thoroughly. If possible, hire a certified lead abatement contractor. Certified contractors will employ qualified workers and follow strict safety rules as set by their state or by the federal government.

Call your state agency for help with locating qualified contractors in your area and to see if financial assistance is available.

Remodeling or Renovating a Home with Lead-based Paint

Take precautions before you begin remodeling or renovations that disturb painted surfaces (such as scraping off paint or tearing out walls):

- Have the area tested for lead-based paint.

- Do not use a dry scraper, belt-sander, propane torch, or heat gun to remove lead-based paint. These actions create large amounts of lead dust and fumes. Lead dust can remain in your home long after the work is done.

- Temporarily move your family (especially children and pregnant women) out of the apartment or house until the work is done and the area is properly cleaned. If you can't move your family, at least completely seal off the work area.

- Follow other safety measures to reduce lead hazards. You can find out about other safety measures by calling 1-800-424-LEAD. Ask for the brochure "Reducing Lead Hazards When Remodeling Your Home." This pamphlet explains what to do before, during, and after renovations.

If you have already completed renovations or remodeling that could have released lead-based paint or dust, get your young children tested and follow the steps outlined above.

If not conducted properly, certain types of renovations can release lead from paint and dust into the air.

Other Sources of Lead

While paint dust, and soil are the most common lead hazards, other lead sources also exist.

Drinking water. Your home might have plumbing with lead or lead solder. Call your local health department or water supplier to find out about testing your water. You cannot see, smell, or taste lead, and boiling your water will not get rid of lead. If you think your plumbing might have lead in it:

- Use only cold water for drinking and cooking.
- Run water for 15 to 30 seconds before drinking it, especially if you have not used your water for a few hours.

The job. If you work with lead, you could bring it home on your hands or clothes. Shower and change clothes before coming home. Launder your clothes separately from the rest of your family's.

Old painted toys and furniture.

Glasses and Dishes. Food and liquids stored in lead crystal or lead-glazed pottery or porcelain can leach lead from the container.

Local industries. Lead smelters or other industries that release lead into the air can distribute lead into your environment.

Crafts and Hobbies. Hobbies that use lead, such as making pottery or stained glass, or refinishing furniture.

Home-made Medicines. Folk remedies that contain lead, such as "greta" and "azarcon" used to treat an upset stomach.

For More Information

The National Lead Information Center

Call 1-800-LEAD-FYI to learn how to protect children from lead poisoning.

For other information on lead hazards, call the center's clearinghouse at 1-800-424-LEAD. For the hearing impaired, call TDD 1-800-526-5456 (FAX: 202-659-1192, Internet: EHC@CAIS.COM).

EPA's Safe Drinking Water Hotline

Call 1-800-426-4791 for information about lead in drinking water.

Consumer Product Safety Commission Hotline

To request information on lead in consumer products, or to report an unsafe consumer product or a product-related injury call 1-800-638-2772. (Internet: info@cpsc.gov). For the hearing impaired, call TDD 1-800-638-8270.

State Health and Environmental Agencies

Some cities and states have their own rules for lead-based paint activities. Check with your state agency to see if state or local laws apply to you. Most state agencies can also provide information on finding a lead abatement firm in your area, and on possible sources of financial aid for reducing lead hazards.

Summary

If you think your home has high levels of lead:

- Get your young children tested for lead, even if they seem healthy.
- Wash children's hands, bottles, pacifiers, and toys often.
- Make sure children eat healthy, low-fat foods.
- Get your home checked for lead hazards.
- Regularly clean floors, window sills, and other surfaces.
- Wipe soil off shoes before entering house.
- Talk to your landlord about fixing surfaces with peeling or chippping paint.
- Take precautions to avoid exposure to lead dust when remodeling or renovating (call 1-800-424-LEAD for guidelines).
- Don't use a belt-sander, propane torch, dry scraper, or dry sandpaper on painted surfaces that may contain lead.
- Don't try to remove lead-based paint yourself.

Chapter 25

Sharing Your Air: Biological Pollutants in Your Home

This chapter will help you understand 1) what indoor biological pollution is, 2) whether your home or lifestyle promotes its development, and 3) how to control its growth and build-up.

Outdoor air pollution in cities is a major health problem. Much effort and money continue to be spent cleaning up pollution in the outdoor air. But air pollution can be a problem where you least expect it, in the place you may have thought was safest, your home. Many ordinary activities such as cooking, heating, cooling, cleaning, and redecorating can cause the release and spread of indoor pollutants at home. Studies have shown that the air in our homes can be even more polluted than outdoor air.

Many Americans spend up to 90 percent of their time indoors, often at home. Therefore, breathing clean indoor air can have an important impact on health. People who are inside a great deal may be at greater risk of developing health problems, or having problems made worse by indoor air pollutants. These people include infants, young children, the elderly, and those with chronic illnesses.

What Are Biological Pollutants?

Biological pollutants are or were living organisms. They promote poor indoor air quality and may be a major cause of days lost from work or school, and of doctor and hospital visits. Some can even damage

American Lung Association. January 1990.

surfaces inside and outside your house. Biological pollutants can travel through the air and are often invisible.

Some common indoor biological pollutants are:

- Animal Dander (minute scales from hair, feathers, or skin)
- Dust Mite and Cockroach parts
- Fungi (Molds)
- Infectious agents (bacteria or viruses)
- Pollen

Some of these substances are in every home. It is impossible to get rid of them all. Even a spotless home may permit the growth of biological pollutants. Two conditions are essential to support biological growth: nutrients and moisture. These conditions can be found in many locations, such as bathrooms, damp or flooded basements, wet appliances (such as humidifiers or air conditioners), and even some carpets and furniture.

Modern materials and construction techniques may reduce the amount of outside air brought into buildings which may result in high moisture levels inside. Using humidifiers, unvented heaters, and air conditioners in our homes has increased the chances of moisture forming on interior surfaces. This encourages the growth of certain biological pollutants.

The Scope of the Problem

Most information about sources and health effects of biological pollutants is based on studies of large office buildings and two surveys of homes in northern U.S. and Canada. These surveys show that 30 percent to 50 percent of all structures have damp conditions which may encourage the growth and build-up of biological pollutants. This percentage is likely to be higher in warm, moist climates.

Some diseases or illnesses have been linked with biological pollutants in the indoor environment. However, many of them also have causes unrelated to the indoor environment. Therefore, we do not know how many health problems relate only to poor indoor air.

Health Effects of Biological Pollutants

All of us are exposed to biological pollutants. However, the effects on our health depend upon the type and amount of biological pollution and the individual. Some people do not experience health reactions from certain biological pollutants, while others may experience one or more of the following reactions:

- Allergic
- Infectious
- Toxic

Except for the spread of infections indoors, ALLERGIC REACTIONS may be the most common health problem with indoor air quality in homes. They are often connected with animal dander (mostly from cats and dogs), with house dust mites (microscopic animals living in household dust), and with pollen. Allergic reactions can range from mildly uncomfortable to life-threatening, as in a severe asthma attack. Some common signs and symptoms are:

- Watery eyes
- Runny nose and sneezing
- Nasal congestion
- Itching
- Coughing
- Wheezing and difficulty breathing
- Headache
- Fatigue

Health experts are especially concerned about people with asthma. These people have very sensitive airways that can react to various irritants, making breathing difficult. The number of people who have asthma has greatly increased in recent years. The number of people with asthma has gone up by 59 percent since 1970, to a total of 9.6 million people. Asthma in children under 16 years of age has increased 41 percent in the same period, to a total of 2.6 million children. The number of deaths from asthma is up by 68 percent since 1979, to a total of almost 4,400 deaths per year.

INFECTIOUS DISEASES caused by bacteria and viruses, such as flu, measles, chicken pox, and tuberculosis, may be spread indoors. Most infectious diseases pass from person to person through physical contact. Crowded conditions with poor air circulation can promote this spread. Some bacteria and viruses thrive in buildings and circulate through indoor ventilation systems. For example, the bacterium causing Legionnaire's disease, a serious and sometimes lethal infection, and Pontiac Fever, a flu-like illness, have circulated in some large buildings.

TOXIC REACTIONS are the least studied and understood health problem caused by some biological air pollutants in the home. Toxins can damage a variety of organs and tissues in the body, including the liver, the central nervous system, the digestive tract, and the immune system.

Talking to Your Doctor

Are you concerned about the effects on your health that may be related to biological pollutants in your home? Before you discuss your concerns with your doctor, you should know the answers to the following questions. This information can help the doctor determine whether your health problems may be related to biological pollution.

- Does anyone in the family have frequent headaches, fevers, itchy watery eyes, a stuffy nose, dry throat, or a cough? Does anyone complain of feeling tired or dizzy all the time? Is anyone wheezing or having difficulties breathing on a regular basis?

- Did these symptoms appear after you moved to a new or different home?

- Do the symptoms disappear when you go to school or the office or go away on a trip, and return when you come back?

- Have you recently remodelled your home or done any energy conservation work, such as installing insulation, storm windows, or weather stripping? Did your symptoms occur during or after these activities?

- Does your home feel humid? Can you see moisture on the windows or on other surfaces, such as walls and ceilings?

- What is the usual temperature in your home? Is it very hot or cold?

- Have you recently had water damage?

- Is your basement wet or damp?

- Is there any obvious mold or mildew?

- Does any part of your home have a musty or moldy odor?

- Is the air stale?

- Do you have pets?

- Do your house plants show signs of mold?

- Do you have air conditioners or humidifiers that have not been properly cleaned?

- Does your home have cockroaches or rodents?

Coping with the Problem

Checking Your Home

There is no simple and cheap way to sample the air in your home to determine the level of all biological pollutants. Experts suggest that sampling for biological pollutants is not a useful problem-solving tool. Even if you had your home tested, it is almost impossible to know which biological pollutant(s) cause various symptoms or health problems. The amount of most biological substances required to cause disease is unknown and varies from one person to the next.

Does this make the problem sound hopeless? On the contrary, you can take several simple, practical actions to help remove sources of biological pollutants, to help get rid of pollutants, and to prevent their return.

Self-inspection: A Walk Through Your Home

Begin by touring your household. Follow your nose, and use your eyes. Two major factors help create conditions for biological pollutants to grow: nutrients and constant moisture with poor air circulation.

- Dust and construction materials, such as wood, wallboard, and insulation, contain nutrients that allow biological pollutants to grow. Firewood also is a source of moisture, fungi, and bugs.

- Appliances such as humidifiers, kerosene and gas heaters, and gas stoves add moisture to the air.

277

- A musty odor, moisture on hard surfaces, or even water stains, may be caused by:

  1. Air-conditioning units

  2. Basements, attics, and crawlspaces

  3. Bathrooms

  4. Carpets

  5. Heating and air-conditioning ducts

  6. Humidifiers and dehumidifiers

  7. Refrigerator drip pans

What You Can Do about Biological Pollutants

Before you give away the family pet or move, there are less drastic steps that can be taken to reduce potential problems. Properly cleaning and maintaining your home can help reduce the problem and may avoid interrupting your normal routine. People who have health problems such as asthma, or are allergic, may need to do this and more. Discuss this with your doctor.

Moisture Control

Water in your home can come from many sources. Water can enter your home by leaking or by seeping through basement floors. Showers or even cooking can add moisture to the air in your home. The amount of moisture that the air in your home can hold depends on the temperature of the air. As the temperature goes down, the air is able to hold less moisture. This is why, in cold weather, moisture condenses on cold surfaces (for example, drops of water form on the inside of a window). This moisture can encourage biological pollutants to grow.

There are many ways to control moisture in your home:

- Fix leaks and seepage. If water is entering the house from the outside, your options range from simple landscaping to extensive excavation and waterproofing. (The ground should slope away from the house.) Water in the basement can result from the lack of gutters or a water flow toward the house. Water leaks in pipes or around tubs and sinks can provide a place for biological pollutants to grow.

- Put a plastic cover over dirt in crawlspaces to prevent moisture from coming in from the ground. Be sure crawlspaces are well-ventilated.

- Use exhaust fans in bathrooms and kitchens to remove moisture to the outside (not into the attic). Vent your clothes dryer to the outside.

- Turn off certain appliances (such as humidifiers or kerosene heaters) if you notice moisture on windows and other surfaces.

- Use dehumidifiers and air conditioners, especially in hot, humid climates, to reduce moisture in the air, but be sure that the appliances themselves don't become sources of biological pollutants.

- Raise the temperature of cold surfaces where moisture condenses. Use insulation or storm windows. (A storm window installed on the inside works better than one installed on the outside.) Open doors between rooms (especially doors to closets which may be colder than the rooms) to increase circulation. Circulation carries heat to the cold surfaces. Increase air circulation by using fans and by moving furniture from wall corners to promote air and heat circulation. Be sure that your house has a source of fresh air and can expel excessive moisture from the home.

- Pay special attention to carpet on concrete floors. Carpet can absorb moisture and serve as a place for biological pollutants to grow. Use area rugs which can be taken up and washed often. In certain climates, if carpet is to be installed over a concrete floor, it may be necessary to use a vapor barrier (plastic sheeting) over the concrete and cover that with sub-flooring (insulation covered with plywood) to prevent a moisture problem.

- Moisture problems and their solutions differ from one climate to another. The Northeast is cold and wet; the Southwest is hot and dry; the South is hot and wet; and the Western Mountain states are cold and dry. All of these regions can have moisture problems. For example, evaporative coolers used in the Southwest can encourage the growth of biological pollutants. In other hot regions, the use of air conditioners which cool the air too quickly may not allow these units to run long enough to remove excess moisture from the air. The types of construction and weatherization for the different climates can lead to different problems and solutions.

Maintain and Clean All Appliances That Come in Contact with Water

- Have major appliances, such as furnaces, heat pumps and central air conditioners, inspected and cleaned regularly by a professional, especially before seasonal use. Change filters on heating and cooling systems according to manufacturer's directions. (In general, change filters monthly during use.) When first turning on the heating or air conditioning at the start of the season, consider leaving your home until it airs out.

- Have window or wall air-conditioning units cleaned and serviced regularly by a professional, especially before the cooling season. Air conditioners can help reduce the entry of allergy-causing pollen. But they may also become a source of biological pollutants if not properly maintained. Clean the coils and incline the drain pans according to manufacturer's instructions, so water cannot collect in pools.

- Have furnace-attached humidifiers cleaned and serviced regularly by a professional, especially before the heating season.

- Follow manufacturer's instructions when using any type of humidifier. Experts differ on the benefits of using humidifiers. If you do use a portable humidifier (approximately 1 to 2 gallon tanks), be sure to empty its tank every day and refill with distilled or demineralized water, or even fresh tap water if the other types of water are unavailable. For larger portable humidifiers, change the water as recommended by the manufacturer. Unplug the appliance before cleaning. Every third day, clean all surfaces coming in contact with water with a 3 percent solution of hydrogen peroxide, using a brush to loosen deposits.

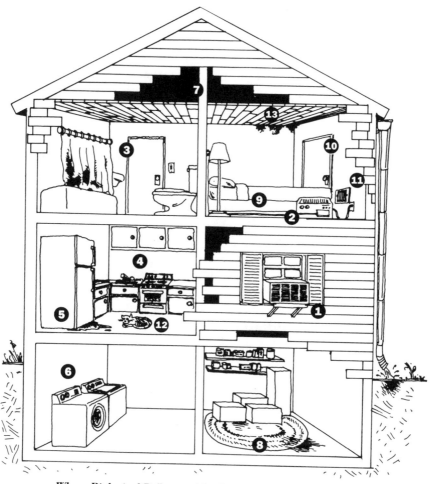

Where Biological Pollutants May Be Found In The Home

1. Dirty air conditioners
2. Dirty humidifiers and/or dehumidifiers
3. Bathroom without vents or windows
4. Kitchen without vents or windows
5. Dirty refrigerator drip pans
6. Laundry room with unvented dryer
7. Unventilated attic
8. Carpet on damp basement floor
9. Bedding
10. Closet on outside wall
11. Dirty heating/air conditioning system
12. Dogs or cats
13. Water damage (around windows, the roof, or the basement)

Figure 25.1. *Where Biological Pollutants Can Be Found in the Home*

Some manufacturers recommend using diluted household bleach for cleaning and maintenance, generally in a solution of one-half cup bleach to one gallon water. When using any household chemical, rinse well to remove all traces of chemical before refilling humidifier.

- Empty dehumidifiers daily and clean often. If possible, have the appliance drip directly into a drain. Follow manufacturer's instructions for cleaning and maintenance. Always disconnect the appliance before cleaning.

- Clean refrigerator drip pans regularly according to manufacturer's instructions. If refrigerator and freezer doors don't seal properly, moisture may build up and mold can grow. Remove any mold on door gaskets and replace faulty gaskets.

Clean Surfaces

- Clean moist surfaces, such as showers and kitchen counters.

- Remove mold from walls, ceilings, floors, and paneling. Do not simply cover mold with paint, stain, varnish, or a moisture-proof sealer, as it may resurface.

- Replace moldy shower curtains, or remove them and scrub well with a household cleaner and rinse before rehanging them.

Dust Control

Controlling dust is very important for people who are allergic to animal dander and mites. You cannot see mites, but you can either remove their favorite breeding grounds or keep these areas dry and clean. Dust mites can thrive in sofas, stuffed chairs, carpets, and bedding. Open shelves, fabric wallpaper, knickknacks, and venetian blinds are also sources of dust mites. Dust mites live deep in the carpet and are not removed by vacuuming. Many doctors suggest that their mite-allergic patients use washable area rugs rather than wall-to-wall carpet.

- Always wash bedding in hot water (at least 130° F) to kill dust mites. Cold water won't do the job. Launder bedding at least every 7 to 10 days.

- Use synthetic or foam rubber mattress pads and pillows, and plastic mattress covers if you are allergic. Do not use fuzzy wool blankets, feather or wool-stuffed comforters, and feather pillows.

- Clean rooms and closets well; dust and vacuum often to remove surface dust. Vacuuming and other cleaning may not remove all animal dander, dust mite material, and other biological pollutants. Some particles are so small they can pass through vacuum bags and remain in the air. If you are allergic to dust, wear a mask when vacuuming or dusting. People who are highly allergy-prone should not perform these tasks. They may even need to leave the house when someone else is cleaning.

Before You Start to Clean

Carefully read instructions for use and any cautionary labeling on cleaning products before beginning cleaning procedures.

- Do not mix any chemical products. Especially, never mix cleaners containing bleach with any product (such as ammonia) which does not have instructions for such mixing. When chemicals are combined, a dangerous gas can sometimes be formed.

- Household chemicals may cause burning or irritation to skin and eyes.

- Household chemicals may be harmful if swallowed, or inhaled.

- Avoid contact with skin, eyes, mucous membranes and clothing.

- Avoid breathing vapor. Open all windows and doors and use an exhaust fan that sends the air outside.

- Keep household chemicals out of reach of children.

- Rinse treated surface areas well to remove all traces of chemicals.

Before You Move

Protect yourself by inspecting your potential new home. If you identify problems, have the landlord or seller correct them before you move in, or even consider moving elsewhere.

283

- Have professionals check the heating and cooling system, including humidifiers and vents. Have duct lining and insulation checked for growth.

- Check for exhaust fans in bathrooms and kitchens. If there are no vents, do the kitchen and bathrooms have at least one window apiece? Does the cook top have a hood vented outside? Does the clothes dryer vent outside? Are all vents to the outside of the building, not into attics or crawlspaces?

- Look for obvious mold growth throughout the house, including attics, basements, and crawlspaces, and around the foundation. See if there are many plants close to the house, particularly if they are damp and rotting. They are a potential source of biological pollutants. Downspouts from roof gutters should route water away from the building.

- Look for stains on the walls, floor or carpet (including any carpet over concrete floors) as evidence of previous flooding or moisture problems. Is there moisture on windows and surfaces? Are there signs of leaks or seepage in the basement?

- Look for rotted building materials which may suggest moisture or water damage.

- If you or anyone else in the family has a pet allergy, ask if any pets have lived in the home.

- Examine the design of the building. Remember that in cold climates, overhanging areas, rooms over unheated garages, and closets on outside walls may be prone to problems with biological pollutants.

- Look for signs of cockroaches.

Correcting Water Damage

What if damage is already done? Follow these guidelines for correcting water damage:

- Throw out mattresses, wicker furniture, straw baskets and the like that have been water damaged or contain mold. These cannot be recovered.

- Discard any water-damaged furnishings such as carpets, drapes, stuffed toys, upholstered furniture and ceiling tiles, unless they can be recovered by steam cleaning or hot water washing and thorough drying.

- Remove and replace wet insulation to prevent conditions where biological pollutants can grow.

Additional Information

Contact your local American Lung Association for copies of: *Indoor Air Pollution Fact Sheets*, *Air Pollution in Your Home* and other publications on indoor air pollution.

Contact the U.S. Consumer Product Safety Commission, Washington, D.C. 20207, for copies of: *The Inside Story: A Guide to Indoor Air Quality and Humidifier Safety Alert*.

To report an unsafe consumer product or product-related health problem, consumers may call the U.S. Consumer Product Safety Commission at 1-800-638-2772. A teletypewriter for the hearing impaired is available at 1-800-8270; the Maryland TTY number is 1-800-492-8104.

Chapter 26

Taking a Breath at Work: Ventilation and Air Quality in Offices

Introduction

Millions of Americans work in buildings with mechanical heating, ventilation, and air-conditioning (HVAC) systems; these systems are designed to provide air at comfortable temperature and humidity levels, free of harmful concentrations of air pollutants. While heating and air-conditioning are relatively straightforward operations, the more complex processes involved in ventilation are the most important in determining the quality of our indoor air.

While many of us tend to think of ventilation as either air movement within a building or the introduction of outdoor air, ventilation is actually a combination of processes which results in the supply and removal of air from inside a building. These processes typically include bringing in outdoor air, conditioning and mixing the outdoor air with some portion of indoor air, distributing this mixed air throughout the building, and exhausting some portion of the indoor air outside. The quality of indoor air may deteriorate when one or more of these processes is inadequate. For example, carbon dioxide (a gas that is produced when people breathe), may accumulate in building spaces if sufficient amounts of outdoor air are not brought into and distributed throughout the building. Carbon dioxide is a surrogate for indoor pollutants that may cause occupants to grow drowsy, get headaches, or function at lower activity levels. There are many potential sources of indoor air pollution, which may singly, or in combination, produce

EPA. Air and Radiation Publication #20A-4002. Revised July 1990.

other adverse health effects. However, the proper design, operation and maintenance of the ventilation system is essential in providing indoor air that is free of harmful concentrations of pollutants.

Sources of Indoor Air Pollution

Indoor air pollution is caused by an accumulation of contaminants that come primarily from inside the building, although some originate outdoors. These pollutants may be generated by a specific, limited source or several sources over a wide area, and may be generated periodically or continuously. Common sources of indoor air pollution include tobacco smoke, biological organisms, building materials and furnishings, cleaning agents, copy machines, and pesticides.

Health Problems and Ventilation

Harmful pollutants from a variety of sources can contribute to building-related illnesses, which have clearly identifiable causes, such as Legionnaire's disease. HVAC systems that are improperly operated or maintained can contribute to sick building syndrome (SBS); SBS has physical symptoms without clearly identifiable causes. Some of these symptoms include dry mucous membranes and eye, nose, and throat irritation. These disorders lead to increased employee sick days and reduced work efficiency.

A committee of the World Health Organization estimates that as many as 30 percent of new or remodelled buildings may have unusually high rates of sick building complaints. While this is often temporary, some buildings have long-term problems which linger, even after corrective action. The National Institute for Occupational Safety and Health reports that poor ventilation is an important contributing factor in many sick building cases.

Controlling Indoor Air Pollution

Control of pollutants at the source is the most effective strategy for maintaining clean indoor air. Control or mitigation of all sources, however, is not always possible or practical. Ventilation, either natural or mechanical, is the second most effective approach to providing acceptable indoor air.

In the past, most buildings had windows that opened; airing out a stuffy room was common practice. In addition, indoor-outdoor air pressure differences provided ventilation by movement of air through leaks in the building shell. Today however, most newer office buildings are constructed without operable windows, and mechanical ventilation systems are used to exchange indoor air with a supply of relatively cleaner outdoor air.

The rate at which outdoor air is supplied to a building is specified by the building code. Supply rates are based primarily on the need to control odors and carbon dioxide levels; carbon dioxide is a component of outdoor air, but its excessive accumulation indoors can indicate inadequate ventilation. Supply rates, hereafter referred to as ventilation rates, are commonly expressed in units of cubic feet per minute per person (cfm/person).

Ventilation Standards and Building Codes

After achieving industry consensus in 1989, the American Society of Heating, Refrigerating, and Air-Conditioning Engineers (ASHRAE) published its "Standard 62-1989: Ventilation for Acceptable Indoor Air Quality." This is a voluntary standard for "minimum ventilation rates and indoor air quality that will be acceptable to human occupants and are intended to avoid adverse health effects." This standard applies to all types of facilities, including dry cleaners, laundries, hotels, dormitories, retail stores, sports and amusement facilities, and teaching, convalescent and correctional facilities. The specified rates at which outdoor air must be supplied to each room within the facility range from 15 to 60 cfm/person, depending on the activities that normally occur in that room.

Standard 62-1989 is a voluntary standard, which means that it becomes enforceable only after a state or locality adopts the standard in its building code. Furthermore, most current building codes pertaining to ventilation are standards only for the way buildings in a particular jurisdiction must be designed; they are not enforceable standards for the way the buildings are operated. A few states, through recently promulgated regulations, pending legislation, labor agreements and other mechanisms, are working to apply existing design codes and standards to building operations.

Ventilation System Problems and Solutions

The processes involved in ventilation provide for the dilution of pollutants. In general, increasing the rate at which outdoor air is supplied to the building decreases indoor air problems. The other processes involved in ventilation however, are equally important. Buildings with high ventilation rates may suffer indoor air problems due to an uneven distribution of air, or insufficient exhaust ventilation. Even in a well-ventilated building there may be strong pollutant sources which impair indoor air quality. The closer such a source is to an exhaust however, the more effective the ventilation; local exhaust ventilation, e.g., a chemical fume hood, is most effective. It is good practice to provide separate exhaust systems in areas where copy machines or solvents are used. Providing localized exhaust for these specific sources can result in a reduction of the amount of overall building exhaust ventilation necessary.

As was mentioned earlier, an HVAC system that is properly designed, installed, operated, and maintained can promote indoor air quality. When proper procedures are not followed, indoor air problems may result. Some common problems, and their solutions, are discussed below.

System Design

Intermittent air flow: Designs that specify HVAC system operation at reduced or interrupted flow during certain portions of the day in response to thermal conditioning needs (as in many variable air volume installations) may cause elevated indoor contaminant levels and impair contaminant removal. Minimum ventilation rates should be defined by air cleanliness and distribution, as well as temperature and humidity.

Distribution of air: Failure to maintain proper temperature, humidity, and air movement in a building can lead occupants to block supply registers if they emit air that is uncomfortably hot or cold; this disrupts air flow patterns. Placement of partitions or other barriers within a space can also impair air movement. In addition, locating air supply and return registers too close together can result in an uneven distribution of fresh air and insufficient removal of airborne contaminants. Precautions must be taken to maintain comfortable thermal conditions, and proper placement of supply and return registers, and furnishings.

Building supply and exhaust locations: Air supply vents that are installed too close to building exhaust vents re-entrain contaminated exhaust air into the building, increasing indoor pollution. Placement of supply vents near outdoor sources of pollution, such as loading docks, parking and heavy traffic areas, chimneys, and trash depots, provides a pathway for contaminants into the building's ventilation system. The location of all air supply vents must be carefully considered.

Proportion of Outdoor Air

To dilute and eventually remove indoor contaminants. HVAC systems must bring in adequate amounts of outdoor air. However, because it is costly to heat cold winter air and to cool hot summer air, some building engineers reduce or eliminate the amount of outdoor air brought into the system during hot and cold spells; this allows contaminated air to accumulate inside, causing pollutant concentrations to increase. Therefore, a continuous supply of fresh air must be provided.

Periods of Operation

An HVAC system that begins to operate after building occupants have arrived, or shuts off before the end of the work day can cause an increase in building- and occupant-generated pollutant levels. Similarly, if the system is off during periods of non-occupancy (e.g., at night and on weekends) building-generated pollutants may accumulate. Therefore, the ventilation system should be turned on several hours prior to occupancy, and shut down only after occupants have left.

Maintenance

HVAC systems must be properly maintained to promote indoor air quality. If this is not done, ventilation systems can become a source of contamination or become clogged and reduce or eliminate air flow. Humidification and dehumidification systems must be kept clean to prevent the growth of harmful bacteria and fungi. Failure to properly treat the water in cooling towers to prevent growth of organisms, such as Legionnella may introduce such organisms into the HVAC supply ducts and cause serious health problems. Accumulations of water anywhere in the system may foster harmful biological growth that can be distributed throughout the building.

Air Cleaners

Air cleaners may be an important part of an HVAC system, but cannot adequately remove all of the pollutants typically found in indoor air. Air cleaners should only be considered as an adjunct to source control and ventilation. Air cleaners that have a high filter efficiency and are designed to handle large amounts of air are the best choice for use in office buildings.

Air cleaners include the simple furnace filter, the electronic air cleaner, and the ion generator. Mechanical filters, either flat or pleated, are generally effective at removing particles; fit filters collect large particles and pleated filters such as the high-efficiency particulate air (HEPA) filters collect the smaller, respirable particles. Electronic air cleaners and ion generators use an electronic charge to remove airborne particles; these devices may also produce ozone, a lung irritant. All air cleaners require periodic cleaning and filter replacement to function properly.

In addition to removing particles, some air cleaners may remove gaseous pollutants; this is possible only if the air cleaner contains special material, such as activated charcoal, to facilitate removal of harmful gases. Although some of the devices which are designed to remove gaseous pollutants may be effective in removing specific pollutants from indoor air, none are expected to adequately remove all of the gaseous pollutants typically present in indoor air. Information is limited on the useful lifetime of these systems; they can be expensive and require frequent replacement of the filter media. (For a more detailed discussion of air cleaners, see the EPA publication 400/1-90-002, Residential Air Cleaning Devices.)

Economic Considerations of Air Quality

It is generally agreed that poor indoor air can adversely affect employee health and productivity. These costs to industry have been estimated to be in the "tens of billions of dollars per year" (*Report to Congress on Indoor Air Quality, 1989*). Improvements in the indoor air environment may substantially increase employee moral and productivity. Therefore, it is important to include indoor air quality controls in operation, maintenance, and energy conservation strategies.

Resolving Air Quality Problems

Building managers and tenants must work together to improve indoor air quality; areas to address include:

HVAC system operation and maintenance: Operate the ventilation system in a manner consistent with its design. Perform maintenance and inspections on a regular basis, as prescribed by the manufacturer.

Record keeping: Maintain records of all HVAC system problems, as well as routine maintenance and inspection activities. Document the nature of complaints concerning the indoor air environment, as well as steps taken to remedy each complaint. These records may be useful in solving future problems.

Pollution control: Identify pollution sources. Implement source removal or special ventilation techniques (including restrictions on smoking).

Occupant activities: Eliminate practices which may restrict air movement (e.g., furniture placement relative to air vents).

Building maintenance activities: Increase ventilation rates during periods of increased pollution, e.g., during painting, renovation, and pesticides use; schedule use of pollutant sources to minimize the impact on indoor air quality.

Ventilation standards and codes: Keep abreast of revisions to ventilation standards and building codes affected by those standards.

Energy conservation: Re-examine energy conservation practices with regard to indoor air quality considerations, employee health, and productivity costs.

Follow-up. Identify areas for follow-up.

Summary

- An HVAC system that is properly designed, installed, maintained, and operated is essential to providing healthful indoor air, a poorly maintained system can generate and disperse air pollutants.

- Control of pollutants at the source is the most effective means of promoting indoor air quality.

- An adequate supply of outdoor air is essential to diluting indoor pollutants.

- In the absence of adequate ventilation, irritating or harmful contaminants can build up, causing worker discomfort, health problems and reduced performance levels.

- Ventilation rates specified in most local building codes are design standards only, and therefore are not enforceable for insuring healthful indoor air quality after the system begins to operate.

- Air cleaning is an important part of an HVAC system, but is not a substitute for source control or ventilation. All air cleaners must be properly sized and maintained to be effective.

- An objective evaluation of indoor air quality, employee health, and productivity costs should be included when considering energy costs and energy-saving strategies.

Additional Information

For more information on topics discussed in this chapter, contact your state or local health department, non-profit agency such as your local American Lung Association, or the following:

U.S. Environmental Protection Agency
Indoor Air Division
Mail Code ANR-445
401 M Street, SW
Washington, D.C. 20460

National Institute for Occupational Safety and Health
U.S. Department of Health and Human Services
4676 Columbia Parkway (Mail Drop R2)
Cincinnati, Ohio 45226

Office of Building and Community Systems
US Department of Energy
CE-13, MS GH-068
1000 Independence Avenue, SW
Washington, D.C. 20585

Public Relations Office American Society of Heating,
Refrigerating, and Air-Conditioning Engineers (ASHRAE)
1791 Tullie Circle, NE
Atlanta, GA 30329

Building Owners and Managers Association International
1250 Eye Street, NW
Washington, D.C. 20005

Copies of this chapter as "Indoor Air Facts Sheet No. 3" and others in
the Indoor Air series are available from:

Public Information Center
U.S. Environmental Protection Agency
Mail Code PM-211B
401 M Street, SW
Washington, D.C. 20460

Chapter 27

Sick Building Syndrome

Introduction

The term "sick building syndrome" (SBS) is used to describe situations in which building occupants experience acute health and comfort effects that appear to be linked to time spent in a building, but no specific illness or cause can be identified. The complaints may be localized in a particular room or zone, or may be widespread throughout the building. In contrast, the term "building related illness" (BRI) is used when symptoms of diagnosable illness are identified and can be attributed directly to airborne building contaminants.

A 1984 World Health Organization Committee report suggested that up to 30 percent of new and remodeled buildings worldwide may be the subject of excessive complaints related to indoor air quality (IAQ). Often this condition is temporary, but some buildings have long-term problems. Frequently, problems result when a building is operated or maintained in a manner that is inconsistent with its original design or prescribed operating procedures. Sometimes indoor air problems are a result of poor building design or occupant activities.

Indicators of SBS include:

- Building occupants complain of symptoms associated with acute discomfort, e.g., headache; eye, nose, or throat irritation; dry

EPA. Air and Radiation Publication EPA ANR-445-W. April 1991.

cough; dry or itchy skin; dizziness and nausea; difficulty in concentrating; fatigue; and sensitivity to odors.

- The cause of the symptoms is not known.

- Most of the complainants report relief soon after leaving the building.

Indicators of BRI include:

- Building occupants complain of symptoms such as cough; chest tightness; fever, chills; and muscle aches.

- The symptoms can be clinically defined and have clearly identifiable causes.

- Complainants may require prolonged recovery times after leaving the building.

It is important to note that complaints may result from other causes. These may include an illness contracted outside the building, acute sensitivity (e.g., allergies), job-related stress or dissatisfaction, and other psycho-social factors. Nevertheless, studies show that symptoms may be caused or exacerbated by indoor air quality problems.

Causes of Sick Building Syndrome

The following have been cited causes of or contributing factors to sick building syndrome:

Inadequate ventilation: In the early and mid 1900s, building ventilation standards called for approximately 15 cubic feet per minute (cfm) of outside air for each building occupant, primarily to dilute and remove body odors. As a result of the 1973 oil embargo, however, national energy conservation measures called for a reduction in the amount of outdoor air provided for ventilation to 5 cfm per occupant. In many cases these reduced outdoor air ventilation rates were found to be inadequate to maintain the health and comfort of building occupants. Inadequate ventilation, which may also occur if heating, ventilating, and air conditioning (HVAC) systems do not effectively distribute air to people in the building, is thought to be an important factor in SBS. In an effort to achieve acceptable IAQ while minimizing energy consumption, the American Society of Heating, Refrigerating and Air-Conditioning Engineers (ASHRAE) recently revised its ventilation standard to provide a minimum of 15 cfm of outdoor air per person (20 cfm/person in office spaces). Up to 60 cfm/person may be required in some spaces (such as smoking lounges) depending on the activities that normally occur in that space (see ASHRAE Standard 62-1989).

Chemical contaminants from indoor sources: Most indoor air pollution comes from sources inside the building. For example, adhesives, carpeting, upholstery, manufactured wood products, copy machines, pesticides, and cleaning agents may emit volatile organic compounds (VOCs), including formaldehyde. Environmental tobacco smoke contributes high levels of VOCs, other toxic compounds, and respirable particulate matter. Research shows that some VOCs can cause chronic and acute health effects at high concentrations, and some are known carcinogens. Low to moderate levels of multiple VOCs may also produce acute reactions. Combustion products such as carbon monoxide, nitrogen dioxide, as well as respirable particles, can come from unvented kerosene and gas space heaters, woodstoves, fireplaces and gas stoves.

Chemical contaminants from outdoor sources: The outdoor air that enters a building can be a source of indoor air pollution. For example, pollutants from motor vehicle exhausts, plumbing vents, and building exhausts (e.g., bathrooms and kitchens) can enter the building through poorly located air intake vents, windows, and other openings. In addition, combustion products can enter a building from a nearby garage.

Biological contaminants: Bacteria, molds, pollen, and viruses are types of biological contaminants. These contaminants may breed in stagnant water that has accumulated in ducts, humidifiers and drain pans, or where water has collected on ceiling tiles, carpeting, or insulation. Sometimes insects or bird droppings can be a source of biological contaminants. Physical symptoms related to biological contamination include cough, chest tightness, fever, chills, muscle aches, and allergic responses such as mucous membrane irritation and upper respiratory congestion. One indoor bacterium, *Legionella*, has caused both Legionnaire's Disease and Pontiac Fever.

These elements may act in combination, and may supplement other complaints such as inadequate temperature, humidity, or lighting. Even after a building investigation, however, the specific causes of the complaints may remain unknown.

A Word about Radon and Asbestos

SBS and BRI are associated with acute or immediate health problems; radon and asbestos cause long-term diseases which occur years after exposure, and are therefore not considered to be among the causes of sick buildings. This is not to say that the latter are not serious health risks; both should be included in any comprehensive evaluation of a building's IAQ.

Building Investigation Procedures

The goal of a building investigation is to identify and solve indoor air quality complaints in a way that prevents them from recurring and which avoids the creation of other problems. To achieve this goal, it is necessary for the investigator(s) to discover whether a complaint is actually related to indoor air quality, identify the cause of the complaint, and determine the most appropriate corrective actions.

An indoor air quality investigation procedure is best characterized as a cycle of information gathering, hypothesis formation, and hypothesis testing. It generally begins with a walk-through inspection of the problem area to provide information about the four basic factors that influence indoor air quality:

- the occupants
- the HVAC system
- possible pollutant pathways
- possible contaminant sources.

Preparation for a walk-through should include documenting easily obtainable information about the history of the building and of the complaints; identifying known HVAC zones and complaint areas; notifying occupants of the upcoming investigation; and, identifying key individuals needed for information and access. The walk-through itself entails visual inspection of critical building areas and consultation with occupants and staff.

The initial walk-through should allow the investigator to develop some possible explanations for the complaint. At this point, the investigator may have sufficient information to formulate a hypothesis, test the hypothesis, and see if the problem is solved. If it is, steps should be taken to ensure that it does not recur. However, if insufficient information is obtained from the walk-through to construct a hypothesis, or if initial tests fail to reveal the problem, the investigator should move on to collect additional information to allow formulation of additional hypotheses. The process of formulating hypotheses, testing them, and evaluating them continues until the problem is solved.

Although air sampling for contaminants might seem to be the logical response to occupant complaints, it seldom provides information about possible causes. While certain basic measurements, e.g., temperature, relative humidity, CO_2, and air movement, can provide a useful "snapshot" of current building conditions, sampling for specific pollutant concentrations is often not required to solve the problem and can even be misleading. Contaminant concentration levels rarely exceed existing standards and guidelines even when occupants continue to report health complaints. Air sampling should not be undertaken until considerable information on the factors listed above has been collected, and any sampling strategy should be based on a comprehensive understanding of how the building operates and the nature of the complaints.

Solutions to Sick Building Syndrome

Solutions to sick building syndrome usually include combinations of the following:

Pollutant source removal or modification is an effective approach to resolving an IAQ problem when sources are known and control is feasible. Examples include routine maintenance of HVAC systems, e.g., periodic cleaning or replacement of filters; replacement of water-stained ceiling tile and carpeting; institution of smoking restrictions; venting contaminant source emissions to the outdoors; storage and use of paints, adhesives, solvents, and pesticides in well-ventilated areas, and use of these pollutant sources during periods of non-occupancy; and allowing time for building materials in new or remodeled areas to off-gas pollutants before occupancy. Several of these options may be exercised at one time.

Increasing ventilation rates and air distribution often can be a cost-effective means of reducing indoor pollutant levels. HVAC systems should be designed, at a minimum, to meet ventilation standards in local building codes; however, many systems are not operated or maintained to ensure that these design ventilation rates are provided. In many buildings, IAQ can be improved by operating the HVAC system to at least its design standard, and to ASHRAE Standard 62-1989 if possible. When there are strong pollutant sources, local exhaust ventilation may be appropriate to exhaust contaminated air directly from the building. Local exhaust ventilation is particularly recommended to remove pollutants that accumulate in specific areas such as rest rooms, copy rooms, and printing facilities. (For a more detailed discussion of ventilation, read the preceding chapter.)

Air cleaning can be a useful adjunct to source control and ventilation but has certain limitations. Particle control devices such as the typical furnace filter are inexpensive but do not effectively capture small particles; high performance air filters capture the smaller, respirable particles but are relatively expensive to install and operate. Mechanical filters do not remove gaseous pollutants. Some specific gaseous pollutants may be removed by adsorbent beds, but these devices can be expensive and require frequent replacement of the adsorbent material. In sum, air cleaners can be useful, but have limited application.

Education and communication are important elements in both remedial and preventive indoor air quality management programs. When building occupants, management, and maintenance personnel fully communicate and understand the causes and consequences of IAQ problems, they can work more effectively together to prevent problems from occurring, or to solve them if they do.

Additional Information

For more information on topics discussed in this chapter, contact your state or local health department, a non-profit agency such as your local American Lung Association, or the following:

National Institute for Occupational Safety and Health
U.S. Department of Health and Human Services
4676 Columbia Parkway (Mail Drop R2)
Cincinnati, Ohio 45226

Public Relations Office American Society of Heating, Refrigerating and Air-Conditioning Engineers (ASHRAE)
1791 Tullie Circle, NE
Atlanta, Georgia 30329

Building Owners and Managers Association International
1250 Eye Street,
NW Washington, D.C. 20005

Copies of this chapter as "Indoor Air Facts Sheet No. 4" and others in the Indoor Air Facts series are available from:

Public Information Center
U.S. Environmental Protection Agency
Mail Code PM-211B
401 M Street, SW
Washington, D.C. 20460

Chapter 28

Beware the Fungus Among Us: Another View of Sick Building Syndrome

Microbes, not materials, may produce irritating emissions in buildings.

In the past few years, "Sick Building Syndrome" has been blamed on a variety of causes from particle board partitions to paints, from carpets to cleaning supplies. Recent research funded by a seed grant from the Georgia Environmental Technology Consortium, a division of the Georgia Research Alliance, indicates that these may be blamed when they are not the primary culprits, however.

The obnoxious emissions that congest our lungs and irritate our eyes may be coming from microbial infestations lurking in the floor beneath us, in the walls around us, and in the ceiling above us. Our buildings may be sicker than we thought.

Dr. Charlene Bayer, principle research scientist and director of Tech's Indoor Environment Research Program, and biologist Sidney Crow of Georgia State University have investigated a number of "sick" buildings. They believe that many of the indoor problems found in the Southeastern United States are caused by volatile organic compounds (VOCs) given off by molds and fungi.

"As molds and fungi grow, they give off metabolic gases that contain VOC emissions," says Bayer."Some of the volatile compounds that we are finding are many of the primary solvents, and we think some of the manufacturers are being blamed for emissions from their products when the emissions may actually be coming from the microbes.

©1995 *Research Horizons*. Summer/Fall 1995. Reprinted with permission.

Because the VOCs have usually been attributed to other types of sources, the source control may be incorrect."

Bayer and Crow collected fungi samples from a number of buildings that were afflicted with microbial contamination. The samples were allowed to grow in the laboratory, and the VOCs released from the microbial broths were collected and identified. These VOCs were then compared to those detected in the ambient air within the buildings.

"Many of the volatile compounds produced by the cultured fungi are identical to those originating from solvent-based building materials and cleaning supplies," says Bayer. "These VOCs included hexane, methylene, chloride, benzene, and acetone."

"The microbial VOCs may contribute heavily to the overall level of ambient VOCs in buildings," says Bayer. In one building the researchers investigated, for example, the microbial contamination was clearly evident on the walls, the carpets, and other locations.

"The concentration of hexane—a solvent commonly used in many cleaning fluids, paints, and adhesives—was extremely high," says Bayer, "but no source of the hexane could be found. The microbiological contamination could have been the source of the hexane."

Lessening the Risk

Cladosporium, Penicillium, and *Aspergillus* are among the host of commonly occurring microbes that can infest our homes, schools, and offices. Usually, the first indication of their presence is a foul, musty odor. When growth runs rampant, then the headaches, itchy eyes, rashes, and respiratory problems begin.

Conditions favorable for microbial growth include heat and moisture, says Bayer. In the Southeast, with its semitropical climate and high humidity, buildings are prime targets for microbial contamination.

Molds and fungi are not particular about what they eat. They will happily devour just about any organic material, including the dirt and dust trapped within our ventilation systems.

What can be done to lessen the risk of microbial contamination? First of all, you can look for ways to reduce the necessary nutrient base. "Under ideal conditions, a building's ventilation system should filter out both the microbes and the dirt they feed upon," says Bayer. "Unfortunately however, many homes, schools, and small office buildings use cheap, throwaway filters in their ventilation systems." Cheap furnace filters are merely "boulder catchers," says Bayer. "They only catch the big stuff—they don't catch the fine dust particles and they don't catch the microbes. So, they really don't do anything to help human health."

Bayer's advice: simply throw away the cheap filters and replace them with higher quality, albeit more expensive, filters.

But the bigger the building, the bigger the problems with ventilation systems become.

In larger office buildings, fiberglass-lined ductwork is often used for noise control, says Bayer. The fibers tend to trap a lot of dirt, and that provides a rich nutrient base for microbes.

"Add a little moisture, and you have a mold garden growing in your ductwork," says Bayer. "The microbes grow and multiply, and then get blown all over the building to infest other areas."

Moisture control is extremely important in preventing microbial contamination, says Bayer. When the humidity goes up, microbial growth can skyrocket.

"Many buildings erected in the Southeast simply were not designed to handle the heavy humidity loads we have particularly during our hot, muggy summers," says Bayer. "And most building owners don't run their ventilation systems continuously."

Schools typically turn their systems off during the summer months (the prime time of year for microbial growth), and most office buildings cycle their systems over nights and weekends, often resulting in an unpleasant "Monday morning cocktail" for workers. Such intermittent operation allows the humidity to increase and the molds to multiply.

Preventative maintenance involves proper filtration, correct moisture control, and periodic cleaning of the entire ventilation system—including the humidifier assembly on residential furnaces.

"Typical reservoir humidifiers are little mold factories," says Bayer. "They are just pools of standing, stagnant water throughout much of the year that allow mold to grow and infiltrate the ducts. They should be cleaned regularly."

Future Work

A great deal of research remains to be done, including identifying individual metabolic gases and their respective odors, and acquiring a better understanding of the microbes that are producing them. Once a knowledge base is developed in these areas, the human response to molds and fungi and the sources of complaints in buildings can be better understood.

"Ultimately, we want to identify the microbial contamination on the basis of the odors which are present," says Bayer. "That way, we will be able to identify the source much more quickly and accurately, and deal with the problem faster and more effectively . . . before it becomes a major problem requiring expensive remediation."

Further information is available from:

Dr. Charlene Bayer.
Georgia Tech Research Institute.
Electro-Optics, Environment and Materials Laboratory.
Georgia Institute of Technology.
Atlanta, GA 30332-0820.
(Telephone 404/894-3825).
(e-mail: charlene.bayer@gtri.gatech.edu)

— by James B. Kloeppel

Part Five

Occupational Risks

Chapter 29

Playing It Safe at Work: Health Hazards in the Workplace

When most people think of workplace hazards, they picture mines, factories, or a construction site. Not many would consider a school gymnasium or a comfortable office an unsafe place to work. However, even the most mundane work environments can pose health hazards that might range from mild discomfort to serious injury or illness. In some cases, the Food and Drug Administration plays a role in limiting these hazards.

Mercury Vapor Lamps

Mercury vapor lamps, most often used to light streets, gymnasiums, sports arenas, banks, and stores must be maintained properly to be safe. These lamps are composed of an inner quartz tube containing the mercury vapor, enclosed by an outer envelope that filters out harmful short wavelength ultraviolet radiation. If the outer envelope is broken and the lamp continues to operate, intense ultraviolet radiation is emitted.

UV exposure at this level has produced photokeratitis (corneal burns) and reddening of the skin, as well as blurred or double vision, headaches, nausea, and diarrhea. Most injuries have occurred in school gymnasiums after the lamps were struck and partially broken by sports equipment.

FDA issued a performance standard for high-intensity mercury vapor discharge lamps on March 7, 1980, allowing the manufacture

FDA Consumer, October 1991.

311

of two types of mercury vapor lamps. One type, marked "T," is equipped with a self-extinguishing device that shuts the lamp off within 15 minutes after the outer envelope is broken. The other type of lamp, marked "R," does not contain a self-extinguishing feature. It may be used only in a fixture with a glass or plastic shield capable of absorbing hazardous ultraviolet radiation, or in areas where people will not be exposed to UV radiation if the outer globe is broken.

A 1980 FDA alert defines labeling that must appear on non-self-extinguishing mercury vapor lamps. This labeling includes the following instructions:

- Check the lamps regularly for missing, broken or punctured outer bulbs. This should be done with the lamps off.

- If a lamp is broken, turn the lamp off immediately.

- Replace lamps only when the lamps are off.

- Persons exposed to ultraviolet radiation from a damaged lamp should see a doctor if symptoms of skin burns or eye irritation occur.

- Report injuries to your state health department and to FDA.

The labeling for self-extinguishing "T" lamps must also state, "This lamp should self-extinguish within 15 minutes after the outer envelope is broken or punctured. If such damage occurs, TURN OFF AND REMOVE LAMP to avoid possible injury from hazardous shortwave ultraviolet radiation."

People near a broken mercury vapor lamp should leave the area immediately while taking steps to limit UV exposure to their eyes and skin by donning outer wear (coats or sweaters, for example) and sunglasses.

Radiation

At the end of World War II, the forerunner of the Nuclear Regulatory Commission was given jurisdiction over all radioactive materials capable of being used to build atomic weapons, including those used for medical diagnosis and treatment. FDA has jurisdiction over products that emit x-rays, overseeing their safety and effectiveness, while individual states have the power to set licensing standards for both facilities using x-rays and the technicians who use such equipment.

Public Law 90-602, enacted in the 1960s, gives FDA jurisdiction over electronic products that emit non-ionizing radiation, such as microwave ovens and color televisions. FDA develops performance standards for these products and provides educational materials for consumers. The National Council on Radiation Protection, with input from experts around the country, formulates guidelines on radiation safety that are nationally accepted.

If you have any questions about radiation safety from ionizing materials, contact your individual state radiation control office. FDA's Center for Devices and Radiological Health's consumer affairs division has consumer information on non-ionizing radiation—such as that from microwave ovens, electric blankets, and televisions—and also has consumer information on products such as lasers (both medical and entertainment), airport x-ray machines, and medical x-rays.

Video Display Terminals

Video display terminals (VDTs) are a staple in today's workplace. While some people use their terminals only intermittently during the day, others face their screens constantly as part of their jobs—making airline or concert reservations, for example. Despite lack of scientific data on serious health hazards, some people still fear that VDTs may cause cancer, immune system irregularities, or miscarriages.

The most common complaints from constant VDT users are dry or burning eyes, eye fatigue, blurred vision, and aches in the neck and back. A few simple steps can alleviate these discomforts:

- Use good room lighting. Adjust the room lighting levels and properly position the computer to get the room lighting that is most comfortable. The typical office lighting may be too bright for computer work.

- Eliminate sources of glare. Use drapes and blinds on windows. Don't sit facing a bright window. If necessary, use screen hoods or glare shields over the screen. Lower light levels in the room may reduce glare.

- Adjust the screen brightness and contrast so that it is comfortable for you.

313

- Rest occasionally during periods of intense concentration. The National Institute of Occupational Safety and Health recommends taking a 15-minute rest break every hour from highly demanding computer tasks. Don't forget to blink frequently to reduce dryness and irritation. Looking at a distant object can relax your eyes. Closing your eyes can also help.

- Maintain a good viewing distance. Close viewing may cause focusing fatigue. Adjust the workstation so that keyboard, screen, and paper copy are an equal distance from the eyes with the screen slightly (about 20 degrees) below eye level. It is helpful to use a copyholder. A good viewing distance is 22 to 26 inches.

- Talk to an eye-care professional about special glasses or an altered prescription. Some people may need special glasses for focusing at the intermediate distance that is neither as long a distance as prescriptions for nearsightedness usually encompass, nor a typical reading distance. This is particularly true if you wear reading glasses or bifocals. Tell your eye-care professional if you use a computer for long periods, and discuss any eye discomfort you have.

- Keep the work environment free of dust. Dust can make the eyes tear, feel gritty, or turn red. Proper humidity and ventilation are important. There are cleaners available to remove dust from the screen.

What about ELF?

Another serious concern associated with VDTs is the extremely low frequency (ELF) electromagnetic fields they produce. Alternating only 60 times a second, the effects of these fields are at the center of a scientific controversy. Some studies of humans exposed to ELF radiation have suggested an association between this exposure and certain types of cancer. But the evidence is not clear. For example, other human studies do not show an increased cancer risk. Even those studies with positive results have not been able to accurately determine how much ELF radiation people in the studies received, making it difficult to determine the risk, if any. And animal experiments have thus far failed to show a cancer-causing effect.

Some studies have also raised the question of an increased risk of miscarriages and other problems during pregnancy among women

Job	Hazard	Protective Eyewear
Chemical handling	splash, acid burns	goggles (eyecup and cover types), face shields for severe exposure
Construction (chipping, grinding machining, masonry riveting, sanding)	flying objects, sand, dirt	safety glasses or goggles, face shields for severe exposure
Furnace operations (pouring, casting, hot dipping, gas cutting, welding)	sparks	goggles and safety glasses, face shields for severe exposure
	splash from molten metals	goggles, face shields
	heat	screen or reflective face shields
Welding electric arc	UV radiation, flying sparks	welding helmets equipped with special filter lenses, welding shields
gas	fumes	welding goggles or welding face shields
Woodworking	dust	goggles (eyecup and cover types)

(Source: Occupational Safety and Health Administration)

Figure 29.1. *Protective Gear. Please note that face shields or welding helmets should be worn over safety glasses or goggles.*

exposed to ELF fields. The evidence for these effects is even more uncertain than that for cancer.

Although existing studies raise concerns about the possibility of health effects from ELF radiation, the scientific evidence is not sufficient at present to warrant regulatory action by FDA. The agency believes that the most prudent course of action is for it to continue to monitor the research in this field and, in the meantime, to work with manufacturers to reduce levels of ELF radiation.

To address these concerns, some VDT manufacturers are beginning to produce terminals that emit less ELF radiation. In the meantime, some people may wish to reduce their exposure, despite the absence of scientific evidence pointing to a clear health hazard by taking three simple steps:

- Turn off the VDT when not in use.

- Position yourself approximately 22 to 28 inches (arm's length) from the screen when using the VDT. If possible, use an adjustable computer shelf so you can position the keyboard further from the screen. ELF emissions fall off drastically after a distance of 28 inches, so sitting at least that far from the screen will reduce exposure.

- Position yourself approximately four feet from the sides and rear of other terminals. ELF emissions are greater from these parts of VDTs than from the front screen.

Carpal Tunnel Syndrome

VDTs have also spawned a rise in carpal tunnel syndrome, or repetitive motion injury. This hand condition results from performing the same motions for hours at a time, as when a terminal operator types continuously. The syndrome is named for the narrow tunnel in the wrist formed by ligament and bone. The tendons that enable the hand to close pass through the carpal tunnel. Injury to this part of the body can cause numbness or weakness, tingling and burning in the fingers and hands, or difficulty opening and closing hands. If the condition is not treated, permanent injury and loss of the use of the hand are possible.

The American Physical Therapy Association recommends several steps to prevent or alleviate the symptoms of carpal tunnel syndrome:

- Keep wrists relaxed and straight, using only finger movements to strike the keys. Your typing table should be slightly higher than your elbows when your arms are held relaxed by your sides. Rest your elbows by your sides or support them with special arm rests now available on some office chairs. Relax your shoulders and keep them level.

- Press keys with the minimum pressure necessary. Make sure the keyboard is kept clean and in good working order to minimize resistance.

- Move your entire hand to press hard-to-reach keys rather than overextending your fingers. Use two hands if necessary to execute combination keystrokes, such as shifting to upper case.

- Break up typing tasks with other activities—such as proofreading, filing, or telephone work—to rest fatigued muscles.

Protective Eyewear

For students and teachers, shop and science-labs pose a danger of eye injuries from foreign objects. Some sports and hobbies can also pose a risk of eye injury. Chemicals or tools can damage unprotected eyes.

Although FDA regulates regular glasses, sunglasses and goggles, the Occupational Safety and Health Administration regulates job-related protective eye equipment. All major component parts of industrial-type eye protectors that conform with the OSHA standard are marked Z87, and the manufacturer's monogram is marked on each lens, Most states require Z87 eyewear for protection for certain occupations.

Choose protective eyewear to shield you from foreign objects, heat, chemicals, dust, and radiation. Safety glasses or goggles with side shields provide protection from frontal and side impact and are designed for such projects as woodworking. These are "primary protectors." For protection against severe hazards such as arc welding or furnace operations, face shields and welding helmets, called "secondary protectors," must be worn in addition to the safety glasses or goggles. (See Figure 29.1)

Our ability to identify deleterious health effects from advancing technology is evolving. As we attempt to keep pace with rapid workplace innovations, some basic safety rules can do much to minimize risk: Keep equipment in good working order, follow directions for use carefully, and use common sense when operating machines.

For More Information

For more information on workplace safety, contact the following organizations:

Food and Drug Administration
Division of Consumer Affairs (HFZ-210)
Center for Devices and Radiological Health
5600 Fishers Lane
Rockville, MD 20857

National Institute for Occupational Safety and Health
1600 Clifton Road, N.E.
Atlanta, GA 30333

National Council on Radiation Protection
7910 Woodmont Ave., Suite 800
Bethesda, Md. 20814

Occupational Safety and Health Administration
200 Constitution Ave., N.W.
Washington, D.C. 20210
(for the free booklet Working Safely with VDTs, send a self-addressed label and a request for publication #3092 to room N3101 at the above address)

The American Physical Therapy Association
1111 North Fairfax St.
Alexandria, Va. 22314
(send a self-addressed, stamped envelope for free brochures on carpal tunnel syndrome and posture and back problems related to VDTs)

—by Jessica Auerbach

Jessica Auerbach is a member of FDA's division of consumer affairs in the Center for Devices and Radiological Health.

Paula Silberberg of the center also contributed to this article.

Chapter 30

Questions and Answers about Asbestos Exposure

What is asbestos?

"Asbestos" is the name given to a group of minerals that occur naturally as masses of strong, flexible fibers that can be separated into thin threads and woven. These fibers are not affected by heat or chemicals and do not conduct electricity. For these reasons, asbestos has been widely used in many industries. Four types of asbestos have been commonly used:

- **Chrysotile,** or white asbestos (curly, flexible white fibers), which accounts for about 90 percent of the asbestos currently used in industry;

- **Amosite** (straight, brittle fibers that are light gray to pale brown in color);

- **Crocidolite,** or blue asbestos (straight blue fibers); and

- **Anthophyllite** (brittle white fibers).

Chrysotile asbestos, with its curly fibers, is in the serpentine family of minerals. The other types of asbestos, which all have needle-like fibers, are known as amphiboles.

National Cancer Institute, NCI Cancerfax, May 1995.

Asbestos fiber masses tend to break easily into a dust composed of tiny particles that can float in the air and stick to clothes. The fibers may be easily inhaled or swallowed and can cause serious health problems.

How is asbestos used?

Asbestos has been mined and used commercially in North America since the late 1800s, but its use increased greatly during World War II. Since then, it has been used in many industries. For example, the building and construction industry uses it for strengthening cement and plastics as well as for insulation, fireproofing, and sound absorption. The shipbuilding industry has used asbestos to insulate boilers, steam pipes, hot water pipes, and nuclear reactors in ships. The automotive industry uses asbestos in vehicle brake shoes and clutch pads. More than 5,000 products contain or have contained asbestos, some of which are listed below:

- Asbestos cement sheet and pipe products used for water supply and sewage piping, roofing and siding, casings for electrical wires, fire protection material, chemical tanks, electrical switchboards and components, and residential and industrial building materials;

- Friction products, such as clutch facings; brake linings for automobiles, railroad cars, and airplanes; and industrial friction materials;

- Products containing asbestos paper, such as table pads and heat-protective mats, heat and electrical wire insulation, industrial filters for beverages, small appliance components, and underlying material for sheet flooring;

- Asbestos textile products, such as packing components, roofing materials, heat- and fire-resistant clothing, and fireproof draperies; and

- Other products, including ceiling and floor tile; gaskets and packings; paints, coatings, and sealants; caulking and patching tape; and plastics.

In the late 1970s, the U.S. Consumer Product Safety Commission banned the use of asbestos in wallboard patching compounds and gas fireplaces because these products released excessive amounts of asbestos fibers into the environment. In addition, asbestos was voluntarily withdrawn by manufacturers of electric hair dryers. These and other regulatory actions, coupled with widespread public concern about the hazards of asbestos, have resulted in a significant annual decline in U.S. use of asbestos: Domestic use of asbestos amounted to about 560,000 metric tons in 1979, but it had dropped to about 55,000 metric tons by 1989.

What are the health hazards of exposure to asbestos?

Exposure to asbestos may increase the risk of several serious diseases:

- **Asbestosis**: a chronic lung ailment that can produce shortness of breath and permanent lung damage and increase the risk of dangerous lung infections;

- **Lung cancer**;

- **Mesothelioma**: a relatively rare cancer of the thin membranes that line the chest and abdomen; and

- **Other cancers**, such as those of the larynx and of the gastrointestinal tract.

Who is at risk?

Since the early 1940s, millions of American workers have been exposed to asbestos dust, including many of the 8.5 million men and women who worked in shipyards during the peak shipbuilding years of World War II. Health hazards from asbestos dust have been recognized in workers exposed in shipbuilding trades, asbestos mining and milling, manufacturing of asbestos textiles and other asbestos products, insulation work in the construction and building trades, brake repair, and a variety of other trades. Demolition workers, drywall removers, and firefighters also may be exposed to asbestos dust. As a result of Government regulations and improved work practices, today's workers (those without previous exposure) are likely to face smaller risks than did those exposed in the past. Although it is known that the risk to workers increases with heavier exposure and longer exposure time, investigators have found asbestos-related diseases in some shipyard workers exposed to high levels of asbestos fibers for only brief periods (as little as one or two months). Even workers who may not have worked directly with asbestos but whose jobs were located near contaminated areas have developed asbestosis, mesothelioma, and other cancers associated with asbestos exposure.

Generally, workers who develop asbestos-related diseases show no signs of illness until many years after first exposure. For examples the time between first exposure to asbestos and the appearance of lung cancer is generally 15 years or more; a lag of 30 to 35 years is not unusual. The lag period for development of mesothelioma and asbestosis is even greater, often as long as 40 to 45 years.

There is also some evidence that family members of workers heavily exposed to asbestos face an increased risk of developing mesothelioma and perhaps other asbestos-related diseases. This risk is thought to result from exposure to asbestos dust brought into the home on the shoes, clothing, skin, and hair of workers.

How great is the risk?

Not all workers exposed to asbestos will develop diseases related to their exposure. In fact, many will experience no ill effects.

Asbestos that is bonded into finished products such as walls, tiles, and pipes poses no risk to health as long as it is not damaged or disturbed (for example, by sawing or drilling) in such a way as to release fibers into the air. When asbestos particles are set free and inhaled, however, exposed individuals are at risk of developing an asbestos-related disease. Once these nearly indestructible fibers work their way into body tissues, they tend to stay there indefinitely.

The risk of developing asbestos-related diseases varies with the type of industry in which the exposure occurred and with the extent of the exposure. In addition, different types of asbestos fibers may be associated with different health risks. For example, results of several studies suggest that crocidolite and amosite are more likely than chrysotile to cause lung cancer, asbestosis, and, in particular, mesothelioma. Even so, no fiber type can be considered harmless, and proper safety precautions should always be taken by people working with asbestos.

How does smoking affect risk?

Many studies have shown that the combination of smoking and asbestos exposure is particularly hazardous. Cigarette smokers, on the average, are 10 times as likely to develop lung cancer as are non-smokers. For nonsmokers who work with asbestos, the risk is about five times greater than for those in the general population. By contrast, smokers who also are heavily exposed to asbestos are as much as 90 times more likely to develop lung cancer than are non-exposed individuals who do not smoke. Smoking does not appear to increase the risk of mesothelioma, however.

There is evidence that quitting smoking will reduce the risk of lung cancer among asbestos-exposed workers, perhaps by as much as half or more after at least five years without smoking. People who were exposed to asbestos on the job at any time during their life or who suspect they may have been exposed **SHOULD NOT SMOKE.** If they smoke, they should stop.

Who needs to be examined?

Individuals who have been exposed (or suspect they have been exposed) to asbestos dust on the job or at home via a family contact should inform their physician of their exposure history and any symptoms. A thorough physical examination, including a chest x-ray and lung function tests, may be recommended. Interpretation of the chest x-ray may require the help of a specialist who is experienced in reading x-rays for asbestos-related diseases. Other tests also may be necessary.

As noted earlier, the symptoms of asbestos-related diseases may not become apparent for many decades after exposure. If any of the following symptoms develop, a physical examination should be scheduled without delay:

- Shortness of breath;
- A cough or a change in cough pattern;
- Blood in the sputum (fluid) coughed up from the lungs;
- Pain in the chest or abdomen;
- Difficulty in swallowing or prolonged hoarseness; and/or
- Significant weight loss.

What are the treatments for asbestos-related diseases?

The key to successful treatment of asbestos-related diseases lies in early detection. The health problems caused by asbestosis are due mainly to lung infections, like pneumonia, that attack weakened lungs. Early medical attention and prompt, aggressive treatment offer the best chance of success in controlling such infections. Depending on the situation, doctors may give a vaccine against influenza or pneumococcal pneumonia as a protective measure.

Treatment of cancer is tailored to the individual patient and may include surgery, anticancer drugs, radiation, or combinations of these therapies. Information about cancer treatment is available from the National Cancer Institute-supported Cancer Information Service, whose toll-free telephone number is 1-800-4-CANCER.

See also Omnigraphics' volumes on cancer, the *Cancer Sourcebook*, the *New Cancer Sourcebook*, and the *Cancer Sourcebook for Women*.

How can workers protect themselves?

Employers are required to follow regulations dealing with asbestos exposure on the job that have been issued by the Occupational Safety and Health Administration (OSHA), the Federal agency responsible for health and safety regulations in the workplace. Regulations related to mine safety are enforced by the Mine Safety and Health Administration (MSHA). Workers should use all protective equipment provided by their employers and follow recommended work practices and safety procedures. Workers who are or who have been exposed to asbestos should not smoke cigarettes.

Workers who are concerned about asbestos exposure in the workplace should discuss the situation with other employees, their union, and their employers. If necessary, OSHA can provide more information or make an inspection. Area offices of OSHA are listed in the "United States Government" section of telephone directories' blue pages (under "Department of Labor"). If no listing is found, workers may call or write to an OSHA regional office. Mine workers may contact MSHA's Office of Standards, Variances, and Regulation at Room 627, 4015 Wilson Boulevard, Arlington, VA 22203; the telephone number is 703-235-1910.

The National Institute for Occupational Safety and Health (NIOSH) is another Federal agency that is concerned with asbestos exposure in the workplace. The Institute conducts asbestos-related research, evaluates work sites for possible health hazards, and makes safety recommendations. In addition, NIOSH distributes publications on the health effects of asbestos exposure and can suggest additional sources of information. The address is Office of Information, National Institute for Occupational Safety and Health, 4676 Columbia Parkway/Mailstop C-19, Cincinnati, OH 45226. The toll-free telephone number is 1-800-35-NIOSH (1-800-356-4674).

What should people who have been exposed to asbestos do?

It is important for exposed individuals to:

- Stop smoking;
- Get regular health checkups;
- Get prompt medical attention for any respiratory illness; and
- Use all protective equipment, work practices, and safety procedures designed for working around asbestos.

Will the Government provide examinations and treatment or pay for such services? What about insurance coverage?

Medical services related to asbestos exposure are available through the Government only for certain groups of eligible individuals. In general, exposed individuals must pay for their own medical services unless they are covered by private or Government health insurance. Medicare may reimburse people with symptoms of asbestos-related diseases for the costs of diagnosis and treatment (following review of medical procedures for appropriateness). General and specific information about benefits is available from the Medicare office serving each state; for the telephone number of the nearest office, call 1-800-772-1213.

People with asbestos-related diseases also may qualify for financial help, including medical payments, under state workers' compensation laws. Because eligibility requirements vary from state to state, workers should contact the workers' compensation program in the state where the last exposure occurred. (The telephone number may be found in the blue pages of a local telephone directory.)

If exposure occurred during employment with a Federal agency (military or civilian), medical expenses and other compensation may be covered by the Federal Employees' Compensation Act. Workers who are or were employed in a shipyard by a private employer may be covered under the Longshoremen and Harbor Workers' Compensation Act. Information about eligibility or how to file a claim is available from the U.S. Department of Labor, Office of Workers' Compensation Programs, Room S-3229, 200 Constitution Avenue NW, Washington, D.C. 20210; the telephone number is 202-219-7552.

Retired military personnel and their eligible dependents may receive health care at any Department of Defense medical facility, Department of Veterans Affairs (VA) hospital, or Public Health Service hospital. Where no Federal facility is available, civilian facilities may be used under the Civilian Health and Medical Program for the Uniformed Services. Those over age 65 may be covered by Medicare. Former members of the military who believe they may have a service-related medical problem may inquire about care at a VA facility or telephone the local VA office.

Workers also may wish to contact their international union for information on other sources of medical help and insurance matters. One organization, the Asbestos Victims Special Fund Trust, provides financial assistance to asbestos victims who have not received workers' compensation or compensation through legal avenues. Information is available from the Trust at Suite M-11, 1500 Walnut Street, Philadelphia, PA 19102; the telephone number is 1-800-447-7590.

Is there a danger of nonoccupational exposure from products contaminated with asbestos particles?

Asbestos is so widely used that the entire population has been exposed to some degree. Air, beverages, drinking water, food, drug and dental preparations, and a variety of consumer products all may contain small amounts of asbestos. In addition, asbestos fibers are released into the environment from natural deposits in the earth and as a result of wear and deterioration of asbestos products.

The U.S. Environmental Protection Agency (EPA) regulates the general public's exposure to asbestos in buildings, drinking water, and the environment. The EPA's Toxic Substances Control Act (TSCA) Assistance Office can answer questions about toxic substances, including asbestos. Printed material is available on a number of topics, particularly on controlling asbestos exposure in schools and other buildings. The TSCA office can provide information about accredited laboratories for asbestos testing and can refer inquirers to other resources on asbestos. Questions may be directed to the TSCA Assistance Office, U.S. Environmental Protection Agency, 7408 M Street SW, Washington, D.C. 20024; the telephone number is 202-554-1404.

The Consumer Product Safety Commission (CPSC) is responsible for the regulation of asbestos in consumer products. The CPSC maintains a toll-free information line on the potential hazards of commercial products; the telephone number is 1-800-638-2772. In addition, CPSC provides information about laboratories for asbestos testing, guidelines for repairing and removing asbestos, and general information about asbestos in the home. Publications are available from the Office of Public Affairs, Consumer Product Safety Commission, 4330

East-West Highway, Bethesda, MD 20816; the telephone number is 301-504-0580.

The U.S. Food and Drug Administration is concerned with asbestos contamination of foods, drugs, and cosmetics and will answer questions on these topics. The address is Office of Consumer Affairs, Food and Drug Administration, HFE-88, 5600 Fishers Lane, Rockville, MD 20857; the telephone number is 301-443-3170.

What other organizations offer information related to asbestos exposure?

The American Lung Association and the American Cancer Society can provide information about lung disease, cancer, and smoking. Local chapters of these organizations are listed in telephone directories. Material about cancer and how to quit smoking is available by calling the National Cancer Institute-supported Cancer Information Service (CIS). The CIS, a program of the National Cancer Institute, provides a nationwide telephone service for cancer patients and their families, the public, and health care professionals. CIS information specialists have extensive training in providing up-to-date and understandable information about cancer and cancer research. They can answer questions in English and Spanish and can send free printed material. In addition, CIS offices serve specific geographic areas and have information about cancer-related services and resources in their region. The toll-free number of the CIS is 1-800-4-CANCER (1-800-422-6237).

Chapter 31

Occupational Risk of Cancer from Pesticides: Farmers' Tales

Studies in the United States and other countries have shown that farmers have a higher risk for certain cancers, particularly cancers of the blood and the immune system (leukemia, non-Hodgkin's lymphoma, and multiple myeloma). The reasons for the increased risks are not clear, and scientists are looking at chemical and other occupational exposures common to farming to identify the possible cause or causes.

Farmers are exposed to a variety of potentially harmful substances during their workday, including pesticides (fungicides, herbicides, insecticides, rodenticides, and others), chemical solvents, fuels and oils, animal viruses, and other microbes. Sore of these agents are known or suspected carcinogens.

In the 1980s, National Cancer Institute (NCI) researchers began several studies of pesticide use by farmers with cancer and by those without the disease (case-control studies). The first of these investigations was a study of Kansas farmers with soft-tissue sarcomas, Hodgkin's disease, and non-Hodgkin's lymphoma (NHL). Published in 1986, this study showed that farmers who used herbicides, especially 2,4-dichlorophenoxyacetic acid (2,4-D), had more cases of NHL than did farmers and non-farmers who did not use these chemicals.

Further, the risk of developing NHL increased with frequency of herbicide use. Farmers who used herbicides on their farms 20 or more days per year had six times the rate of NHL seen for non-farmers. Within the high-exposure group, farmers who mixed and applied the

National Cancer Institute. *Cancer Facts*. May 1995.

herbicides themselves had an eight-fold greater rate. Soft-tissue sarcomas and Hodgkin's disease were not linked with use of herbicides.

Scientists at NCI have completed case-control studies of NHL among farmers in eastern Nebraska and leukemia among farmers in Iowa and Minnesota. Each study included all cases of these cancers occurring in a specific geographic area. Hospital records and pathology slides from the cases were carefully reviewed by pathologists to verify the cancer diagnoses.

Study subjects, or their next-of-kin, were interviewed for details about the subjects' use of agricultural pesticides and other factors that might be associated with these cancers. Pesticide exposure reported by the cancer patients was compared with exposure reported by randomly selected men without those cancers who lived in the same area.

Non-Hodgkin's Lymphoma

Sheila Hoar Zahm, Sc.D., and collaborators at NCI and the University of Nebraska Medical Center studied 201 men living in 66 counties in eastern Nebraska who developed NHL between 1983 and 1986. The researchers compared the pesticide exposures of these men with exposures of 725 men from the general population who did not have this cancer. Although there was no overall excess of NHL among farmers, the NHL rate for farmers who mixed or applied 2,4-D was 50 percent higher than for the general population. The rate of NHL also increased with frequency of 2,4-D use. Farmers who used the pesticide for 20 or more days per year had a threefold higher rate than those not exposed to the chemical.

The longer farmers waited to change into clean work clothes after a pesticide application, the higher their rate of NHL. The rate of NHL among farmers who changed out of work clothes immediately after completing a single application was similar to that among non-farmers. Farmers who continued to use these work clothes the following day or longer had nearly five times the NHL rate of non-farmers.

The investigators also looked at the possible effects of pesticides other than 2,4-D and other factors that might be associated with NHL, such as other agricultural exposures, medical conditions, exposure to radiation, and tobacco use. In other reports, non-2,4-D pesticides, particularly organophosphate insecticides, have also been shown to increase the risk of NHL. The NCI study results suggest that 2,4-D and organophosphate insecticides have independent influences on the risk of cancer. Further evaluation of organophosphate insecticides is necessary to quantify any possible risks associated with their use.

The association of 2,4-D and NHL in Nebraska farmers is consistent with results of the NCI study conducted in Kansas. Pesticide exposures that occurred many years in the past are difficult to assess accurately and tend to cause an underestimation of the cancer risk. Dr. Zahm and her collaborators believe the evidence suggests that the use of 2,4-D in the agricultural setting increases the risk of NHL among persons handling this pesticide frequently.

Leukemia

Linda Morris Brown, M.P.H., and colleagues at NCI, the University of Iowa, and the University of Minnesota studied a total of 578 cases of leukemia diagnosed in men in Iowa and Minnesota between 1981 and 1984 (293 cases in Iowa and 285 cases in Minnesota). To compare the effects of pesticide exposure, 1,245 men without the disease were selected at random from the general population.

The researchers found a slight excess of leukemia, especially chronic lymphocytic leukemia, among farmers. Exposure to specific fungicides, herbicides (including 2,4-D), or crop insecticides did not increase the rate.

The leukemia rate was significantly elevated for farmers who used certain pesticides to inhibit insects on animals rather than on crops. The insecticides were the organophosphates crotoxyphos (11 times greater rate), dichlorvos (2 times), and famphur (2 times); the natural product pyrethrin (4 times); and the chlorinated hydrocarbon methoxychlor (2 times).

The rate of leukemia did not increase consistently with frequency of use for any pesticide. However, the highest rate for farmers was seen in those using the chemicals on animals 10 or more days a year. The leukemia rate was even higher for farmers who had used insecticides at least 20 years before the study.

The investigators improved the accuracy of the risk estimate from individual pesticides by accounting for the cancer risk from smoking, non-farming occupational and chemical exposures, family history of cancer, and other factors. Larger studies are still needed to fully evaluate the effect of any single pesticide on leukemia risk. The higher cancer risk from animal insecticides than from crop pesticides may result from closer proximity to animals on a regular basis. Animal insecticides need to be carefully scrutinized in future studies.

For More Information

The Cancer Information Service (CIS), a program of the National Cancer Institute, is a nationwide telephone service for cancer patients and their families, the public, and health care professionals. CIS information specialists have extensive training in providing up-to-date and understandable information about cancer. They can answer questions in English and Spanish and can send free printed material. In addition, CIS offices serve specific geographic areas and have information about cancer-related services and resources in their region. The toll-free number of the CIS is 1-800-4-CANCER (1-800-422-6237).

Chapter 32

Danger in the Dust: Agricultural Environmental Hazards

In contrast to widely held images of urban pollution and blight the persistence of an "agrarian myth" that associates life on the farm with healthful, bucolic joys ignores a fundamental reality agriculture can be a dangerous occupation. In agriculture, a large proportion of acute traumatic injury and death comes from accidents involving farm machinery. Farm equipment also inflicts chronic injuries upon workers including noise-induced hearing loss and vibration-associated diseases of the back. Agrichemicals pose a risk for direct toxicity and possibly cancer. Dermatologic diseases including cancers, among farmers and farm workers are often linked to ultraviolet light exposure, contact dermatitis, and zoonosis. But the most prevalent agricultural hazard involves the respiratory tract. Says Marc B. Schenker, medical epidemiologist and director of the Center for Occupational and Environmental Health at the University of California, Davis, "Despite this litany of significant occupational health problems, respiratory disease remains one of the most common and important issues for those working in the agricultural field." Indeed, occupational mortality studies from the United States, England, and Scandinavia reveal higher respiratory disease mortality rates among farmers than the general population.

The farming population in the United States includes approximately three million Americans fully engaged in agricultural production and as many as nine million more who are seasonal and migrant

Environmental Health Perspectives Volume 104, Number 1. January 1996.

workers, part-time farmers, and farm family members, the latter often considerably active in farm work.

Schenker points out that agriculture is different from many occupations that give rise to respiratory disease. "You have a whole range of respiratory hazards. This isn't like asbestos where you're looking for those fibers, or sandblasting when you're just measuring quartz." Schenker's list of potential respiratory hazards includes gases at potentially lethal concentrations (chlorine, hydrogen sulfide, ammonia), diesel exhaust, solvents, welding fumes, infectious agents and viral diseases from animals, and organic and inorganic dusts, "which can exacerbate any of the others," Schenker says.

Written in the Dust

"It is organic dust that accounts for the most common exposure leading to agricultural respiratory disease," says James Merchant, director of Iowa University's Environmental Health Sciences Research Center. "Virtually everybody who works in agriculture gets exposed to some organic dust."

Indeed, studies indicate that the risk associated with developing respiratory disease appears to be more than threefold greater among those who are heavily exposed to inhalable dust generated in the agricultural environment. According to pulmonologist David A. Schwartz of the University of Iowa College of Medicine, asthma and bronchitis are the main diseases.

"Between 5 and 20 percent of individuals in aggregate will develop some airway disease as a result of agricultural dust exposures," he says.

"The major health effect is airway inflammation, and that extends from the nose to the terminal bronchiole," says Merchant. These dusts and their components are highly respirable, under 10 microns in aerodynamic diameters, so they can penetrate to the terminal bronchiole. "We see an effect in all levels of the airway, but the basic mechanism is airway inflammation, which is manifested clinically as rhinitis, either allergic or irritant; bronchitis, asthma, which can be allergic or irritant; and hypersensitivity pneumonitis."

Agricultural workers encounter a variety of airborne organic dusts generally containing 30-40 percent of particles in the respirable range. These include molds, pollens, and dusts generated in silos, barns, and grain elevators. Organic dusts measured in enclosed settings such as dairy, poultry, and swine buildings are particularly biologically active.

Along with suspended inorganic matter (primarily silicates), they contain plant material (feed and bedding), animal-derived particles (skin, hair, feathers, droppings, urine), bacteria and fungi, mites and other arthropods, insects and insect fragments, feed additives (including antibiotics), pesticides and microbial toxins (including glucans from molds, fungal mycotoxins, and endotoxin, the lipopolysaccharide traction of certain bacterial cell walls).

"One thing that's really important is that farmers in general have a relatively low prevalence of cigarette smoking in comparison to the general population," says Schwartz. "And given that, it's really striking that they have such major problems with airway disease. So even if it turns out not to be endotoxin or grain dust, there's something in the environment that's causing them to have major problems with airway disease in comparison with other groups."

By Any Other Name

In the early 18th century, the Italian physician Bernardo Ramazzini recorded his observations associating respiratory disorders with worker exposure to dusts from vegetable fibers and grain. Only in the 20th century has careful study of these phenomena occurred.

Among the factors that may have accounted for this lack of study was the rise of manufacturing. Victorian-era social concerns were focused on factories with their concentrations of workers and related issues of workplace conditions, safety, and child labor. Agriculture was still individual in nature in that people worked for themselves, on their own farms, and in small groups. The art and literature of the day painted a healthy and wholesome picture of agrarian life in contrast to highly publicized industrial disasters such as mine cave-ins, factory explosions, and sweatshop fires. "Occupational health, since its inception, has largely ignored agriculture, even though agriculture was the source of some of the earliest recognized occupational diseases," Schenker observes.

Still, the Industrial Revolution did help draw some attention to adverse health effects of exposure to agricultural dusts. As NIOSH Senior Medical Epidemiologist Robert M. Castellan points out, "The increasingly regular work schedule associated with the Industrial Revolution and its concentrations of workers in manufacturing facilities led to the recognition of a peculiar 'Monday phenomenon' among cotton textile workers. This was characterized by symptoms of chest tightness and other breathing difficulties occurring predominately on the first day back to work after Sunday break." In 1877, the term "byssinosis," derived from the Latin byssus, meaning "a fine cotton or linen," first entered the scientific literature.

Since then, adverse health effects arising from exposures to many other agricultural dusts have been described and documented, but myriad syndromes such as silo unloader's syndrome, bark stripper's disease, farmer's lung and grain fever have caused confusion among clinicians and epidemiologists. "People thought they were looking at many diseases, all of which needed to be attacked separately. But essentially they're the same, except one was diagnosed, say, in mushroom growers, the other in British pigeon handlers," says NIOSH physiologist Vincent Castranova. "The most recent understanding of the situation is that there are acute and chronic forms of agricultural dust disease in general, or responses to either isolated or multiple exposures to organic dust." For example, Castranova explains that the flu-like mill fever among cotton workers that follows initial, intense exposures to cotton dust is not present after repeated exposures, though chronic exposures can result in byssinosis, with its symptoms of chest tightness, decline in lung function, and bronchitis.

Acute responses to isolated exposures have been lumped under the term organic dust toxic syndrome (ODTS). ODTS typically occurs in the presence of large amounts of airborne, organic dust. The syndrome often occurs in small clusters and is characterized by fever occurring 4-12 hours after exposure and flu-like symptoms such as general weakness, headache, chills, body aches, and cough. Chest tightness and shortness of breath may also occur.

Chest examination usually reveals normal breathing sounds, although lung crackles and wheezing may be present. Chest X-rays are usually normal. Pulmonary function may be impaired, and an increase in the number of white blood cells (leukocytosis) is common. Circulating blood antibodies to the specific dust are usually not present. ODTS usually disappears within 24 hours to a few days following removal from the exposure. However, repeated ODTS episodes can occur after reexposure to the organic dust. An estimated 30-40 percent of workers exposed to organic dusts will develop ODTS. Grain fever, pulmonary mycotoxicosis, silo unloader's syndrome, inhalation fever, and mill fever in cotton textile workers are all included under ODTS.

A 1988 case reported by NIOSH researchers exemplifies a typical cluster of ODTS. Eleven male workers, aged 15-60, moved 800 bushels of oats from a poorly ventilated storage bin. The oats were reported to contain pockets of powdery, white dust. Work conditions were described as extremely dusty, and all workers wore disposable masks while inside the bin. The workers shoveled oats for 8 hours in groups of two or three in shifts of 20-30 minutes. Within 4-12 hours, all nine men who worked inside the bin became ill with fever and chills, chest discomfort, weakness, and fatigue. Eight reported shortness of breath, six had nonproductive coughs, five complained of body aches, and four developed headaches. Upon medical examination, crackle sounds in the lungs were found in two workers, wheezing in one. No symptoms developed in the two workers who remained outside the storage bin. Symptoms in all affected workers disappeared within 2-12 days.

"As to the chronic response," Castranova explains, "symptoms would be similar. But you would have a history of prior exposure, presence of serum antibodies to that dust, and the response in the lung is lymphocytic [an accumulation of specific white blood cells that participate in cell-mediated immune responses]."

Farmer's lung disease (an immunologic lung response involving antibodies to the fungi found in moldy hay), mushroom worker's lung, bark stripper's disease, and allergic alveolitis are examples of chronic responses and are synonymous with hypersensitivity pneumonitis. Symptoms often become progressively worse with increasing exposure and may lead to chronic bronchitis, shortness of breath, loss of appetite, and severe reductions in lung volume and diffusing capacity (the volume of gases that move through lung tissue membranes). Five to eight percent of workers exposed to organic dusts develop hypersensitivity pneumonitis. Although it has been studied for more than 25 years, the precise pathological mechanism of hypersensitivity pneumonitis remains unknown.

The conceptual road from acute to chronic responses to organic dusts may not be so clear. According to Castranova, if dust exposure levels are high enough, an affected worker may have neutrophils and lymphocytes in the lungs typical of both acute inflammatory and immunologic reactions. "It's never quite as simple as we'd like to make it," he says.

From Acute to Chronic

In his five-year longitudinal study of 611 workers employed at six cotton mills, biomedical engineer Henry Glindmeyer of Tulane University Medical Center's environmental medicine section reported a significant association between the acute and chronic effects of cotton dust exposure. Cotton dust exposure levels and acute pulmonary function changes measured across workshifts were predictive of annual declines in lung function. Moreover, an inverse exposure-response relationship was found. Yarn production workers in the initial manufacturing process were exposed to lower dust levels (below OSHA permissible exposure limits of 200 micrograms/ cubic meter of air [µg/ m³]) than workers exposed to the higher permissible levels (750 µg/ m³) in their slashing and weaving jobs in the later production process. Yet yarn production workers showed a greater annual decline in lung function, a finding which Glindmeyer and his colleagues interpreted as a dust potency effect, possibly due to endotoxin.

Early processing includes bringing the cotton into the warehouse, opening the bales, then manufacturing the cotton into long yarn. "Slashing and weaving is, number one, generally less dusty, but more importantly, tends to have a less potent dust," Glindmeyer explains. "Whatever might be in the dust is generally scrubbed out in the early process."

He adds, "In yarn manufacturing we were able to pick up a dose-response relationship at the 200 µg/m³ level. But we were not able to find one in the slashing and weaving area." The slashing and weaving area of the mill, he points out, does not necessarily have cleaner air. "In fact, it can have more dust, but it's less potent."

In this study, smoking proved also to be a significant determinant of decline in lung function. The Tulane researchers say their findings support lowering cotton dust exposures and excluding smokers from working in yarn manufacturing.

The implications of this and other recent longitudinal studies were summarized by McGill University epidemiologist Margaret Becklake. "There is some uncertainty as to whether the acute responses are always in the causal pathway for chronic responses or are independently related to exposure, or whether both mechanisms operate," she said. However, she points to similar findings for exposure to grain dust among grain elevator workers in Vancouver, British Columbia. These studies, she says, indicate a much broader role for occupational exposures in the development of chronic obstructive pulmonary disease than has been previously assumed.

In Keokuk County, Iowa, Merchant is directing a large-scale longitudinal rural health study. Begun just four years ago, this study comparing farm families, rural non-farm families, and urban families is still in the first round of data collection. It involves children and adults and focuses particularly on effects on the elderly and women. "We are taking a hard look at not only symptoms, but pulmonary function, airway responsiveness, and immunological factors in terms of lung disease risk," he says. The study is aimed at assessing and quantitating the risk to a variety of rural, agricultural, and other environmental exposures ranging from farm equipment to pesticides and agricultural dusts.

Endotoxin: A Critical Component?

Endotoxins are a combination of lipid (lipid A) and polysaccharide side chains and are integral components of the outer membrane of gram negative bacteria. Endotoxins are released into the surrounding environment during active cell growth or breakdown (lysis), or when bacterial cells are engulfed by immune cells called phagocytes.

In the 1930s and early 1940s, widespread outbreaks were reported of an acute, self-limited respiratory illness that appears to have been clinically identical to mill fever, but that also included chest tightness and cough much like symptoms of byssinosis. But rather than textile mill workers, those affected were poor rural families making mattresses for personal use from surplus, low-grade, stained cotton provided by a federally sponsored program.

"With our current knowledge, staining would be indicative of microbial growth on that cotton," says Castellan. "And on subsequent investigation, it was found that this cotton was highly contaminated, much more than it normally is, with an enterobacter species, a gram negative bacteria." The U.S. Public Health Service investigation of this outbreak resulted in the first scientific evidence suggesting that gram negative bacteria or its products are a likely cause of mill fever and possibly also a contributing factor in the etiology of acute and chronic pulmonary effects associated with byssinosis.

Endotoxins have been known to cause profound inflammation of any tissue exposed to them, including lung tissue. "Exposure to endotoxins causes an influx of inflammatory cells into the lungs," says NIOSH immunologist Stephen A. Olenchock. "They bring with them and they release various agents called cytokines, which cause swelling, exudate, or seepage, from blood vessels. These are very potent inflammatory agents."

Initially, the response to endotoxin may seem to be allergic. But unlike allergy, the active component is lipid A, and not an antigenic protein. "This is not an allergy at all,"

Olenchock explains. "Allergy involves a type of antibody associated with a specific antigen. Here, there is an absence of antibody. Endotoxins activate the complement system, which causes inflammation and then removal of foreign agents."

Occupational inhalation of endotoxins induces fever and constriction of airways. According to Castranova, endotoxins tend to upregulate the activity of lung phagocytes, encouraging pulmonary inflammation. "Many studies seem to show that if you put lung phagocytes in a test tube and add endotoxin, not much happens," he explains. "But if you add endotoxin and then add a second stimulus, the [phagocytic] response to that second stimulus is greater than if the endotoxin weren't there. The second stimulus could be the dust, the particulate matter."

In vitro studies of animal lung phagocytes reveal that endotoxins may initiate this response following a single dose, but decline in ability to do so after multiple doses. Castranova says this may explain the Monday phenomenon in cotton textile workers with byssinosis. "The cells are more responsive to endotoxin given once. After that they downregulate. Their receptors are internalized with the cell wall and are not available to respond again. After a weekend period of no exposures those receptors are externalized on the cell surface and are ready to respond to endotoxin again."

In the 1980s, controlled experimental exposures of human volunteers to cotton dusts contaminated with endotoxins provided insight into the roles of endotoxins in eliciting acute respiratory responses. Castellan and his colleagues reported a highly correlated relationship between acute changes in pulmonary function and endotoxin concentrations.

Experimental human exposure studies have been aimed at closely mimicking dust conditions experienced by mill workers. These results show decreases in lung function, such as forced expiratory volume (FEV), to be associated more strongly with endotoxin content than with mass exposures of dust. Moreover, studies involving cotton that was washed to lower its endotoxin content showed such cotton dust to be a less potent inducer of airway obstruction.

In one experiment, Castellan and colleagues investigated acute respiratory responses (FEV) to a wide range of cotton dust types— cotton raised in different parts of the country and of differing grades. "We note there is a much stronger dose-response relationship using endotoxin as the index of exposure, and in fact, no dose-response relationship [for] gravimetric dust." Gravimetric dust is measured by a device called a vertical elutriator designed to collect lint-free samples of aerodynamic size corresponding to inhaled dust particles deposited at or below an individual's trachea.

Signs and symptoms of respiratory exposures to dusts contaminated with endotoxins have also been reported for grain workers and those involved in animal production, including swine and poultry. Attempting to identify the role of endotoxin in grain dust-induced lung disease, Schwartz and his colleagues conducted a population-based, cross-sectional investigation comparing a cohort of grain handlers and postal workers in eastern Iowa After controlling for age, gender, and cigarette-smoking status, the researchers found that occupational exposure to grain dust was associated with acute and chronic respiratory symptoms, objective measures of diminished airflow, and enhanced bronchial reactivity (hyperresponsiveness). While it wasn't shown that endotoxin causes airway disease in grain handlers, airway disease appeared to be more pronounced in those exposed to higher concentrations of airborne endotoxin in the work setting.

"Other exposures associated with microbial contamination of grain dust may be involved here," Schwartz says. "Endotoxin may serve as a good surrogate marker for the more pathogenic components. We don't know whether it's the cause, but it seems to be."

In studying workers in swine confinement buildings, which are minimally ventilated, Schwartz found decreases in lung function that were independently associated with greater cross-shift changes (a measure of a worker's respiratory function over a specific workshift) in FEV and higher concentrations of airborne endotoxins. Moreover, acute declines in lung airflow across the workshift and higher concentrations of endotoxin were linked to accelerated declines in airflow during the period of observation, about two years. According to Schwartz, this indicates that acute airway responses are predictive of chronic changes in airflow.

Animal models have been developed that mimic the fever and acute pulmonary response reactions to organic dust inhalation. These studies have also exhibited a strong correlation between endotoxin levels and lung responses to organic dusts, including grain and cotton dusts. Schwartz used genetic strains of endotoxin-sensitive and endotoxin-resistant mice to perform corn dust inhalation studies. Endotoxin-sensitive mice showed a more profound inflammatory response in the lower respiratory tract to inhaled corn dust than the endotoxin-resistant mice. Endotoxin-sensitive mice that were made tolerant to endotoxins showed a significantly diminished inflammatory response to inhaled corn dust.

In experiments with guinea pigs, in which airway reactivity to organic dust closely mimics that of humans, Castranova demonstrated that changes in breathing pattern—the "Monday accentuation" response—depended on the endotoxin content of cellulose, which when untreated with endotoxin did not alter respiratory responses in the animals.

341

"In general, more work needs to be done with animal models," Castranova says. "The importance of various mediators has been brought out, including tumor necrosis factor, a product of lung phagocytes. If one gives the animal antibody to that, so that it's no longer active, the animal's acute pulmonary response to organic dust is mitigated."

Beyond the Tip of the Iceberg

The interaction between environmental and physiological factors may play a significant role in exposure to organic dusts, but the specifics remain to be clarified. As Schenker observes, "The determinants of the hypersensitivity pneumonitis response remain poorly understood. Initiation [of this response] in farmers who may have had similar exposures for years without pulmonary problems is unexplained."

Cigarette smoking is associated with diminished lung function responses to cotton and grain dusts, but the prevalence of hypersensitivity pneumonitis is higher in nonsmokers than in smokers. Some investigators point to cigarette-mediated immune alterations such as reduced cytokine production by lung macrophages. Others suggest that smokers are generally less susceptible to irritants, which may be a factor in why they smoke.

Clarification of environment and host interactions is often complicated by another element: "the healthy worker effect." Rates of long-term ill effects may be reduced because of early departure of sensitized workers from an industry. In grain workers, for example, smoking, mite allergy, and nonspecific bronchial hyper-reactivity may increase departure rates.

Studies in the cotton industry have shown that mill workers may still have accelerated declines in lung function related to cotton dust in the absence of symptoms characteristic of the Monday syndrome. "To many of us, that's not surprising," says Castellan. "The more we study the phenomena of occupational respiratory disease, the more we realize that the gross symptoms and gross findings are the tip of the iceberg. There's much more going on in terms of very subtle effects."

Minimizing Health Risks

Prevention, ventilation, and avoidance of exposures appear to be key recommendations for workers facing occupational health risks from agricultural dusts. According to some authorities, primary prevention through dust control, though more readily applicable in some agricultural industries such as cotton, is difficult elsewhere. "Dust presents a challenge because of its ubiquity," says Schenker.

In many situations there are steps that can effectively prevent dust generation," he said. Some of the steps he outlines for specific work practices include reducing levels of microorganisms in cut grasses to be used for feed or bedding via adequate drying in the field before baling, adding fat to the diet of animals in confinement facilities and using covered feed troughs filled through enclosed spouts to reduce ambient dust levels, capping silage materials to reduce spoilage, and pouring a quart of water on the cut surface of a hay bale prior to use in a bedding chopper, which can reduce dust levels by 85 percent.

In terms of ventilation, NIOSH recommends local exhaust ventilation for barns and confinement houses. NIOSH Alert, an agency publication, advises agricultural workers and employers on a number of practices aimed at minimizing risk of exposure to dusts, including wearing respirators with the highest assigned protection factor. In accordance with the OSHA respiratory protection standard, employers must train and monitor personnel in the use of respiratory protection equipment, as well as how to maintain, inspect, store, and clean it.

Cotton dust is the only specific agricultural dust that currently has an OSHA standard, although the main regulatory requirements apply only to regulated cotton industries and processes. Growing, harvesting, ginning, classing, warehousing, and knitting of cotton are not currently regulated. Handling and processing of woven or knitted cotton fabrics are also not regulated. Several different exposure limits ranging from 200 $\mu g/m^3$ to 750, $\mu g/m^3$ apply in textile mill operations. The cotton dust standard also requires medical examinations for new employees as well as periodic monitoring for all workers exposed to cotton dust. OSHA also has a standard for nonspecific dusts: 15 $\mu g/m^3$ for total dust and 5 $\mu g/m^3$ for respirable dust.

Future Needs

The extent of risks associated with dust exposures needs to be refined. Specific agents within agricultural dusts that are responsible for toxic and immunologic responses remain in question, as do methods for quantifying these components. Research is also needed to elucidate susceptibilities to these exposures. And more work is needed in the area of education and intervention to develop sound strategies aimed at preventing acute and chronic respiratory symptoms for a widespread and varied population of agricultural workers.

—by Leslie Lang

Chapter 33

In Answer to Your Questions about Agent Orange

Agent Orange was a mixture of herbicides used between 1963 and 1971 during the Vietnam War. Named for the orange-striped containers in which it was stored, Agent Orange was employed mainly to defoliate forest trees. It also was used to destroy the enemy's crops. Agent Orange contained two chlorophenoxy herbicides: 2,4,5-trichlorophenoxyacetic acid (2,4,5-T) and 2,4,5-dichlorophenoxyacetic acid (2,4-D). These herbicides were first used in the United States in the mid-l960s to control broadleaf weeds in cereal grain fields, pastures, and turf. They also were used to remove unwanted plants from rangeland, forests, non-cropland, and waterways. By the mid-1960s, chlorophenoxy herbicides had become the most important class of herbicides in the United States

During the 1970s, health concerns about the herbicides brought about Government restrictions that caused a sharp decrease in the manufacture and use of 2,4,5-T. Since 1983, the use of 2,4,5-T has been prohibited in the United States. Many other countries also have ended its use. Of additional concern is a contaminant commonly called dioxin (2,3,7,8-tetrachlorodibenzo-*p*-dioxin, or TCDD), which often forms when 2,4,5-T is manufactured. Of the approximately 75 chemicals in the dioxin family, TCDD is the most toxic. It can cause chloracne, a skin disease, and is suspected to cause some kinds of cancer. The TCDD level in Agent Orange varied from 0.02 to 54 micrograms per gram of 2,4,5-T.

National Cancer Institute. NCI Cancerfax. May 1995.

Farmers, forestry workers, and Vietnam veterans exposed to chlorophenoxy herbicides have been studied to see whether they had a higher incidence of cancer than would be expected. The results of these studies have been conflicting and inconclusive.

In 1984, Congress mandated that studies be conducted to determine whether service in Vietnam could be related to adverse health effects. In one study, scientists investigated the long-term health effects of military service in Vietnam; another study focused specifically on the health effects of exposure to Agent Orange in Vietnam; and a third study looked at the increased risk, if any, that Vietnam veterans would develop any of six specific kinds of cancer.

In March 1990, the Centers for Disease Control and Prevention (CDC) released the results of the last of its studies. The investigators reported a 50-percent higher incidence of non-Hodgkin's lymphoma (NHL), a cancer of the immune system, among Vietnam veterans than among veterans who did not serve in Vietnam. However, the studies could not show that this increased incidence is related to exposure to Agent Orange. For example, Navy veterans who served on vessels off the coast of Vietnam tended to have a higher rate of NHL than did veterans based on land, and veterans who served in the region of heaviest Agent Orange use tended to have a somewhat lower incidence than veterans who served in other regions of Vietnam. The CDC could not determine why the Navy veterans had an increased incidence of NHL. No increased incidence was found for the other five cancers in the study (soft tissue and other sarcomas, Hodgkin's disease, and nasal, nasopharyngeal, and liver cancers). Following the release of the results of the CDC studies, the Secretary of the Department of Veterans Affairs (VA) announced that VA would begin awarding compensation to Vietnam veterans with NHL. Vietnam veterans with NHL will receive monthly disability payments for the rest of their lives. A short time later, it was announced that Vietnam veterans with soft tissue sarcomas are eligible for disability payments even though the CDC studies failed to show that they are at increased risk for this kind of cancer. Vietnam veterans suffering from chloracne and peripheral neuropathy, a nerve disease, also are eligible for benefits. The VA recently stated that no connection between exposure to Agent Orange and the development of lung cancer has been shown and denied disability benefits for Vietnam veterans with this disease.

In 1990, National Cancer Institute researchers reported the results of a study showing an increased risk of testicular tumors in military working dogs who served in Vietnam during the conflict there.

Because the carcinogenic (cancer-causing) risk to dogs can be a useful indicator of carcinogenic risk to humans, another study was initiated to determine whether Vietnam service led to an increased risk of testicular cancer in humans. The results of this study showed a twofold increased risk of testicular cancer in Vietnam veterans. However, identification of specific factors, such as exposure to Agent Orange, could not be implicated as the cause of this increase.

For additional information about Agent Orange, contact:

Centers for Disease Control and Prevention
1600 Clifton Road NE
Mail Stop F16
Atlanta, GA 30333
404-488-4460

U.S. Department of Veterans Affairs
Environmental Medicine Office
1-46A
810 Vermont Avenue NW
Washington, D.C. 20420
202-535-8175

Disabled American Veterans
807 Maine Avenue SW
Washington, D.C. 2002
202-554-3501

The Cancer Information Service (CIS), a program of the National Cancer Institute, is a nationwide telephone service for cancer patients and their families, the public, and health care professionals. CIS Information specialists have extensive training in providing up-to-date and understandable information about cancer. They can answer questions in English and Spanish and can send free printed material. In addition, CIS offices serve specific geographic areas and have information about cancer-related services and resources in their region. The toll-free number of the CIS is 1-800-4-CANCER (1-800-422-6237).

Chapter 34

The Persian Gulf Experience and Health

Introduction

Following the return of U.S. and coalition forces from the complex environment of the Persian Gulf region during Operations Desert Shield and Desert Storm and the operational conditions of the military deployment, a variety of health effects have been reported. Many troops were exposed to potentially adverse substances and experiences present in this wartime environment—fumes and smoke from military operations, oil well fires, diesel exhaust, toxic paints, pesticides, sand, depleted uranium, infectious agents, chemoprophylactic agents, and multiple immunizations; some troops are convinced they were exposed to chemical or biological weapons. Few combat casualties occurred, but substantial transient gastrointestinal and respiratory symptoms were seen during the troop buildup and immediately after the short conflict. Since then, there have been increasing reports of illness from troops who were participants in these operations, and many attribute their health problems to these experiences. Many of the cases include combinations of nonspecific symptoms of fatigue, skin rash, muscle and joint pain, headache, loss of memory, shortness of breath, and gastrointestinal and respiratory symptoms, which may not fit readily into a common diagnosis. In the absence of clear and complete diagnosis and effective treatment of all symptoms, the concept of a distinct syndrome that is peculiar to the Gulf War theater of operations has been suggested. Some veterans have reported illnesses

NIH Publication *Technology Assessment Statement*. April 1994.

in their spouses and birth defects in children conceived after the conflict and are concerned about the spread of disease as a public health issue.

A number of governmental responses have been initiated as a result of the Gulf War veterans' complaints. The Department of Defense and the Department of Veterans Affairs have begun registration of Persian Gulf veterans. Special referral centers for clinical evaluation of complaints have been established by the Department of Veterans Affairs, and research proposals have been solicited to better understand their cause, diagnosis, and treatment. The intent of this Technology Assessment Workshop was to examine the information provided to the panel on these reports of illness, to assess the types and extent of environmental exposures of troops serving in the Persian Gulf, to determine the adequacy of information on the prevalence and incidence of unusual illnesses, and to attempt to develop working case definitions for those illnesses. In addition, plausible etiologies and biological explanations for the illnesses were considered, and recommendations for future research were made.

After 1 1/2 days of medical, scientific, and Government presentations by academic and Federal investigators, testimony of Gulf War veterans, and questioning and discussion by a public audience, this independent, non-Federal panel weighed the objective and subjective evidence and wrote a statement in response to the following key questions:

1. What is the evidence for an increased incidence of unexpected illnesses attributable to service in the Persian Gulf War?

2. If unexpected illnesses have occurred, what are the components of the most practical working case definition(s) based on the existing data?

3. If unexpected illnesses have occurred, what are the plausible etiologies and biological explanations for these unexpected illnesses?

4. What future research is necessary?

This workshop was sponsored by the NIH Office of Medical Applications of Research, the U.S. Department of Health and Human Services, the U.S. Department of Defense, the U.S. Department of Veterans Affairs, and the U.S. Environmental Protection Agency.

Question 1: What is the evidence for an increased incidence of unexpected illnesses attributable to service in the Persian Gulf War?

Definition of Unexpected Illness

Under conditions of the Persian Gulf War, certain infectious diseases, such as acute viral, bacterial, and parasitic respiratory and gastrointestinal infections due to crowded living conditions, as well as endemic infectious diseases such as leishmaniasis, schistosomiasis, and malaria, were expected. Noninfectious respiratory conditions including reactive airways diseases, interstitial lung diseases, and diminished lung function were not expected but are explainable and diagnosable. Other expected conditions include post-traumatic stress disorders and various skin disorders such as hypersensitivity dermatitis and chemical dermatitis. In this report, unexpected illnesses are defined as previously unrecognized and unanticipated symptom complexes or illnesses that do not fit traditional diagnostic categories.

An Assessment of the Incidence of the Unexpected Illnesses

The available data are too limited to draw any conclusions regarding the incidence of unexpected illnesses in this population. In general, all the data presented are numbers of individuals reporting symptoms, and those studied to date may not be representative of all individuals at risk for developing these symptoms. Since all Gulf War veterans or a representative sample of these veterans has not been surveyed for presence of symptoms, it is not possible to calculate the incidence of unexpected illnesses. In addition, we do not have comprehensive information on the dates of onset of illness. Such information is needed to estimate incidence and trends over time in the occurrence of illness.

Nevertheless, the data that were provided to the panel suggest that deployed active-duty personnel and deployed reservists reported more symptoms than did their non-deployed counterparts. Veterans of the Gulf War reported more illnesses than other veterans. Data on the symptom profile reported in the Gulf War Registry were also compared with those reported for Vietnam veterans in the Agent Orange Registry. Fatigue, muscle and joint pain, headache, and shortness of breath were more frequent among those who served in the Persian Gulf area; skin rash was less frequent. Since data were not collected in a comparable fashion for the two registries, only limited conclusions can be drawn from this study.

In the case of leishmaniasis, a novel and unexpected manifestation of the disease was identified—viscerotropic leishmaniasis. Because this disease is difficult to diagnose, its true incidence is unknown. The cases reported are minimum estimates of the true number of infected people.

Although congenital malformations have been reported in the offspring of people who served in the Persian Gulf area, the currently available data are not sufficient to determine whether the incidence is increased and thus may be unexpected.

Question 2: If unexpected illnesses have occurred, what are the components of the most practical working case definition(s) based on the existing data?

It appears from the information presented that some Persian Gulf veterans have symptoms that are not readily explained by using established disease categories. Under these circumstances, it would be helpful to establish a single case definition to assist in evaluating and managing these veterans. However, a single case definition may not be sufficient, Since there may be more than one disease category. Therefore, an evolving case definition might be more appropriately used in developing a research strategy.

In order to describe better the particular symptom complex needed for a case definition or definitions, other cohorts of veterans should be evaluated and compared with the Persian Gulf veterans. These cohorts would consist of veterans who were deployed to other foreign locations for combat and noncombat situations and/or veterans who were not deployed. Information should be obtained from these veterans using standardized and symptom-specific evaluations. These evaluations could be conducted in conveniently accessible regional centers, with monitoring and analysis of data at a single location. In addition, evaluation of Persian Gulf veterans should be continued at these same locations using identical standardized protocols. Case definitions could then be developed by means of these comparisons.

For the above reasons, it is impossible at this time to establish a single case definition. Furthermore, a premature attempt to establish a case definition for this illness may be misleading and inaccurate. Eligibility for medical care need not depend on case definition.

Question 3: If unexpected illnesses have occurred, what are the plausible etiologies and biological explanations for these unexpected illnesses?

The Persian Gulf War was an experience of unprecedented stress for our military and their families. Reserve and National Guard units were rapidly mobilized to join 500,000 active-duty troops in southwest Asia. The military command anticipated that chemical and/or biological weapons would be used. Detectors signaled the presence of chemical weapons on several occasions that caused increased anxiety. As many as 50,000 casualties were expected in a full-scale 15-day war with Iraq. Tactical strategy demanded secrecy. Troops could not be informed about the timing and objectives of their actual assignments. Public knowledge that Iraq had stockpiles and capabilities of delivering chemical and biological weapons contributed to mass anxiety.

The complex set of exposures and stressors made the Persian Gulf tour unique. Individuals who were deployed had severe psychological stresses upon entering the area. All had multiple vaccines and medications administered during this period, worked long hours, and lived in crowded and often unsanitary conditions among flies, snakes, spiders, and scorpions. The chemical contaminants from oil fires, burning dumps (feces and trash), fuels, and solvents were ubiquitous. The climate exhibited temperature extremes in a sand/dust environment. The threat of biological and chemical warfare was omnipresent. In this report, no single or multiple etiology or biological explanation for the reported symptoms was identified from the data available to the panel. In this setting, standard dose-and-effect relationships may be altered. Possible causative or contributing factors to the unexplained symptoms are reviewed below.

Leishmaniasis

Thirty-one proven cases of leishmaniasis were diagnosed by parasite identification. These cases probably represent a small subset of the expected population of infected persons. Visceral leishmaniasis can present with typical manifestations (hepatosplenomegaly, fever, weight loss, pancytopenia) and/or vague, nonspecific symptoms (fatigue, low-grade fever, gastrointestinal symptoms); or it may be subclinical. The finding of visceral involvement by *Leishmania tropica* in one report is novel; it would constitute a new disease entity that could be missed by conventional diagnostic procedures. The natural history of this so-called viscerotropic leishmaniasis is unknown.

Many of the proven cases of leishmaniasis had nonspecific symptoms, including chronic fatigue, gastrointestinal symptoms, and low-grade fever-symptoms shared by Persian Gulf veterans with unexplained symptoms. The delayed onset and prolonged duration of leishmaniasis are also compatible with the symptom patterns of some Gulf War veterans. Certainly, some of the illnesses of the veterans could be attributable to this form of leishmaniasis.

The standard diagnostic tests (bone marrow, skin tests, serology) may not be sensitive enough to detect infection in this disease, and therefore, other methods need to be applied. These methods should be made available as rapidly as possible and include (1) T cell proliferation assay in response to *L. tropica* antigens, (2) cytokine profile analysis, and (3) detection of *L. tropica* DNA in bone marrow based on polymerase chain reaction (PCR). The underlying prevalence is likely to be substantially higher than reported and, thus, should be part of the primary Veterans Affairs (VA) diagnostic protocol(s).

Petroleum

Exposure to petroleum vapors, solvents, and combustion products was common during the Persian Gulf War. Inhalation was evidently the dominant route of exposure, but ingestion and dermal exposures were important in some circumstances. Petroleum (kerosene, diesel fuels, and leaded gasoline) was used for heating. Petroleum products including diesel fuels were used as sand/dust suppressants. Mobile armament and vehicles used diesel and gasoline fuels. Oil well fires resulted in exposures to carbonaceous particulates composed of metals, as well as unburned and partially pyrolyzed hydrocarbons. Oil on surfaces was partially volatilized, resulting in the distillation of lighter weight hydrocarbons. Where crude oil was burned or deposited, inorganic gases (SO_2, NO_2, CO, CO_2, H_2S, reduced sulfur compounds) were released. Engine exhaust, burning, and evaporating petroleum would also result in increased exposures to aromatics, aliphatic and aldehyde gaseous compounds, and a great number of semi-volatile organic compounds. Exposures to petroleum-related pollutants occurred throughout the Persian Gulf. For many military personnel, both chronic and acute exposures to respiratory irritants, carcinogens, and neurotoxic compounds were highest during winter-time encampments in Saudi Arabia. Beginning in late February, military personnel in Kuwait and eastern Saudi Arabia were exposed to gases and particulate soot from the oil well fires. Exposures were more frequent and severe for those in closer proximity to the sabotaged wells.

The practices of spreading oily dust suppressants, burning trash and human waste, and using gasoline and diesel fuels for unvented heaters are documented. There were no reported measurements of ambient or indoor pollutants. On the basis of published reports on residential kerosene heater studies, elevated concentrations of SO_2, NO_2, HNO_2, H_2SO_4, NH_4HSO_4, CO, lead, respirable particulates, and other pollutants would be expected. Elevated concentrations lasting throughout the winter nights would have been repeated occurrences in tents where non-issued fuels were used. Exposures could have exceeded Federal standards and World Health Organization (WHO) health guidelines. Elevated blood lead levels, increased airway resistance, and persistent wheezing and coughing, as well as respiratory infections, might be expected. Repeated and chronic exposures to these combustion pollutants could result in permanent impairment.

Open burning of fuels, with the exception of the oil wells, would have produced localized plumes. Diesel exhaust from electric generators could be reentrained into ventilation systems. The spreading of fuels for dust suppression as well as refueling operations would certainly have resulted in petroleum vapor exposures. Transient levels of benzene, toluene, ethylbenzene, and xylene exceeding one ppm could have occurred. Prolonged exposures to these vapor compounds may result in symptoms of light-headedness, mucosal irritation, fatigue, and cognitive dysfunction. Since benzene and some polycyclic aromatic hydrocarbons are known human carcinogens, some exposures might increase long-term cancer risk.

Oil well fires produced dense clouds of soot, liquid aerosols, and gases. Particulate concentrations between 500 and 2,000 $\mu g/m^3$ would have occurred during fumigation. Hydrogen sulfide, sulfur dioxide, and reduced sulfur compounds, together with the organic carbon and metals in the particulate phase, would cause pulmonary irritations. It is possible that prolonged exposure might lead to sinusitis, bronchiolitis, pneumonitis, asthma, or chronic obstructive pulmonary disease. Comprehensive air monitoring did not start until early May 1991 and it missed the most severe exposures to ground troops in Kuwait.

Sand Dust

Desert sand can be eroded by wind and mechanical disruption by vehicles. Troops experienced a dusty environment where ambient concentrations have been measured as high as a few milligrams per cubic meter. Inhalation of finely ground sand and associated dust certainly could have irritated upper airways of many and could possibly have exacerbated asthma. Long-term effects of inhaling resuspended sand are unknown, but are not likely to be associated with the complex of symptoms reported by Persian Gulf veterans.

Depleted Uranium

Depleted uranium in an aerosolized form, resulting from impacts and burning of the metal, provided a source of exposure for individuals in certain localized areas. The radioactivity associated with these operations was described as mostly below U.S. standards for acceptable exposure. The quantitation of radiation exposures that occurred should be attempted and the information made available so that any diseases arising in the future that may be connected with this exposure can be properly evaluated. Because of the latent period for most cancers, it is too soon to see significant increases.

Uranium, a heavy metal, causes kidney damage and, when inhaled, can accumulate in the lungs, but no pulmonary toxicity has been reported. The symptoms reported among the Persian Gulf veterans do not appear to be related to the heavy metal, uranium.

Pyridostigmine

Pyridostigmine was fielded as "pretreatment" for nerve agent poisoning in anticipation of chemical warfare. All personnel were provided with pyridostigmine bromide at doses of 30 mg in blister packs of 21 tablets each. The drug was ordered for self-administration by the major commanding officer when attack was thought to be imminent. The drug was self-administered every eight hours for up to seven days or until orders were given for discontinuation. Other coalition troops also used the drug. It is likely that a great majority of ground personnel received at least one dose and probably up to the full 21 tablets dispensed. However, there are reports that some personnel received repeated courses of the drug.

Pyridostigmine inhibits acetylcholinesterase. Short-term adverse drug effects were noted in some personnel including nausea, vomiting, genitourinary effects, headache, rhinorrhea, dizziness, tingling of the extremities, abdominal cramping, and dizziness. Reported side effects ranged from 5 to 50 percent in treated troops. These effects resulted in a medical visit in less than 1 percent of the cases. Pyridostigmine is eliminated primarily in the urine and does not enter the brain. It has an average plasma half-life of approximately 3.7 hours. When given at the prescribed dose and dose frequency, significant plasma or tissue accumulation is unlikely. However, numerous reports suggest that more severe acute effects occurred in Persian Gulf personnel.

Generally considered safe, pyridostigmine has been used in clinical medicine for decades in patients with myasthenia gravis, in doses up to 6,000 mg/day for life. No significant long-term adverse effects have been noted in these patients. Significant drug interactions that might heighten acute or chronic toxicity were not documented in the U.S. forces. Exposure to pesticides might enhance acute effects of pyridostigmine, but are unlikely to have chronic effects at these doses.

Pesticides

Pesticides and rodenticides approved by the Environmental Protection Agency were used in vector-borne or rodent disease prevention and control efforts. Application records for these agents do not exist, but their use was unrestricted. Relative quantities of pesticides available for use in operations are available from supply records, but total available tonnage was not available to the panel. Common pesticides used include d-phenothrin, chlorpyrifos, resmethrin, malathion, methomyl, lindane, pyrethroids, azamethiphos, and DEET. Potential acute adverse effects of organophosphates include headache, diarrhea, dizziness, blurred vision, weakness, nausea, cramps, discomfort in the chest, nervousness, sweating, miosis (pinpoint pupils), tearing, salivation, pulmonary edema, uncontrollable muscle twitches, convulsions, coma, and loss of reflexes and sphincter control. Nausea, incoordination, and eye and skin irritation can occur following acute pyrethroid exposure. Polyneuropathy can occur two to three weeks following high-level exposure to some organophosphates (malathion, chlorpyrifos).

Acute biological responses to pesticides in the Gulf War were not reported. Chronic responses to organophosphates are considered unlikely Because of the absence of reported polyneuropathy among the examined veterans.

Chemical Agent Resistant Coatings

Vehicles and equipment were painted with chemical agent resistant coatings (CARCs), either before being shipped to the Persian Gulf or at the port in Dammam/Dhahran. It was reported that CARC painting was conducted by civilian workers and a guard unit from Florida. CARCs contain toluene diisocyanate, which could lead to sensitization of the lung, including asthma. The exposures are considered to be limited to a small number of veterans.

Biological and Chemical Warfare Agents

Exposure to chemical and biological warfare agents remains controversial. Many veterans report that exposures occurred. There were numerous sightings of dead animals. The Czechs reported detection of both sarin and mustard gas in separate incidents. The Department of Defense reported no evidence of exposures. The preliminary report of the Department of Defense's "Defense Science Board," which was specifically charged to evaluate chemical and biological warfare, was not provided to the panel. Until it can be unequivocally established that chemical and/or biological weapons were not used and that troops were not exposed to plumes of destroyed stockpiles, the possibility remains that some symptoms are chronic manifestations of such exposure.

Vaccines

The Persian Gulf War participants were vaccinated against expected infectious diseases, as well as against two agents of biological warfare-anthrax and botulinum toxin. All the vaccines, except for the latter two, are standard reagents administered to all enlisted personnel and are also routinely given to civilians. The anthrax and botulinum vaccines, which are produced by the Michigan State Public Health Department, have been available for many years and have been given to thousands of civilian and military personnel. No long-term adverse effects have been documented.

Stressors

The stresses of the Persian Gulf experience have been of such a nature that the form of symptoms reported as a post-traumatic stress disorder (PTSD) needs to be understood in light of the unique types of stresses presented by that experience. The stresses include sudden mobilization for military service in a hot, sandy, strange southwest Asian desert; exposure to the largest, most dramatic oil well fires in history, which spilled smoke and oil over a vast area; and potential chemical and biological warfare. Although warfare has always been stressful and fear-inducing, the Persian Gulf War was the first combat experience in which the real threat of chemical and biological warfare was known to troops before entering the combat area.

The symptoms reported by veterans of the Persian Gulf War are multisystemic, often unassociated with objective signs of pathology, and not easily distinguished from other multisystem symptom complexes that have been described in the 9th International Classification of Diseases, such as chronic fatigue, fibromyalgia, and somatiform disorders. A variety of symptoms of unknown etiology have developed in some Persian Gulf veterans, accompanied by what appears to be a posttraumatic stress disorder that is distinct from or overlapping with classic PTSD. Perhaps the clinicians who applied standard criteria for PTSD from: *Third Edition, Revised the Diagnostic and Statistical Manual of Mental Disorders* = (DSM-III-R), such as numbing and flashbacks, may not have documented or paid sufficient attention to high body concerns and high physical symptom conditions in Persian Gulf veterans that reflect a post-traumatic stress disorder not emphasized by classic PTSD criteria. Some Persian Gulf veterans' behavioral responses, far from being numbed, are active, vivid anxiety manifestations expressed as multisystem physical symptoms. It is possible that the expression of post-traumatic distress may be distinct in the Persian Gulf experience and may take the form of somatic and multisystem symptoms rather than classic PTSD numbness and flashbacks. We are not suggesting that there is no physical basis for the reported symptoms, but that expression of the reported symptoms of posttraumatic stress disorder represents a psychophysiological response that needs to be evaluated.

Question 4: What future research is necessary?

- It is important that a more accurate estimate of the symptom prevalence be established. A short health questionnaire could be sent to all 700,000 veterans, or to a representative sample, including dates of service and a symptom checklist including illness in family members.

- A coordinated Department of Veterans Affairs and Department of Defense hospital-based case assessment protocol should be developed to provide a uniformly thorough assessment, diagnosis, and treatment of all Persian Gulf veterans with multisystem illness. An assessment strategy modeled after the Centers for Disease Control and Prevention (CDC) protocol for chronic fatigue syndrome is recommended. Such systematic diagnosis and evaluation would ensure the identification of specific treatable disease, would minimize the likelihood of misdiagnosis and inappropriate treatment, and would lead to a case definition needed for clinical, epidemiological, and other purposes.

- Only by comparing symptom rates among population groups can true underlying differences and unusual illnesses be revealed. Cohort studies are needed in which deployed and non-deployed soldiers are compared. Comparison populations should include those deployed elsewhere. Also needed are well-designed case-control studies that include detailed exposure information for those reporting symptoms and for appropriately selected controls. Case-control studies will permit the evaluation of specific exposures as possible etiologic agents for the illnesses reported by Gulf War veterans. Family studies should be included when appropriate.

- Pulmonary symptomatology is the most common reason for disability applications. Pulmonary functions of combat and support troops can be determined directly. The military should, therefore, conduct a retrospective cohort study to investigate pulmonary function related to oil fire plume exposures.

- The military should simulate the indoor situations associated with unvented heaters and other exposure scenarios involving petroleum, insecticides, and spray paints among others. Physical and mathematical modeling is a reasonable approach to estimating concentrations in situations representative of those experienced in the Persian Gulf operation. The exposure estimates obtained from these simulations should be used in conjunction with questionnaires to estimate individual exposure in the case-control and cohort studies described above.

- Research is needed to establish the relationship of stressors of deployment and combat to the constellation of symptoms afflicting some Gulf War veterans. The Department of Defense should anticipate how specific features of contemporary deployment and combat may contribute to acute and delayed psychophysiological dysfunction and should develop educational, training, and instructional protocols that reduce deployment and combat stress.

- The Department of Veterans Affairs should develop more responsive and effective approaches to diagnosis and therapy of veterans affected by stress-related or stress-exacerbated illness. Attention should be devoted to multidisciplinary research and clinical approaches that identify treatable conditions, provide objective assessments of physiological and neuropsychological dysfunction, and lead to interventional strategies to limit disability due to stress-related symptoms.

- The panel found that few data are available regarding the troops who served in the Persian Gulf and their exposures during that period of service and that data collection that was carried out was initiated only after a considerable delay. The panel therefore strongly recommends that the Department of Defense develop plans for prompt collection of high-quality, relevant data at any time U.S. forces are deployed in the future. The data collected should include baseline data regarding the pre-deployment health status of the troops, the environmental characteristics of their surroundings, their exposures during deployment, and their health status both at the end of deployment and subsequently. Plans for such data collection should be developed by a multidisciplinary group including clinicians, occupational physicians, epidemiologists, and industrial hygienists, among others. Input from outside the Department of Defense should be solicited before the plan is finalized, and the final plan should be reviewed and revised periodically thereafter. From the time this planning effort is initiated, the group or individuals who will be responsible for its successful implementation should be clearly designated.

- A previously unrecognized manifestation of leishmaniasis—viscerotropic leishmaniasis—was identified among some veterans suffering from symptoms compatible with the unexplained illness. Research that would facilitate more sensitive diagnosis, as well as identifying appropriate treatment and management of this disease, should be a high priority. A standard evaluation protocol should be established at all VA hospitals to screen veterans suffering from an unexplained illness for this infection.

Conclusions

- The complex biological, chemical, physical, and psychological environment of the Persian Gulf theater of operations appears to have produced complex adverse health effects in the primary military personnel.

- No single disease or syndrome is apparent, but rather there are multiple illnesses with overlapping symptoms and causes. Some of these diseases or illnesses can be sorted out by rigorous diagnostic, medical, and epidemiological procedures. Others may only be characterized after further research is conducted.

- A collaborative government-supported program has not been established. Evaluation of undiagnosed Persian Gulf illnesses has not followed a uniform protocol across military branches, VA facilities, and civilian physicians.

- This has led to imprecise description of diseases and/or symptoms, uncertainties about underlying prevalence rates, and inconsistent treatments. Well-designed epidemiological studies have not been conducted to link the illnesses of the military personnel with exposures in the Persian Gulf theater of operations. The absence of such studies has hampered the development of an appropriate case definition.

- Chronic symptoms of viscerotropic leishmaniasis and posttraumatic stress disorders were found to be compatible with some of the cases of unexplained illnesses. The proportion of these illnesses attributable to leishmaniasis and PTSD is unknown at this time, however.

Part Six

Chemicals and Poisons

Chapter 35

Citizen's Guide to Pesticides

Knowing Your Options

They're there. Whether you see them or not, you know they're there—in your home, your vegetable garden, your lawn, your fruit and shade trees, your flowers, and on your pets. They are pests—insects, weeds, fungi, rodents, and others. American households and their surrounding grounds are frequent hosts to common structural pests (termites, cockroaches, fleas, rodents), as well as a wide array of pests that are usually associated with agriculture. Because pests are all around—sometimes creating a nuisance but sometimes causing severe financial loss—consumers have turned increasingly to pesticides to control them. Just as "pests" can be anything from cockroaches in your kitchen to algae in your swimming pool, pesticides include insecticides, herbicides, fungicides, rodenticides, disinfectants, and plant growth regulators—anything that kills or otherwise controls a pest of any kind. The first and most important step in pest control is to identify the pest. Some pests, or signs of them, are unmistakable. Others are not. For example, some plant "diseases" are really indications of insufficient soil nutrients.

Three information sources are particularly helpful in identifying pests and appropriate pest control methods: reference books (such as insect field guides or gardening books), the County Extension Service, and pesticide dealers.

EPA. Pesticides and Toxic Substances (H7506C). Publication No. 22T-1002. November 1991.

The next step is to decide what level of treatment you want. Is anyone in the family or neighborhood particularly sensitive to chemical pesticides? Does your lawn really need to be totally weed-free? Do you need every fruit, vegetable, or flower you grow, or could you replace certain pest-prone species or varieties with hardier substitutes? Will you accept some blemished produce? In other words, do you need to eliminate all weeds and insects, or can you tolerate some pests?

Remember that total pest elimination is virtually impossible, and trying to eradicate pests from your premises will lead you to more extensive, repeated chemical treatments than are required for pest control. Remember, too, that to manage any pest effectively, you must use each method (or combination of methods) correctly. Finally, you must also abide by all pertinent local, state, and federal regulations.

Prevention

There is another important question to ask in making pest control decisions: is there something on your premises that needlessly invites pest infestations? The answer to this question may lead you to take some common-sense steps to modify pest habitat:

- **Remove water sources.** All pests, vertebrate or invertebrate, need water for survival. Fix leaky plumbing and do not let water accumulate anywhere in your home. This means no water in trays under your houseplants overnight if you have a cockroach infestation.

- **Remove food sources** (if the pest's food is anything other than the plant or animal you are trying to protect). For example, this could mean storing your food in sealed glass or plastic containers, avoiding the habit of leaving your pet's food out for extended periods of time, and placing your refuse in tightly covered, heavy-gauge garbage cans.

- **Remove or destroy pest shelter.** Caulk cracks and crevices to control cockroaches; remove piles of wood from under or around your home in order to avoid attracting termites; remove and destroy diseased plants, tree prunings, and fallen fruit that might harbor pests.

- **Remove breeding sites.** The presence of pet manure attracts flies, litter encourages rodents, and standing water provides a perfect breeding place for mosquitoes.

- **Remove sources of preventable stress to plants** (flowers, trees, vegetable plants, and turf). Plant at the optimum time of year. Use mulch to reduce weed competition and maintain even soil temperature and moisture. Provide adequate water.

- **Use preventive cultural practices,** such as careful selection of disease-resistant seed or plant varieties, companion planting to exploit the insect-repellent properties of certain plants, strategic use of "trap" crops to lure pests away from crops you wish to protect, crop rotation and diversification, and optimum use of spacing. Make sure you have good drainage and soil aeration.

Non-chemical Controls

If you practice preventive techniques such as those mentioned above, you will reduce your chances, or frequency, of pest infestation. However, if you already have an infestation, are there any pest control alternatives besides chemical pesticides?

The answer is an emphatic "yes." One or a combination of several non-chemical treatment alternatives may be appropriate. Your best strategy depends on the pest and the site where the pest occurs.

Non-chemical alternatives include:

- **Biological treatments,** including predators such as purple martins, praying mantises, and lady bugs; parasites; and pathogens such as bacteria, viruses (generally not available to home-owners), and other microorganisms like *Bacillus thuringiensis* and milky spore disease. There is no way to be certain how long predators will stay in target areas. Contact your County Extension Service for information about how to protect desirable predators.

- **Mechanical treatments,** including cultivating to control weeds, hand-picking weeds from turf and pests from plants, trapping to control rodents and some insects, and screening living space to limit mosquito and fly access.

Non-chemical pest control methods really work. They do have some disadvantages: the results are not immediate, and it requires some work to make a home or garden less attractive to pests. But the advantages of non-chemical methods are many. Compared to chemical pesticide treatments, such methods are generally effective for longer periods of time. They do not create hardy, pesticide-resistant pest populations. And they can be used without safeguards, because they pose virtually no hazards to human health or the environment.

Chemical Controls

If you decide that chemical treatment can provide the best solution to your pest problem, and you want to control the pests yourself rather than turning the problem over to a professional pest control operator, then you have an important decision to make: which product to choose. Before making that decision, learn as much as you can about a product's active ingredient—its biologically active agent. Is it "broad-spectrum" in its mode of action (effective against a broad range of pests), or is it "selective" (effective against only a few pest species)? How rapidly does the active ingredient break down once it is introduced into the environment? Is it suspected of causing chronic health effects? Is it toxic to non-target wildlife and house pets? Is it known, or suspected, to leach through soil into ground water?

Here again, your County Extension Service, reference books, pesticide dealers, your state pesticide agency, or your regional EPA office may be able to provide assistance.

When you have narrowed your choices of active ingredients, you are ready to select a pesticide product. Choose the least toxic pesticide that can achieve the results you desire. Read the label. It lists active ingredients, the target pests (for example, mites, flies, Japanese beetle grubs, broad-leafed weeds, algae, etc.), and the sites where the product may be used (for example, lawns, specific vegetable crops, roses, swimming pools, etc.). Be sure the site of your pest problem is included among the sites listed on the label.

Pesticide active ingredients are formulated in many ways. Choose the formulation best suited to your site and the pest you are trying to control. The most common types of home-use pesticide formulations include:

- **Solutions,** which contain the active ingredient and one or more additives, and readily mix with water.

- **Aerosols,** which contain one or more active ingredients and a solvent. They are ready for immediate use as is.

- **Dusts,** which contain active ingredients plus a very fine dry inert carrier such as clay, talc, or volcanic ash. Dusts are ready for immediate use and are applied dry.

- **Granulars,** which are similar to dusts, but with larger and heavier particles for broadcast applications.

- **Baits,** which are active ingredients mixed with food or other substances to attract the pest.

- **Wettable powders,** which are dry, finely ground formulations that generally are mixed with water for spray application. Some also may be used as dusts.

Depending on the type of formulation you choose, you may need to dilute or mix the product. Prepare only the amount that you need for each application; don't prepare larger amounts to store for possible future use. (See "Determining Correct Dosage.")

Once you have identified the pest, selected the right pesticide, and determined proper dosage, you are ready to use the product. Application technique and timing are every bit as important as the material used, so read the label for directions. That advice—to read the label—is repeated so often in this guide that it may become tiresome. But in fact, the advice cannot be repeated often enough. Read the label before you buy a product, and again before you mix it, before you apply it, before you store it, and before you throw it away. The directions on a label are there for a very good reason: to help you achieve maximum benefits with minimum risk. But these benefits depend upon proper use of the products.

Chemical pesticides also have their disadvantages. They must be used very carefully to achieve results while protecting users and the environment. The results are generally temporary, and repeated treatments may be required.

Therefore, to achieve best results when you do use chemical pesticides, use preventive and non-chemical treatments along with them. This will reduce the need for repeated applications.

You should always evaluate your pesticide use, comparing pre-treatment and post-treatment conditions. You should weigh the benefits of short-term chemical pesticide control against the benefits of long-term control using a variety of techniques. Knowledge of a range of pest control techniques gives you the ability to pick and choose among them. Pests, unfortunately, will always be around us, and, if you know about all pest control options, you will know what to do the next time THEY'RE THERE.

Tips for Handling Pesticides

Pesticides Are Not "Safe." They are produced specifically because they are toxic to something. By heeding all the following tips, you can reduce your risks when you use pesticides.

- All pesticides legally marketed in the United States must bear an EPA-approved label; check the label to make sure it bears an EPA registration number.

- Before using a pesticide, read the entire label. Even if you have used the pesticide before, read the label again—don't trust your memory. Use of any pesticide in any way that is not consistent with label directions and precautions is subject to civil and/or criminal penalties.

- Do not use a "restricted use" pesticide unless you are a formally trained, certified pesticide applicator. These products are too dangerous to be used without special training.

- Follow use directions carefully. Use only the amount directed, at the time and under the conditions specified, and for the purpose listed. Don't think that twice the dosage will do twice the job. It won't. What's worse, you may harm yourself, others, or whatever you are trying to protect.

- Look for one of the following signal words on the front of the label. It will tell you how hazardous a pesticide is if swallowed, inhaled, or absorbed through skin.

"DANGER" means highly poisonous;
"WARNING" means moderately hazardous;
"CAUTION" means least hazardous.

- Wear the items of protective clothing the label requires: for example, long sleeves and long pants, impervious gloves, rubber (not canvas or leather) footwear, hat, and goggles. Personal protective clothing usually is available at home building supply stores.

- If you must mix or dilute the pesticide, do so outdoors or in a well-ventilated area. Mix only the amount you need and use portions listed on the label.

- Keep children and pets away from areas where you mix or apply pesticides.

- If a spill occurs, clean it up promptly. Don't wash it away. Instead, sprinkle with sawdust, vermiculite, or kitty litter; sweep into a plastic garbage bag; and dispose with the rest of your trash.

- Remove pets (including birds and fish) and toys from the area to be treated. Remove food, dishes, pots, and pans before treating kitchen cabinets, and don't let pesticides get on these surfaces. Wait until shelves dry before refilling them.

- Allow adequate ventilation when applying pesticides indoors. Go away from treated areas for at least the length of time prescribed by the label. When spraying outdoors, close the windows of your home

- Most surface sprays should be applied only to limited areas; don't treat entire floors, walls, or ceilings

- Never place rodent or insect baits where small children or pets can reach them.

- When applying spray or dust outdoors, cover fish ponds, and avoid applying pesticides near wells. Always avoid over-application when treating lawn, shrubs, or gardens. Runoff or seepage from excess pesticide usage may contaminate water supplies. Excess spray may leave harmful residues on home-grown produce.

- Keep herbicides away from non-target plants. Avoid applying any pesticide to blooming plants, especially if you see honeybees or other pollinating insects around them. Avoid birds' nests when spraying trees.

- Never spray or dust outdoors on a windy day.

- Never smoke while applying pesticides. You could easily carry traces of the pesticide from hand to mouth. Also, some products are flammable.

- Never transfer pesticides to containers not intended for them, such as empty soft drink bottles. Keep pesticides in containers that clearly and prominently identify the contents. Properly refasten all childproof caps.

- Shower and shampoo thoroughly after using a pesticide product. Wash the clothing that you wore when applying the product separately from the family laundry. To prevent tracking chemicals inside, also rinse boots and shoes before entering your home.

- Before using a pesticide product, know what to do in case of accidental poisoning.

- To remove residues, use a bucket to triple rinse tools or equipment, including any containers or utensils used to mix the chemicals. Then pour the rinse water into the pesticide container and reuse the solution by applying it according to the pesticide product label directions.

- Evaluate the results of your pesticide use.

Determining Correct Dosage

So much information is packed onto pesticide labels that there is usually no room to include examples of each dilution applicable to the multitude of home-use situations. As a result, label examples may inadvertently encourage preparation of more pesticide than is needed. The excess may contribute to overuse, safety problems related to storage and disposal, or simply wasted costs of unused pesticide.

Determining the correct dosage for different types of pesticides requires some simple calculations. The following information can help you to prepare the minimum quantity of pesticide needed for your immediate use situation.

For example, the product label says, "For the control of aphids on tomatoes, mix eight fluid ounces of pesticide into 1 gallon water and spray until foliage is wet." Your experience has been that your six tomato plants require only one quart of pesticide to wet all the foliage. Therefore, only two fluid ounces of the pesticide should be mixed into 1 quart of water. Why? Because a quart is one-fourth of a gallon, and two fluid ounces mixed into 1 quart make the same strength spray recommended by the label, but in a quantity that can be used up all at once.

Consumers can solve problems similar to this one with careful arithmetic, good measurements, and intelligent use of the information provided here.

How to Measure

If you need to determine the size of a square or rectangular area, such as a lawn for herbicide application, measure and multiply the length and width. For example, an area 10 feet long by 8 feet wide contains 80 square feet. Common area measurements may involve square yards (one square yard = nine square feet) or square feet (one square foot = 144 square inches).

If you need to determine the volume of a space such as a room, measure and multiply the room's length, width, and height. For example, a space 10 feet long, 8 feet wide, and 8 feet high contains a volume of 640 cubic feet. You would use this procedure, for instance, for an aerosol release to control cockroaches.

Most residential-use pesticides are measured in terms of volume. Some common equivalents are:

1 gallon (gal.)
    = 128 fluid ounces (fl. oz.)
    = 4 quarts (qt.)
    = 8 pints (pt.)
    = 16 cups

1 qt.
    = 32 fl. oz.
    = 2 pt.
    = 4 cups

1 pt.
> = 16 fl. oz.
> = 2 cups

1 cup
> = 8 fl. oz.

1 tablespoon
> = 1/2 fl. oz.
> = 3 teaspoons

1 teaspoon
> = 1/6 fl. oz.

In measuring teaspoons or tablespoons of pesticide, use only level spoonfuls, and never use the same measuring devices for food preparation.

The following table provides examples to help you convert label information to your specific use situations. "Amount" can be any measure of pesticide quantity. However, the same unit of measure must be used on both sides of the chart. For example, eight fluid ounces per gallon of water is equivalent to two fluid ounces per quart of water.

Not all dosage rates are included in the examples given here. For rates not included, remember that, for pesticides not diluted with water, proportionally change both the quantity of pesticide and the area, volume, or number of items treated. For example, one-half pound per 1,000 square feet is equivalent to one-quarter pound per 500 square feet. For a pesticide that is diluted with water, proportionally change the quantity of pesticide, the quantity of water, and the area, volume, or number of items treated. For example, one-half pound of pesticide in 1 gallon of water applied to 1,000 square feet is equivalent to 1 pound of pesticide in 2 gallons of water applied to 2,000 square feet.

There is a point at which measurements needed for smaller quantities of pesticides are too minute to be accurately measured with typical domestic measuring devices. In such cases, the user can either mix the larger volume, realizing that there will be leftover material; obtain a more accurate measuring device, such as a graduated cylinder or a scale which measures small weights; or search for an alternative pesticide or less concentrated formulation of the same pesticide.

Pesticide Label Says Mix			Amount of Pesticide Per	
Amount Pesticide	Per		1 qt. Water	1 pt. Water
8 units	1 gal. water	EQUALS	2 units	1 unit
16 units	1 gal. water	EQUALS	4 units	2 units
32 units	1 gal. water	EQUALS	8 units	4 units
128 units	1 gal. water	EQUALS	32 units	16 units

Pesticide Label Says Apply			Amount of Pesticide Per		
Amount Pesticide	Per		20,000 sq. ft.	10,000 sq. ft	500 sq. ft.
1 unit	1,000 sq. ft.	EQUALS	20 units	10 units	½ unit
2 units	1,000 sq. ft.	EQUALS	40 units	20 units	1 unit
5 units	1,000 sq. ft.	EQUALS	100 units	50 units	2½ units
10 units	1,000 sq. ft.	EQUALS	200 units	100 units	5 units

Pesticide Label Says Release			Cans Per		
Aerosol Cans	Per		20,000 cu. ft.	10,000 cu. ft.	5,000 cu. ft.
1	10,000 cu. ft.	EQUALS	2	1	don't use
1	5,000 cu. ft.	EQUALS	4	2	1
1	2,500 cu. ft.	EQUALS	8	4	2

Table 35.1.

Correct Storage and Disposal

The following tips on home storage and disposal can help you handle pesticides correctly.

Storage

- Buy only enough product to carry you through the use season, to reduce storage problems.

- Store pesticides away from children and pets. A locked cabinet in a well-ventilated utility area or garden shed is best.

- Store flammable liquids outside living quarters and away from an ignition source.

- Never put pesticides in cabinets with, or near, food, medical supplies, or cleaning materials. Always store pesticides in their original containers, complete with labels that list ingredients, directions for use, and antidotes in case of accidental poisoning. Never transfer pesticides to soft drink bottles or other containers that children may associate with something to eat or drink. Always properly refasten child-proof closures or lids.

- Avoid storing pesticides in places where flooding is possible, or in open places where they might spill or leak into the environment. If you have any doubt about the content of a container, dispose of it with your trash.

Disposal

- The best way to dispose of a small, excess amount of pesticide is to use it—apply it according to directions on the product label. If you cannot use it, ask your neighbor whether he/she can use it. If all the pesticide cannot be used, first check with your local health department or solid waste management agency to determine whether your community has a household hazardous waste collection program or any other program for handling disposal of pesticides.

- If no community programs exist, follow label directions regarding container disposal. To dispose of less than a full container of a liquid pesticide, leave it in the original container, with the cap securely in place to prevent spills or leaks. Wrap the container in several layers of newspapers and tie securely. Then place the package in a covered trash can for routine collection with municipal refuse. If you do not have a regular trash collection service, take the package to a permitted landfill (unless your municipality has other requirements).

  Note: No more than one gallon of liquid pesticide should be disposed of in this manner.

- Wrap individual packages of dry pesticide formulations in several layers of newspaper, or place the package in a tight carton or bag, and tape or tie it closed. As with liquid formulations, place the package in a covered trash can for routine collection.

  Note: No more than 5 pounds of pesticide at a time should be disposed of in this manner.

- Do not pour leftover pesticides down the sink or into the toilet. Chemicals in pesticides could interfere with the operation of wastewater treatment systems or could pollute waterways, because many municipal systems cannot remove all pesticide residues.

- An empty pesticide container can be as hazardous as a full one because of residues remaining inside. Never reuse such a container. When empty, a pesticide container should be carefully rinsed and thoroughly drained. Liquids used to rinse the container should be added to the sprayer or to the container previously used to mix the pesticide and used according to label directions.

    Empty product containers made of plastic or metal should be punctured to prevent reuse. (Do not puncture or burn a pressurized product container it could explode.) Glass containers should be rinsed and drained, as described above, and the cap or closure replaced securely. After rinsing, an empty mixing container or sprayer may also be wrapped and placed in the trash.

- If you have any doubts about proper pesticide disposal, contact your state or local health department, your solid waste management agency, or the regional EPA office.

How to Choose a Pest Control Company

Termites are chomping away at your house. Roaches are taking over your kitchen. Mouse droppings dot your dresser drawer. You've got a pest control problem, and you've decided that it's too serious for you to solve on your own. You've decided you need a professional exterminator.

If you find yourself in a situation like this, what can you do to be sure that the pest control company you hire will do a good job? Here are some questions you can ask:

1. Does the company have a good track record?

    Don't rely on the company salesman to answer this question; research the answer yourself. Ask around among neighbors and friends; have any of them dealt with the company before? Were they satisfied with the service they received? Call the Better Business Bureau or local consumer office; have they received any complaints about the company?

2. Does the company have insurance? What kind of insurance? Can the salesman show some documentation to prove that the company is insured?

   Contractor's general liability insurance, including insurance for sudden and accidental pollution, gives you as a homeowner a certain degree of protection should an accident occur while pesticides are being applied in your home. Contractor's workmen's compensation insurance can also help protect you should an employee of the contractor be injured while working in your home. In most states, pest control companies are not required to buy insurance, but you should think twice before dealing with a company that is uninsured.

3. Is the company licensed?

   Regulatory agencies in some states issue state pest control licenses. Although the qualifications for a license vary from state to state, at a minimum the license requires that each company have a certified pesticide applicator present in the office on a daily basis to supervise the work of exterminators using restricted-use pesticides. (Certified applicators are formally trained and "certified" as qualified to use or supervise the use of pesticides that are classified for restricted use.) If restricted-use pesticides are to be applied on your premises, make sure the pest control operator's license is current. Also ask if the company's employees are bonded.

   You may want to contact your state lead pesticide agency to ask about its pesticide certification and training programs and to inquire if periodic recertification is required for pest control operators.

   In addition to the licenses required in some states, some cities also issue pest control licenses. Again, qualifications vary, but possession of a city license—where they are available—is one more assurance that the company you are dealing with is reputable and responsible.

4. Is the company affiliated with a professional pest control association?

   Professional associations—whether national, state, or local—keep members informed of new developments in pest control methods, safety, training, research, and regulation. They also have codes of ethics that members agree to abide by. The fact that a company, small or large, chooses to affiliate itself with a professional association signals its concern for the quality of its work.

5. Does the company stand behind its work? What assurances does the company make?

You should think twice about dealing with a company unwilling to stand behind its work. Be sure to find out what you must do to keep your part of the bargain. For example, in the case of termite control treatments, a guarantee may be invalidated if structural alterations are made without prior notice to the pest control company.

6. Is the company willing, and able, to discuss the treatment proposed for your home?

Selecting a pest control service is just as important as selecting other professional services. Look for the same high degree of competence you would expect from a doctor or lawyer. The company should inspect your premises and outline a recommended control program, including what pests are to be controlled; the extent of the infestation; what pesticide formulation will be used in your home and why; what techniques will be used in application; what alternatives to the formulation and techniques could be used instead; what special instructions you should follow to reduce your exposure to the pesticide (such as vacating the house, emptying the cupboards, removing pets, etc.); and what you can do to minimize your pest problems in the future.

Contracts should be jointly developed. Any safety concerns should be noted and reflected in the choice of pesticides to be used. These concerns could include allergies, age of occupants (infants or elderly), or pets. You may want to get two to three bids from different companies—evaluate them by value, not price. What appears to be a bargain may merit a second look.

Even after you have hired a company, you should continue your vigilance. Evaluate results. If you have reason to believe that something has gone wrong with the pesticide application, contact the company and/or your state/lead pesticide agency. Don't let your guard down, and don't stop asking questions.

How to Reduce Your Exposure to Pesticides

Because chemical pesticides are so widely used in our society, and because of the properties of many of the chemicals, low levels of pesticide residues are found throughout the environment. Pesticides reach us in a variety of ways—through food, water, and air.

In regulating pesticides, EPA strives to ensure that lawful use of these products will not result in harmful exposures. Proper use of registered products should yield residue levels that are well within established safety standards. Therefore, the average American's exposure to low-level residues, though fairly constant, should not cause alarm.

Still, many people want to learn what choices they can make to further reduce their exposure to any potential risks associated with pesticides. By limiting your exposure to these products, you can keep your risks to a minimum.

Below you will find descriptions of the main pathways of human exposure to pesticides, as well as suggestions on ways to reduce overall exposure and attendant risks. If, however, you suspect that you suffer from serious chemical sensitivities, consult an expert to develop a more personally tailored approach to managing this problem.

Exposure Through Food

Commercial Food. Throughout life—beginning even before birth—we are all exposed to pesticides. A major source of exposure is through our diets. We constantly consume small amounts of pesticides. Fruits and vegetables, as well as meat poultry, eggs, and milk, are all likely to contain measurable pesticide residues.

EPA sets standards, called tolerances, to limit the amount of pesticide residues that legally may remain in or on food or animal feed marketed in U.S. commerce. Both domestic and imported foods are monitored by the Food and Drug Administration (FDA) and the U.S. Department of Agriculture (USDA) to ensure compliance with these tolerances. Further, since pesticide residues generally tend to degrade over time and through processing, residue concentrations in or on most foods are well below legal tolerance levels by the time the foods are purchased.

Although EPA does limit dietary pesticide exposure through tolerances, you may wish to take extra precautions. You can take several steps to reduce your exposure to residues in purchased food.

- Rinse fruit and vegetables thoroughly with water; scrub them with a brush and peel them, if possible. Although this surface cleaning will not remove "systemic" pesticide residues taken up into the growing fruit or vegetable, it will remove most of the existing surface residues, not to mention any dirt.

- Cook or bake foods to reduce residues of some (but not all) pesticides.

- Trim the fat from meat and poultry. Discard the fats and oils in broths and pan drippings, since residues of some pesticides concentrate in fat.

Home-grown Food. Growing some of your own food can be both a pleasurable activity and a way to reduce your exposure to pesticide residues in food. But, even here, there are some things you may want to do to assure that exposure is limited.

- Before converting land in an urban or suburban area to gardening, find out how the land was used previously. Choose a site that had limited (or no) chemical applications and where drift or runoff from your neighbor's activities will not result in unintended pesticide residues on your produce. Choose a garden site strategically to avoid these potential routes of entry, if possible.

  If you are taking over an existing garden plot, be aware that the soil may contain pesticide residues from previous gardening activities. These residues may remain in the soil for several years, depending on the persistence of the pesticides that were used. Rather than waiting for the residues to decline naturally over time, you may speed the process.

- Plant an interim, non-food crop like annual rye grass, clover, or alfalfa. Such crops, with their dense, fibrous root systems, will take up some of the lingering pesticide residues. Then discard the crops—don't work them back into the soil—and continue to alternate food crops with cover crops in the off season.

- During sunny periods, turn over the soil as often as every two to three days for a week or two. The sunlight will help to break down, or photodegrade, some of the pesticide residues.

  Once you do begin gardening, develop strategies that will reduce your need for pesticides while maintaining good crop yields.

- Concentrate on building your garden's soil, since healthy soil grows healthy plants. Feed the soil with compost, manure, etc., to increase its capacity to support strong crops.

- Select seeds and seedlings from hardy, disease-resistant varieties. The resulting plants are less likely to need pesticides in order to flourish.

- Avoid monoculture gardening techniques. Instead, alternate rows of different kinds of plants to prevent significant pest problems from developing.

- Don't plant the same crop in the same spot year after year if you want to reduce plant susceptibility to over-wintered pests.

- Become familiar with integrated pest management (IPM) techniques, so that you can manage any pest outbreaks that do occur without relying solely on pesticides.

- Mulch your garden with leaves, hay, grass clippings, shredded/chipped bark, or seaweed. Avoid using newspapers to keep down weeds, and sewage sludge to fertilize plants. Newsprint may contain heavy metals; sludge may contain heavy metals and pesticides, both of which can leach into your soil.

Food from the Wild. While it might seem that hunting your own game, catching your own fish, or gathering wild plant foods would reduce your overall exposure to pesticides, this isn't necessarily so. Wild foods hunted, caught, or gathered in areas where pesticides are frequently used outdoors may contain pesticide residues. Migratory species also may contain pesticide residues if these chemicals are used anywhere in their flyways.

Tolerances generally are not established or enforced for pesticides found in wild game, fowl, fish, or plants. Thus, if you consume food from the wild, you may want to take the following steps to reduce your exposure to pesticide residues.

- Because wild game is very lean, there is less fat in which pesticides can accumulate. However, avoid hunting in areas where pesticide usage is very high.

- Avoid fishing in water bodies where water contamination is known to have occurred. Pay attention to posted signs warning of contamination.

- You may want to consult with fish and game officials where you plan to hunt or fish to determine whether there are any pesticide problems associated with that area.

- When picking wild plant foods, avoid gathering right next to a road, utility right-of-way, or hedgerow between farm fields which probably have been treated (directly or indirectly) with pesticides. Instead, seek out fields that have not been used to produce crops, deep woods, or other areas where pesticide use is unlikely.

- When preparing wild foods, trim fat from meat, and discard skin of fish to remove as many fat-soluble pesticide residues as possible. For wild plant foods, follow the tips provided for commercial food.

Exposure Through Water

Whether it comes from surface or ground water sources, the water flowing from your tap may contain low levels of pesticides.

When pesticides are applied to land, a certain amount may run off the land into streams and rivers. This runoff, coupled with industrial discharges, can result in low-level contamination of surface water. In certain hydrogeologic settings—for example, sandy soil over a ground water source that is near the surface-pesticides can leach down through the soil to the ground water.

EPA's Water Program sets standards and provides advisory levels for pesticides and other chemicals that may be found in drinking water. Public municipal water systems test their water periodically and provide treatment or alternate supply sources if residue problems arise. Private wells generally are not tested unless the well owner requests such analysis.

If you get your drinking water from a private well, you can reduce the chance of contaminating your water supply by following these guidelines:

- Be cautious about using pesticides and other chemicals on your property, especially if the well is shallow or is not tightly constructed. Check with your EPA regional office or County Extension Service before using a pesticide outdoors, to determine whether it is known or suspected to leach to ground water. Never use or mix a pesticide near your well head.

- To avoid pesticide contamination problems, be sure your well extends downward to aquifers that are below, and isolated from, surface aquifers, and be sure the well shaft is tightly sealed. If you have questions about pesticide or other chemical residues in your well water, contact your state or county health department.

- If your well water is analyzed and found to contain pesticide residue levels above established or recommended health standards, you may wish to use an alternate water source such as bottled water for drinking and cooking. The best choice is distilled spring water in glass bottles. Ask your local bottler for the results of a recent pesticide analysis.

Exposure Through Air

Outdoors, air currents may carry pesticides that were applied on adjacent property or miles away. But there are steps you can take to reduce your exposure to airborne pesticide residue, or drift, outdoors. To reduce your exposure to airborne pesticides:

- Avoid applying pesticides in windy weather (when winds exceed 10 miles per hour).

- Use coarse droplet nozzles to reduce misting.

- Apply the spray as close to the target as possible.

- Keep the wind to your side so that sprays and dusts do not blow into your face.

- If someone else is applying pesticides outdoors near your home, stay indoors with your pets and children, keeping doors and windows closed. If it is very windy during the pesticide application, stay inside for an hour or two.

- If pesticides are applied frequently near your home (if you live next to fields receiving regular pesticide treatment), consider planting a buffer zone of thick-branched trees and shrubs upwind to help serve as a buffer zone and windbreak.

- Many local governments require public notification in advance of area-wide or broad-scale pesticide spray activities and programs—through announcements in newspapers, letters to area residents, or posting of signs in areas to be treated. Some communities have also enacted "right to know" ordinances which require public notification, usually through posting, of lawn treatments and other small-scale outdoor pesticide uses. If your local government does not require notifications, either for large- or small-scale applications, you may want to work with local officials to develop such requirements.

  Indoors, the air you breathe may bear pesticide residues long after a pesticide has been applied to objects in your home or office, or to indoor surfaces and crawl spaces. Pesticides dissipate more slowly indoors than outdoors. In addition, energy efficiency features built into many homes reduce air exchange, aggravating the problem. To limit your exposure to indoor pesticide residues:

- Use pesticides indoors only when absolutely necessary, and then use only limited amounts. Provide adequate ventilation during and after application. If you hire a pest control company, oversee its activities carefully.

- If pesticides are used inside your home, air out the house often, since outdoor air generally is fresher and purer than indoor air. Open doors and windows, and run overhead or whole-house fans to exchange indoor air for outside air rapidly and completely.

- If pesticides have been used extensively and an indoor air contamination problem has developed, clean—scrub—all surfaces where pesticides may have settled, including cracks and crevices.

Consult a knowledgeable professional for advice on appropriate cleaning materials if soap and water are insufficient.

Exposure Through Home Usage

Over a lifetime, diet is the most significant source of pesticide exposure for the general public. However, on a short-term basis, the most significant exposure source is personal pesticide use.

An array of pesticide products, ranging widely in toxicity and potential effects, is available "off the shelf" to the private user. No special training is required to purchase or use these products, and no one is looking over the users' shoulder, monitoring their vigilance in reading and following label instructions. Yet many of these products are hazardous, especially if they are stored, handled, or applied improperly.

To minimize the hazards and maximize the benefits that pesticides bring, exercise caution and respect when using any pesticide product.

- Consider pesticide labeling to be what it is intended to be: your best guide to using pesticides safely and effectively.

- Pretend that the pesticide product you are using is more toxic than you think it is. Take special precautions to ensure an extra margin of protection for yourself, your family, and pets.

- Don't use more pesticide than the label says. You may not achieve a higher degree of pest control, and you will certainly experience a higher degree of risk.

- If you hire a pest control firm to do the job, ask the company to use the least toxic or any chemical-free pest control means available that will do the job. For example, some home pest control companies offer an electro-gun technique to control termite and similar infestations by penetrating infested areas and "frying" the problem pests without using any chemicals.

- And remember: sometimes a non-pesticidal approach is as convenient and effective as its chemical alternatives. Consider using such non-pesticidal approaches whenever possible.

"Someone's Been Poisoned. Help!"

What to Do in a Pesticide Emergency

The potential for a pesticide to cause injury depends upon several factors:

- **Toxicity of the active ingredient.** Toxicity is a measure of the inherent ability of a chemical to produce injury Some pesticides, such as pyrethrins, have low human toxicity while others, such as sodium fluoroacetate, are extremely toxic.

- **Dose.** The greater the dose of a specific pesticide, i.e., the amount absorbed, the greater the risk of injury. Dose is dependent upon the absolute amount of the pesticide absorbed relative to the weight of the person. Therefore, small amounts of a pesticide might produce illness in a small child while the same dose of the same pesticide in an adult might be relatively harmless.

- **Route of absorption.** Swallowing a pesticide usually creates the most serious problem. In practice, however, the most common route of absorption of pesticides is through the skin and the most toxic pesticides have resulted in death through this route of exposure.

- **Duration of exposure.** The longer a person is exposed to pesticides, the higher the level in the body. There is a point at which an equilibrium will develop between the intake and the output. Then, the level will no longer continue to increase. However, this point may be either above or below the known toxic level.

- **Physical and chemical properties.** The distribution and the rates of breakdown of pesticides in the environment significantly alter the likelihood that injury might occur.

- **Population at risk.** Persons who run the greatest danger of poisoning are those whose exposure is highest, such as workers who mix, load, or apply pesticides. However, the general public also faces the possibility of exposure.

Recognizing Pesticide Poisoning

Like other chemicals, pesticides may produce injury externally or internally.

External irritants may cause contact-associated skin disease primarily of an irritant nature—producing redness, itching, or pimples—or an allergic skin reaction, producing redness, swelling, or blistering. The mucous membranes of the eyes, nose, mouth, and throat are also quite sensitive to chemicals. Stinging and swelling can occur.

Internal injuries from any chemical may occur depending upon where a chemical is transported in the body. Thus, symptoms are dependent upon the organ involved. Shortness of breath, clear saliva, or rapid breathing may occur as the result of lung injury. Nausea, vomiting, abdominal cramps, or diarrhea may result from direct injury to the gastrointestinal tract. Excessive fatigue, sleepiness, headache, muscle twitching, and loss of sensation may result from injury to the nervous system. In general, different classes of pesticides produce different sets of symptoms.

For example, organophosphate pesticides may produce symptoms of pesticide poisoning affecting several different organs, and may progress rapidly from very mild to severe. Symptoms may progress in a matter of minutes from slight difficulty with vision to paralysis of the diaphragm muscle, causing inability to breathe.

Therefore, if someone develops symptoms after working with pesticides, seek medical help promptly to determine if the symptoms are pesticide-related. In certain cases, blood or urine can be collected for analysis, or other specific exposure tests can be made. It is better to be too cautious than too late.

It is always important to avoid problems by minimizing your exposure when mixing and applying pesticides by wearing gloves and other protective clothing.

The appropriate first aid treatment depends upon which pesticide was used. Here are some tips for first aid that may precede, but should not substitute for, medical treatment:

- **Poison on skin.** Drench skin with water and remove contaminated clothing. Wash skin and hair thoroughly with soap and water. Dry victim and wrap in blanket. Later, discard contaminated clothing or thoroughly wash it separately from other laundry.

- **Chemical burn on skin.** Drench skin with water and remove contaminated clothing. Cover burned area immediately with loose, clean, soft cloth. Do not apply ointments, greases, powders, or other drugs. Later, discard or thoroughly wash contaminated clothing separately from other laundry.

- **Poison in eye.** Eye membranes absorb pesticides faster than any other external part of the body; eye damage can occur in a few minutes with some types of pesticides. Hold eyelid open and wash eye quickly and gently with clean running water from the tap or a hose for 15 minutes or more. Do not use eye drops or chemicals or drugs in the wash water.

- **Inhaled poison.** Carry or drag victim to fresh air immediately. (If proper protection is unavailable to you, call for emergency equipment from the Fire Department.) Loosen victim's tight clothing. If the victim's skin is blue or the victim has stopped breathing, give artificial respiration and call rescue service for help. Open doors and windows so no one else will be poisoned by fumes.

- **Swallowed poison.** A conscious victim should rinse his mouth with plenty of water and then drink up to one quart of milk or water to dilute the pesticide. Induce vomiting only if instructions to do so are on the label. If there is no label available to guide you, do not induce vomiting. Never induce vomiting if the victim is unconscious or is having convulsions.

In dealing with any poisoning, act fast; speed is crucial.

First Aid for Pesticide Poisoning

First aid is the first step in treating a pesticide poisoning. Study the "Statement of Treatment" on the product label before you use a pesticide. When you realize a pesticide poisoning is occurring, be sure the victim is not being further exposed to the poison before calling for emergency help. An unconscious victim will have to be dragged into fresh air. Caution: do not become poisoned yourself while trying to help. You may have to put on breathing equipment or protective clothing to avoid becoming the second victim.

After giving initial first aid, get medical help immediately. This advice cannot be repeated too often. Bring the product container with its label to the doctor's office or emergency room where the victim will be treated; keep the container out of the passenger space of your vehicle. The doctor needs to know what chemical is in the pesticide before prescribing treatment (information that is also on the label). Sometimes the label even includes a telephone number to call for additional treatment information.

A good resource in a pesticide emergency is NPTN, the National Pesticide Telecommunications Network, a toll-free telephone service. Operators are on call 24 hours a day, 365 days a year, to provide information on pesticides and on recognizing and responding to pesticide poisonings. If necessary they can transfer inquiries directly to affiliated poison control centers.

National Pesticide
Telecommunications Network
Call Toll-Free 1-800-858-7378

NPTN operators answer questions about animal as well as human poisonings. To keep your pets from being poisoned, follow label directions on flea and tick products carefully, and keep pets off lawns that have been newly treated with weed killers and insecticides.

EPA is interested in receiving information on any adverse effects associated with pesticide exposure. If you have such information, contact Frank Davido, Pesticide Incident Response Officer, Field Operations Division (H-7506C), Office of Pesticide Programs, EPA, 401 M Street, SW., Washington, D.C. 20460. You should provide as complete information as possible, including any official investigation report of the incident and medical records concerning adverse health effects. Medical records will be held in confidence.

The Environmental Protection Agency (EPA) "registers" (licenses) thousands of pesticide products for use in and around homes. No pesticide may legally be sold or used in the United States unless its label bears an EPA registration number. The Federal Insecticide, Fungicide, and Rodenticide Act (FIFRA), which governs the registration of pesticides, prohibits the use of any pesticide product in a manner that is inconsistent with the product labeling.

Chapter 36

Conversations about Breast Cancer Risk and Environmental Exposures

Studies Under Way To Assess Environmental Exposures and Risk of Breast Cancer

NCI Cancerfax. May 1995.

A study in the April 21, 1993 issue of the *Journal of the National Cancer Institute* (JNCI) showed that women with high blood levels of DDE, a chemical from the pesticide DDT, had an increased risk of breast cancer. The women who participated in the study were from New York City, which is in an area of the United States where breast cancer rates are higher than expected. This report adds to a growing body of research that raises concern about the potential risk of breast cancer from exposure to fat-seeking halogenated chemicals such as the now-banned DDT (dichlorodiphenyltrichloroethane, an organochlorine pesticide) and PBBs (polybrominated biphenyls).

While some of the regional variation in breast cancer death rates may be due to differences in the prevalence of known breast cancer risk factors, such as beginning menstruation before age 12 and bearing children after age 30, concerns remain that environmental hazards are partially to blame. In addition to pesticides such as DDT, questions have been raised about the possible effects of polychlorinated biphenyls (PCBs), vehicle exhaust, contaminated drinking water, extremely low frequency electromagnetic fields, chemicals formed

National Cancer Institute and EPA.

in food by high temperature cooking methods, and many other occupational and environmental exposures.

The National Cancer Institute (NCI) has set breast cancer as a major research priority and will spend $196.6 million for research on the disease in 1993. NCI and NCI-funded scientists across the country are exploring a wide variety of issues related to the causes, detection and diagnosis, treatment, rehabilitation, and prevention of the disease. Several studies assessing exposures to organochlorines and other fat-seeking halogenated compounds are expected to provide vital information on potential breast cancer risk factors in the environment.

Northeast Studies

Scientists at NCI are surveying populations with high breast cancer mortality in the Northeast and mid-Atlantic regions of the United States and areas of low breast cancer mortality in the South to obtain detailed information on known risk factors and selected environmental exposures. In conjunction with researchers from the National Institute of Environmental Health Sciences (NIEHS), NCI researchers will support research to determine how recognized risk factors and specific environmental exposures may be contributing to the excess breast cancer deaths. Some of the environmental exposures researchers are being encouraged to look at are electromagnetic fields, pesticides, and contaminants in the food and water supply.

California Health Maintenance Study

NCI-funded researchers are also studying women enrolled in the Kaiser Permanente prepaid health maintenance plan in California. Using previously collected samples of serum and newly collected breast biopsies and breast tumor tissue, the researchers will look for mutations of the p53 gene, which normally prevents a cell from turning cancerous. In collaboration with scientists from the NIHES, the researchers will also search for residues of fat-seeking chemicals, such as organochlorine pesticides.

Michigan Study

In the mid-1970s, contamination of animal feed with PBBs on about 600 farms in Michigan led to widespread contamination of farm animals, milk, and residents in the area. Since 1978, NCI has been collaborating with the Centers for Disease Control and Prevention and the Michigan Department of Public Health to monitor the health effects of this exposure and to collect blood samples from the 4,000 residents with the highest exposures. These people are being evaluated in several case-control studies, including one in which the researchers will compare the levels of PBB residues from breast fat of women who are diagnosed with breast cancer to the level of residues from women without cancer.

Alabama Survey

Another group of individuals exposed to high levels of the pesticide DDT from about 1947 to 1971 live in a rural area in Alabama. During that time, a chemical company discharged tons of DDT waste into a nearby river. Residents in the area regularly ate fish from this river. This exposure was discovered in 1979 which led the CDC to investigate. CDC found that blood levels of DOE were 10 times higher in this group than the average level elsewhere in the country. This group is under medical surveillance and a health survey is being completed for all residents in the area. The NCI is planning to utilize the survey results in developing a case-control study to compare DOE residues in breast fat and blood of women with breast cancer to residues in individuals without cancer. In collaboration with the University of Alabama School of Nursing, NCI is developing a screening mamography program for the residents.

Turkish Cohort

A group of about 4,000 people in southeast Turkey accidentally ingested extremely high levels of the grain fumigant hexachlorobenzene (HCB). The result was an epidemic of severe HCB poisoning between 1955 and 1961. At one time, the neonatal death rate reached 100 percent because HCB is selectively taken up by the breast and secreted into breast milk. The NCI is having difficulties beginning a study in this group because of military activity and civil unrest in the area where the group lives.

Farmer Study

The Agricultural Health Study, a contract-supported intramural research project being carried out in collaboration with NIEHS and the Environmental Protection Agency, is the largest study ever undertaken to evaluate the relationship between exposures characteristic of an agricultural lifestyle and risk for cancer. The study will involve about 100,000 farmers, their spouses, and their children, and will assess exposures to such agents as pesticides, chemical solvents, engine exhausts, animal viruses, and sunlight. Cancer risks associated with diet, cooking practices, and the chemicals resulting from the cooking process will also be examined.

Earlier this year, 5-year contracts were awarded to the University of Iowa College of Medicine, Iowa City, and Survey Research Associates, Durham, North Carolina, to carry out the study in their respective states. Iowa and North Carolina have large populations of farmers and pesticide applicators. The cohort will be followed for more than a decade to compare actual cancer cases and deaths to expected rates. As cancer cases are diagnosed, breast cancer compare will be incorporated into special studies to collect even more detailed information on possible exposures and risk factors.

The Cancer Information Service (CIS), a program of the National Cancer Institute, is a nationwide telephone service for cancer patients and their families, the public, and health care professionals. CIS information specialists have extensive training in providing up-to-date and understandable information about cancer. They can answer questions in English and Spanish and can send free printed material. In addition CIS offices serve specific geographic areas and have information about cancer-related services and resources in their region. The toll-free number of the CIS is 1-800-4-CANCER (1-800-422-6237).

The study in *JNCI* is entitled "Blood Levels of Organochlorine Residues and Risk of Breast Cancer" by Mary S. Wolff and colleagues.

DDT and Breast Cancer

NCI Cancerfax. May 1995.

In a study reported in the April 20, 1994 issue of the *Journal of the National Cancer Institute, (JNCI)* researchers conclude that their data do not support the hypothesis that DDT is associated with breast cancer. [Note: The article is "Breast Cancer and Serum Organochlorines: A Prospective Study Among White, Black, and Asian Women," Nancy Krieger, Mary S. Wolff, Robert A. Haitt et. al. *JNCI*, April 20, 1994.]

The finding, reported by Nancy Krieger, Ph.D., at the Kaiser Foundation Research Institute, Oakland, Calif., and colleagues runs counter to two recent studies, but is similar to other studies and supports the concept that further research is needed to clarify the relationship, if any, of DDT and breast cancer. [Note: The other studies are "Pesticides and Polycholorinated Biphenyl Residues in Human Breast Lipids and Their Relation to Breast Cancer," Frank Falck, Jr., Andrew Ricci, Jr., Mary S. Wolff et al. *Archives of Environmental Health*, March/April 1992 and "Blood Levels of Organochlorine Residues and Risk of Breast Cancer," Mary S. Wolff, Paolo G. Toniolo, Eric W. Lee et al. *JNCI*, April 21, 1993.]

DDT was banned in the United States in 1972, but because it was ubiquitous in the food chain and has a long half life, residues still persist in the environment. In recent years, the pesticide, which is stored in human fat and is released slowly, has been detected in breast tissue and breast milk. Thus far, only a handful of epidemiologic investigations on the possible DDT-breast cancer connection have been completed, but the question is of considerable research interest.

In Krieger's study, stored blood samples that were taken from women in the late 1960s as part of health examinations were analyzed. A random sample of 50 white women, 50 black women, and 50 Asian women in California who developed breast cancer six months or more after the examinations were studied. Each woman was matched by age, sex, and race, with a woman who did not develop cancer and followed through the 1980s.

When data on the three racial groups were combined, no strong association was seen between DDE, the compound to which DDT is metabolized in the body, and increased risk for breast cancer. For whites, there was an increasing risk with increasing level of DDE which was not statistically significant; that is, the increases could be due to chance. For blacks, there was evidence of a slight trend—a "borderline" statistically significant increased risk associated with increased blood levels of DDE. And for Asian women, there was a decreased risk associated with increasing blood levels of DDE that was not statistically significant.

Analyzing the data according to lowest, middle, and highest DDE blood levels, there was an increase in relative risk between white women in the lowest tertile of exposure and the middle level, but a smaller increase in risk to the highest level. But for black women, the increase in risk was consistently higher with each level of DDE exposure.

A limitation of the study was lack of availability of information on breast feeding. Breast feeding can reduce levels of DDE and could be protective against cancer.

Commenting on the study, Robert Hoover, M.D., Sc.D., chief of the Epidemiology Branch, National Cancer Institute, said, "The study is somewhat provocative in that there is a positive dose-response relationship in blacks and whites." Sometimes too much can be made of statistical significance when looking for clues, he added.

"I disagree not with the analysis, which is a fine analysis, but the interpretation. I wouldn't have written it so strongly negative," said Hoover.

In addition to DDE, Krieger analyzed data on PCB (polychlorinated biphenyls) blood levels, but she did not find an association with breast cancer. Study results have been conflicting, with more evidence on the side of findings of no association with increased risk for the cancer. Some researchers suggest, however, that certain types of PCBs may increase risk. PCBs are a group of more than 200 chemicals, some of which are anti-estrogenic and nay be protective against cancer, and others are estrogenic. PCBs were once used in the manufacture of electric capacitors and transformers, and in cutting oils, lubricants, and plasticizers.

NCI, in collaboration with the National Institute of Environmental Health Sciences, is funding six epidemiologic studies involving environmental exposures, including DDT, and breast cancer risk in the Northeast and mid-Atlantic regions of the United States. In much of the Northeast and many mid-Atlantic states, breast cancer rates are above the national average. The NCI-funded Long Island Breast Cancer Project also is investigating environmental exposures, including DDT and its metabolites and numerous other potential risk factors.

Breast Cancer, Other Hormonal Effects and Pesticides

United Sates Environmental Protection Agency. Prevention, Pesticides, and Toxic Substances. (7505C). October 1993.

The incidence rates of breast cancer have been steadily increasing over the last 20 years, yet the causes are not well understood. The disease is produced by a complex interaction of many factors, including hormonal status, genetic susceptibility, smoking, environmental and dietary exposures. Although some risk: factors for breast cancer are known, these account for only some of these cancers. Environmental exposure and its association with breast cancer is another potential risk factor which needs to be fully examined. Recent news articles have reported on scientific studies which link exposure to organochlorine pesticides with breast cancer.

Certain organochlorine pesticides represent a distinct pesticidal class that are known to persist in the environment, and to accumulate in human fat tissue. Many of these pesticides were registered in the 1950s and 1960s before modern data requirements and evaluation techniques were in place. As concerns regarding a number of these pesticides surfaced, many of them were canceled or withdrawn from the market. These include DDT, chlordane, aldrin, dieldrin, kepone, mirex, heptachlor, endrin and toxaphene. Some organochlorine pesticides are still registered. These include endosulfan, lindane, methoxychlor, and dicofol. All of these pesticides are undergoing reregistration.

Recent Epidemiologic Studies

A recent study conducted at the Mount Sinai School of Medicine in New York City, supported by the National Cancer Institute (NCI) and the National Institute of Environmental Health Sciences (NIEHS) and published in the *Journal of the National Cancer Institute*, indicates a link: between breast cancer and organochlorine pesticides. It specifically looked at levels of DDE, which is a stable metabolite of DDT, and PCBs. This study analyzed blood samples and found that 58 women who later developed breast cancer had significantly higher levels of DDE when compared to 171 matched controls. Another study in Israel found a 10-percent drop in breast cancer during the same time period in which there was a decline of levels of organochlorine pesticides in human and cow milk, This study focused on DDE and lindane or its isomers

A third study in Connecticut found that breast cancer cases had higher levels of some highly chlorinated hydrocarbons—specifically, PCBs, DDT and DDE—than did the control group, suggesting an association with breast cancer.

In addition, there is laboratory evidence that a number of pesticides—organochlorine pesticides that are similar to DDT—may cause estrogenic effects in cell cultures (in vitro) and in animals (in vivo), including developmental effects on young animals. These findings raise questions not only about cancers that are related to estrogen hormone status (e.g., breast cancer), but also other estrogen related end points (e.g., development of the reproductive system).

Scientific Uncertainties

Taken individually, or as a whole, these studies, while suggestive, do not conclusively draw the direct link between pesticide exposure and breast cancer. However, these studies are very useful in identifying future areas for more research about environmental factors and their association with human breast cancer. Because breast cancer is a major public health problem, EPA will welcome opportunities to take steps to prevent exposures to any causative agents that might be found.

Current Activity

EPA is working with NCI, NIEHS, and the Centers for Disease Control on a large multi-year prospective epidemiological study of pesticide exposure and potential health risks, including cancer. Given the potential for other hormone-related health effects, EPA is conducting considerable research to evaluate the non-cancer health effects of organochlorine pesticides, particularly reproductive and developmental effects.

EPA has begun a project with the Risk Science Institute of Life Sciences, a non-profit scientific organization concerned with food safety and nutrition issues, based in Washington, D.C. The project will examine the usefulness of the occurrence of mammary tumors in rodents (particularly, rats) as an indicator of human cancer risk. In addition, the initiative will survey the state-of-the-science with respect to the mechanism(s) by which rodent mammary tumors develop, particularly with respect to whether or not a threshold to this effect exists. A research agenda for future activity on this project to clarify these issues is also expected.

In addition, we are continuing to assess the carcinogenic potential of the registered organochlorine pesticides through our reregistration review process.

Chapter 37

EBDC Is Becoming a Household Word

"Say the secret 'woid' and you'll win a hundred dollars," Groucho Marx promised contestants on his 1950s television show "You Bet Your Life." Wiggling his bushy eyebrows and puffing his cigar, Groucho explained that at the mention of a certain common household word, a toy duck would fall from the ceiling, signaling the win. The duck would not have appeared for a word like "ethylenebisdithiocarbamates." EBDCs, as they are called, may never be a household word, but more American consumers are becoming aware of these chemicals as attention focuses on their possible carcinogenicity (cancer-causing potential) in humans.

EBDCs have been used in the United States since the mid-1940s to control mold, mildew, and other fungal diseases in crops. This class of chemicals, which includes mancozeb, maneb and metiram, has been under review by the Environmental Protection Agency because animal studies show that ethylenethiourea (ETU), a breakdown product of the chemicals, causes cancer of the liver and thyroid in laboratory animals.

On Dec. 4, 1989 EPA proposed to cancel the use of EBDCs on 45 of the 55 crops for which they are now registered. (EPA approves, or registers, pesticides for use on raw agricultural products and sets tolerance levels for residues of each pesticide. A tolerance is the maximum amount of residue permitted on a product.)

Although other fungicides have been developed since EBDCs came on the market, the older products have remained in wide use because

---

FDA Consumer, March 1990.

they work against a broad spectrum of organisms and are relatively inexpensive. Some 12 million to 18 million pounds of the chemicals are used annually in the United States, and about 150 million pounds worldwide, particularly in areas where humid conditions are more conducive to the growth of fungus. The principal uses of EBDCs in this country have been on apples, potatoes, tomatoes, melons, cabbage, and spinach.

EBDCs are relatively unstable compounds. They degrade during production, storage, application, cooking, and heat processing. EPA has classified ethylenethiourea—a breakdown product of EBDC—as a probable human carcinogen, and scientists are concerned that the chemical can cause birth defects and possible damage to the thyroid gland as well, particularly in those who mix, load and apply the fungicide.

FDA Monitoring

The Food and Drug Administration monitors pesticide residue levels in domestic and imported foods and enforces tolerances on food shipped in interstate commerce (except for meat, poultry, and egg products, which are the responsibility of the U.S. Department of Agriculture). FDA has monitored for EBDCs and ETU for more than 10 years.

Between Oct. 1, 1987, and Sept. 6, 1989, FDA analyzed more than 100 different food commodities for EBDC or ETU residues. Ninety percent of the 2,156 samples tested had no detectable residues, and only 1 percent contained residues exceeding EPA tolerances.

"When FDA finds that a food shipment contains a residue that exceeds a tolerance or is otherwise illegal, we try to prevent that product from reaching the consumer," explains Pat Lombardo, associate director of FDA's division of contaminants chemistry. "The initial sampling is done at the wholesale level. If violative residues are found, we go back to the source—the grower or shipper—inform them of the problem, put a hold on the product if it's still available, and collect and analyze follow-up samples. In that way, we can turn off the problem at the source."

If necessary, the agency will initiate legal action, such as seizure or injunction, to prevent the product from reaching consumer channels. For imports, the food shipments may be refused entry into the country.

Domestic products that are not shipped out of state do not fall within FDA's jurisdiction. In cases of violations not involving interstate commerce, the agency alerts the state to the problem so that it can take appropriate action.

Additional data on ETU residues are now being gathered from FDA's Total Diet Study, also referred to as the Market Basket Study, for which agency personnel purchase foods from local supermarkets and grocery stores throughout the country four or five times a year. Each of the market baskets comes from a different geographic region and is a composite of foods collected in three cities in that region. Different cities are selected each year. Each market basket contains 234 food items that have been chosen, based on nationwide dietary surveys, to represent the diet of eight different U.S. age-sex population groups. Agency personnel prepare the foods to be table-ready—from peeling bananas to making beef and vegetable stew. They then analyze the foods for pesticide residues.

Under an interagency agreement with FDA, USDA's Gulfport, Miss., facility is also analyzing several commodities for ETU, primarily processed fruits and vegetables. In addition, USDA will determine ETU residue levels in 60 processed baby foods to enable scientists to better assess the exposure of children to the fungicide.

Regulatory History

EPA initiated a special review of EBDCs in 1977 to determine what action, if any, it needed to take to protect the public. The resulting "decision document," issued in 1982, imposed protective clothing requirements for workers who apply the chemicals. The report concluded, however, that the scientific data then available were inadequate to evaluate the potential for EBDCs to cause cancer. EPA, therefore, postponed addressing this risk until the agency could acquire more complete information.

In 1984, following settlement of a suit brought against EPA by the Natural Resources Defense Council, the agency agreed to issue "data call-ins," requiring EBDC manufacturers to submit extensive product information for EPA to use in reassessing the risk of the chemicals. The manufacturers were directed to provide information relating to metabolism, skin absorption, ability to cause birth defects, residues and dietary exposure, ground water contamination, and long-term feeding and inhalation.

In 1987 EPA began a second special review, focusing on cancer risk from dietary exposure and risks of thyroid damage and birth defects for persons applying the pesticide.

In September 1989, the leading manufacturers of EBDCs—Rohm and Haas Corporation, E.I. du Pont de Nemours & Company, BASF Corporation, and Pennwalt Corporation—announced that they had asked EPA to amend the registrations for the chemicals to eliminate their use on all but 13 crops. Under the manufacturers' proposal, the fungicides would still be sold for use on almonds, asparagus, bananas, corn, cranberries, figs, grapes, onions, peanuts, potatoes, sugar beets, tomatoes, and wheat.

Linda Fisher, EPA assistant administrator for the Office of Pesticides and Toxic Substances, was quoted in the Oct. 30 *Food Chemical News* as saying that EPA has "enough concern about the dietary risks of the remaining EBDC uses to proceed with issuing a proposed regulatory action" despite the cutback in these uses. Fisher said EPA is examining "possible increased costs to farmers and consumers if EBDC fungicide registrations are cancelled, the availability of alternative pest control methods, and the possibility that the loss of the uses of EBDCs could result in incidents of human poisoning by produce infected with fungi." This would be in addition to evaluating the potential risk from eating treated foods or from handling or applying EBDC pesticides.

"Pesticide Reduction Pledge"

Four days after the EBDC manufacturers' announcement, several consumer and environmental groups had a press conference in Washington, D.C., to promote a food retailer "pesticide reduction pledge." At that conference, according to the Sept. 18 *Food Chemical News*, five small supermarket chains and one food distributor formally agreed with the Consumer Pesticide Project of the National Toxics Campaign Fund to reduce pesticide residues, including EBDCs, on produce sold in their stores. Their stated goal is to stop selling—by Jan. 1, 1995—any fruits or vegetables treated with probable cancer-causing pesticides, as defined by EPA.

EPA's Fisher expressed concern about the environmental consumer coalition's program. "We are concerned that the coalition's campaign could cause confusion for consumers and unnecessary economic hardship for both consumers and American farmers," she said. Fisher noted that the present law requires EPA to balance the value to society with the risks that may be presented by pesticides, and that decisions must be based on "top quality science."

In early November, United Press International reported that some of Florida's largest produce growers had stopped using EBDCs, fearing the kind of "food safety scare that hit apple growers in February during the Alar controversy." The wire service reported growers' fears that vulnerable crops, such as lettuce, cucumbers and green peppers, would not survive Florida's warm, humid winter, adding that, according to the Florida Fruit and Vegetable Association, there is no alternative fungicide for some crops, such as lettuce.

Risk Assessment

Then, on Dec. 4, based on review of the data available to the agency, EPA decided that the current use of EBDCs presented an unreasonable cancer risk. The theoretical lifetime total dietary cancer risk from the EBDCs used on the 13 crops was calculated to be two cancer cases per 100,000 population. However, according to EPA, this risk estimate does not take into account the rapid degradation of EBDCs, but is based on residue data close to harvest and assumes the highest allowable application rates.

Because these 13 crops are not always treated with EBDCs, because the maximum applications are not always used, and because residues may dissipate significantly before the food reaches the consumer, the agency maintains that if grocery store exposure estimates were used, the risks for most crops would be significantly lower. Therefore, EPA has required manufacturers to conduct a grocery store level study and furnish results in September 1990.

In the meantime, EPA has proposed to cancel use of all EBDCs on 45 crops. These include the 42 crops that the manufacturers had requested be deleted from the registrations, as well as three others: bananas, potatoes and tomatoes. The lifetime cancer risk of continuing use of the chemicals on the 10 remaining crops—almonds, asparagus, cranberries, figs, grapes, onions, peanuts, sugar beets, sweet corn, and wheat—is estimated at three in a million, and benefits from their use at $13 million to $26 million.

EPA maintains that EBDC residue levels on food are low and can be reduced further by washing and peeling fruits and vegetables. The chemicals remain on the surface of the produce; they don't penetrate. FDA also recommends peeling away outer leaves, skin or rinds and scrubbing certain vegetables such as potatoes and carrots.

—by Marian Segal

Marian Segal is a member of FDA's public affairs staff.

Chapter 38

Deciding about Dioxins: The Chlorine Debate

Even though paperboard milk cartons may leach dioxin into milk, it is only a trace amount and milk is presently safe to drink, the Food and Drug Administration advised American consumers last fall.

A close look at the agency's investigation of the problem can provide insight into how FDA assesses risks when it comes to foods.

The Tipoff

Bleached paper—including the paperboard used for milk cartons—can contain minuscule amounts of chlorinated dioxins and furans, chemicals that are formed as byproducts of certain processes, such as incineration, manufacture of certain pesticides, and chlorine treatment of wood pulp during paper manufacture. In the case of bleached paper milk cartons, dioxins and furans may leach into milk.

The "tipoff" implicating the paper bleaching process came when a 1987 EPA analysis revealed dioxins in river sediment and fish downstream from some paper mills, says Michael Callahan, director of the exposure assessment group at the Environmental Protection Agency's Office of Research and Development. This finding prompted EPA to conduct a joint study with the American Paper Institute, a trade association representing the pulp and paper industry. The study identified the chlorine bleaching process as the source of dioxins in the fish.

Shortly afterwards, Health and Welfare Canada, Canada's national health agency, reported finding trace levels of dioxins and furans in

FDA Consumer, February 1990.

paper-packaged milk samples collected in the Halifax region. This study, although limited in scope, served as a signal for FDA to look more closely at milk in this country.

FDA's subsequent sampling of chlorine-bleached milk cartons found that they did leach dioxins into milk. However, the dioxin levels in the milk sampled were minuscule—well below one part per trillion (ppt). One ppt is approximately equal to one large grain of sand on the surface of Daytona Beach. No one has ever demonstrated that such minute amounts of dioxin pose a health hazard. In fact, before its milk study for dioxins, FDA had never analyzed foods for such low levels of a chemical contaminant.

Dioxins and Furans

Dioxin actually is chemical shorthand for a large family of compounds called chlorinated dibenzo-p-dioxins. One of these compounds, 2,3,7,8-TCDD (short for 2,3,7,8-tetrachlorodibenzo-p-dioxin), has been proven to cause cancer in animals. TCDD frequently is accompanied by a compound in the furan family—TCDF (short for 2,3,7,8-tetrachlorodibenzofuran), which is about one-tenth as toxic as TCDD.

When TCDD was first discovered in 1957, chemists were able to detect the compound in concentrations of a few parts per million. At that time, scientists linked heavy exposure with a serious skin disease called chloracne suffered by workers in a West German firm that manufactured a herbicide now known as Agent Orange. TCDD is a contaminant in this herbicide.

Since the 1970s, however, detecting equipment has improved a million-fold. Now scientists can detect TCDD in concentrations of less than one part per trillion. (One trillion is a million multiplied by a million.)

FDA's Milk Study

FDA's Chicago district laboratory modified the agency's analytical method for determining TCDD in fish so that the method could be used to detect the minute quantities reported in milk (see below). With the new procedure, FDA scientists were able to determine concentrations of TCDD as low as 0.02 ppt and of TCDF at or above 0.1 ppt.

The scientists then collected milk in half-pint paperboard cartons from 15 milk packaging plants throughout the country. The cartons were from all five U.S. companies that make paperboard for milk cartons.

FDA included only whole milk in the study because TCDD and TCDF collect in milk fat. After collection, the milk was stored refrigerated for 14 days, the shelf life for milk, to allow for the greatest contact of the carton with the milk.

In 4 of 15 samples of milk from cartons, FDA chemists found TCDD in concentrations ranging from 0.02 to 0.07 ppt. TCDF was detected in 7 of these 15 samples at levels from 0.14 to 0.62 ppt. Neither TCDD nor TCDF was found in milk from one-gallon glass containers, leading the chemists to conclude that TCDD and TCDF in the milk migrated from the paper carton containers.

Is It Safe?

Once FDA determined that packaged milk may contain dioxins and furans, the agency faced a more difficult challenge—deciding whether milk packaged in bleached paperboard cartons is safe to drink.

This question is fraught with uncertainties. Intelligent guesses based on existing data are often the cornerstone of risk decisions. Robert Scheuplein, Ph.D., acting director of FDA's office of toxicological sciences, underlines the dilemma FDA regulators faced regarding milk safety by pointing to the differing estimates U.S. agencies and foreign countries have made about dioxin's dangers. FDA considers a chemical to present a cancer risk when it may cause more than one additional case of cancer for every 1 million persons over a 70-year lifetime. This benchmark figure was selected because it is insignificant compared to cancer risks encountered in daily life.

Investigators, however, have used different methods to estimate the level at which dioxin may cause toxicity in humans. In applying results from laboratory test animals to humans, FDA adjusts for relative weight; EPA's projections are based on body surface. Scientists in Canada, Germany and Switzerland use still other methods (which leads those countries to permit higher amounts of dioxin in the diet).

The dioxin issue is especially complicated because, while on one hand the chemical is known to be extremely carcinogenic (cancer causing) in some test animals, it has not been shown to cause cancer in humans. So, in estimating cancer risk from dioxin, scientists must rely entirely on extrapolation of animal data to humans.

But results in animals cannot always be easily translated to humans. In fact, results among animal species vary greatly. For instance, experiments show that guinea pigs are 1,900 times more sensitive than hamsters to toxic effects of dioxin. Besides cancer, dioxin has been shown to cause liver degeneration, spleen and thymus damage, toxicity to the immune system, and birth defects in test animals.

TCDD is stored unmetabolized in the body and is a tumor promoter in animals. This has led some scientists to believe that TCDD acts only as a tumor promoter, rather than a direct cause of cancer, and has a threshold below which there is no carcinogenic effect.

The effect of dioxin on humans remains unclear. Vernon Houk, M.D., director of the Center of Environmental Health and Injury Control at the U.S. Centers for Disease Control, says that studies from the 1976 industrial accident at Seveso, Italy, suggest that risks from dioxin "are not as bad as once thought." In the Seveso incident, an explosion in an unattended chemical reactor at a manufacturing plant just north of the city exposed people living nearby to high levels of dioxin. Research is now being planned to retest the blood levels of the Seveso residents. The only known lasting effect on these victims was chloracne. However, immediately following the chemical release, the Seveso residents had 5,000 times the average amount of dioxin in their blood—the normal U.S. blood level is 5 to 10 ppt.

Other known effects on humans from dioxin exposure following major industrial accidents include stomach upset, headaches, and muscle and joint pains. These effects, however, have been temporary.

Reaching a Conclusion

Because of the uncertainties surrounding the potential dangers of dioxin, EPA has agreed to assess, by April 1990, the health risks from the production of dioxins and furans in chlorine-bleached wood pulp. The paper industry will provide data on the amount of dioxins contained in paper products. FDA and the Consumer Product Safety Commission will use these data to determine exposure based on consumption of food and use of household products, and then they will perform risk estimates. James Benson, FDA's acting commissioner, testified before the House of Representatives' health and environment subcommittee last September that the levels of dioxin found in milk could represent 5 to 30 percent of a person's total dietary exposure to dioxin.

"If findings of carcinogenicity in test animals have a parallel in humans, FDA has tentatively estimated that the cancer risk of consuming milk for a lifetime, packaged in cartons such as those sampled, would be less than five in a million," Benson said.

Because the paper industry is in the process of reducing the use of chlorine in bleaching paperboard to lower dioxin levels, the lifetime intake of dioxin consumption from milk will be below the amounts in the above estimate. Therefore, FDA has concluded that there is no health hazard from drinking milk from paper cartons until the technology changeover is accomplished. "Even if milk contained levels that we found in our survey for the next three to five years, the risk would be less than one in a million," Benson said, adding that the principal concern is long-term, not short-term, exposure.

Industry Changes

Red Cavaney, the president of the American Paper Institute, also testified at the September 1989 congressional hearing. He outlined changes the paper industry is making to reduce the amount of dioxin in paper.

In addition to its use in making paper white, chlorine also helps separate the lignin (a natural material) from cellulose in the wood. Paper manufacturers are modifying the delignification step so that less chlorine gas is used. "Mills are now manufacturing, on a regular production basis for the market, milk carton board with reported dioxin levels that are at or below two ppt," said Cavaney. These levels, says Cavaney, represent a 60 to 90 percent reduction—depending on the mill—in the past year. (The concentration of two ppt dioxin in paperboard is higher than the concentrations in milk because all the dioxin from the paper does not leach into the milk.)

At the hearing, environmental groups urged the industry to stop using bleached paper to package milk. But, according to Cavaney, unbleached paper "imparts a distinct taint and malodor to milk." He cited consumer complaints in Sweden (where some packagers have been using unbleached paper) about "off-taste" and "smell" in the milk.

If industry is able to modify its techniques to reduce the amount of dioxins in bleached paper, changing to unbleached paper milk cartons may require an unnecessarily costly and time-consuming overhaul of paper production.

FDA officials have met regularly since last year with makers of paperboard products to monitor the industry's progress in reducing the amount of chlorine—and dioxins—in manufacturing paper. Already more than 75 percent of milk carton stock being produced in the United States is new board, said Cavaney. And he promised that "before year-end, virtually all U.S. output will be new board, and by the following year-end [1990], 100 percent of U.S. production will be fully converted."

A Prudent Approach

FDA's attention has turned not just to milk cartons, but to all bleached paper products that come in direct contact with food or humans. These include coffee filters, containers for microwave dinners, juice containers, and tampons. Changes in packaging procedures will not address the extent of the dioxin concern, and paper manufacture has become the focus of government efforts.

EPA and the National Council of the Paper Industry for Air and Stream Improvement (the American Paper Institute's research arm) are investigating bleaching lines at 25 paper mills to identify elements important in the formation of dioxin. The study is part of the government and industry effort to further enhance safety in paper manufacturing techniques.

FDA believes that the current nonstop research and changes already being made in paper manufacture represent the most "prudent" approach until April 1990, when EPA will announce the results of the interagency dioxin risk assessment.

FDA's New Method

When FDA learned that whole milk packaged in bleached paperboard cartons might be contaminated with low levels of dioxin (TCDD) and furan (TCDF), the agency immediately made plans to test milk for these chemicals. In fall 1988, FDA's Chicago district laboratory was assigned to develop a method for detecting TCDD and TCDF in milk.

The assignment delivered a double challenge. First, the anticipated levels of TCDD and TCDF in milk were minuscule—nearly 1,000 times smaller than researchers were used to analyzing. They relied on an established method for detecting dioxin and furan contained in Great Lakes fish. But, in fish, scientists looked at TCDD and TCDF levels of 25 to 50 parts per trillion (ppt), while in milk they needed to detect TCDD and TCDF levels of less than one ppt. (Although dioxin may be present in milk only in trace amounts, people consume much larger amounts of milk than fish.)

Second, the quantity of milk required to detect and measure such small levels of TCDD and TCDF contains about 10 times as much animal fat as the current method was designed to handle.

The Chicago district scientists got to work. They began by studying ways to adapt the established method used for fish. At the same time, they evaluated a method used by their counterparts to the north at Health and Welfare Canada, Canada's national health agency. The Chicago team decided to continue with the established FDA fish method, using one modification from the Canadian method and fine-tuning with a step from the U.S. Fish and Wildlife Service analytical procedure.

The bulk of the detection process involves a series of steps to isolate TCDD and TCDF from the milk. The scientists begin by using a technique called extraction to combine 1,000 grams (a little more than a quart) of milk with hexane and a large volume of acetone, two organic solvents. When mixed vigorously, these liquids separate and form two layers. Dioxin and furan—along with fat and fat-soluble chemicals—dissolve in hexane, however, and these substances separate with the hexane from the rest of the milk, which is mostly water.

To remove most of the fat, the Chicago team developed a step in which they poured the hexane extract through a glass column or tube containing a relatively powerful acid (sulfuric) suspended on a powdery material called silica gel. The acid chemically breaks up fat.

The scientists further purified the dioxin-containing substance by passing it through glass tubes containing powdery materials such as Florisil and aluminum oxide. Florisil absorbs the TCDD and TCDF, allowing other substances to pass through the tube. Other powdery materials isolate the chemicals by trapping interfering substances while the dioxin and furan pass through.

The Chicago team then used high performance liquid chromatographs (HPLC), sophisticated laboratory instruments, to more precisely isolate the TCDD and TCDF. By the time they finished the HPLC procedure, the solvent had concentrated to a volume of five microliters (a drop of liquid less than the size of the head of a pin). If the procedure was successful, that solvent should contain the TCDD and TCDF that previously was dispersed throughout the quart of milk.

The scientists then used a gas chromatograph/mass spectrometer to see whether they could detect the TCDD and TCDF. This instrument can measure and identify extremely minute amounts of a chemical. The Chicago team found the milk contained TCDD and TCDF in quantities of less than one part per trillion.

The entire process took six 10-hour days. "When working with chemicals at such small levels, we need to handle the sample and clean the laboratory equipment very carefully," says Chicago supervisory chemist Roy Brosdal. "One minor slip in those six days could contaminate the sample, and we would have to start the procedure all over again."

—by Dale Blumenthal

Dale Blumenthal is a member of FDA's public affairs staff.

Chapter 39

Multiple Chemical Sensitivity: A Sensitive Issue

Dianne Wiganowsky heard an unusual noise outside her house in Cheyenne, Wyoming, in September 1992, so she went to look out her screen door. She did not expect the potent stream of lawn chemicals that struck her in the face, nor could she know that, at that moment her health would begin to decline to the point that most of her time is spent monitoring pain.

What hit Wiganowsky was a strong mix of active agricultural organophosphates and fungicides that a lawn care company was spraying, carelessly, with a bullet nozzle on a neighbor's shrubs and trees. The powerful stream hit Wiganowsky at the door with such velocity that the chemical mixture ran down the rear wall of her living room.

Two days later she had "the worst flu in the world," followed by lethargy so severe she couldn't get out of bed, succeeded by pneumonia. She visited five different doctors, all of whom couldn't find anything wrong, and all of whom referred her to a psychiatrist. When Wiganowsky, 54, went outside, her eyes turned red and bloodshot, her lips cracked and bled, and pain roamed her body, settling in different areas.

Eventually, Wiganowsky got sick after bathing because of chlorine in her water, and she stopped using her favorite shampoo when it burned her scalp. She can't stand the prickly pain she experiences after using deodorant or lipstick, and a whiff of perfume makes her

Environmental Health Perspectives. Volume 102, Number 9, September 1994.

nauseated and sick. After sitting on the carpet in a friend's new home, Wiganowsky got blisters on her thighs. She is now engaged in an unhappy struggle to avoid nearly everything.

Until recently, most physicians, like the ones Wiganowsky first saw, would refer such patients to a psychiatrist. Many still do. But a segment of the medical profession is giving more and more credence to evidence suggesting that Wiganowsky and others are victims of an illness that has been variously dubbed environmental illness, total allergy syndrome, chemical AIDS, and, most commonly, multiple chemical sensitivity (MCS). Some patients and physicians call MCS "20th-century illness" because they believe it is caused by a growing environmental load of chemicals in the modern world. To someone who has become sensitized to these chemicals, sniffs of such common products as hair spray and laundry soap produce myriad symptoms, including headaches, rashes, depression, confusion, and fatigue.

After talking with all the experts she could find, including the Centers for Disease Control, Wiganowsky now knows that MCS is not recognized by many physicians. So, to control her constant pain, Wiganowsky throws away anything that causes her pain. But what bothers her most, she says, is that many people with symptoms like hers are dismissed by some as wackos. "There can't be so many people that are crazy in a similar way. All I ask for is a benefit of the doubt," she said. That may be as much as the scientific community is willing to give. MCS is perhaps medicine's most controversial disorder—if it can even be called a disorder.

Recognition of a Problem

The malady is one that baffles medical experts. They disagree whether MCS is real, and they argue over its definition, etiology, and treatment. Detractors point out that most who suffer from MCS have a lifelong history of medical problems which usually includes depression, and they wonder why it seems to strike mostly white, middle-aged, middle-class women. Most academic allergists and immunologists reject an MCS diagnosis as unconventional and unproven, pointing to little evidence of immune system dysfunction. Patients who can't find solace in the hands of establishment medicine turn to a breed medical practitioners called "clinical ecologists" who believe that single or multiple exposures to a wide range of chemicals, even foods, can cause supersensitivity. More than 20 patient-support newsletters are published annually, and some of the terms they use to describe themselves are "universal reactors," "chemies" and "canaries." Other patients, wary of the controversy, tell their friends they suffer from a more politically correct disorder, chronic fatigue syndrome, which some people believe overlaps with MCS.

The scientific debate centers around this question: is MCS a real clinical condition, a form of psychiatric illness, or, as has been recently proposed, a combination of both? There is a growing number of clinical observations concerning patients who report multiple chemical sensitivities and investigators who might propose a mechanism or model to explain this syndrome, but few of these observations or models have been confirmed.

Although ecologists and skeptics are still far apart, the issue of the health consequences of exposure to the onslaught of chemicals has been further addressed in the public, to the point of some acceptance.

Advertisers now tout dishwashing detergent that contains no perfumes or dyes. In June, the U.S. Department of Transportation asked foreign countries not to spray pesticides on airplanes that land in their countries because passengers were getting sick. The State of California proposed a bill to ban perfume in the workplace. And the popular television show "Northern Exposure" featured a chemically sensitive attorney who lived in a toxic-free geodesic dome in Alaska, isolated from the toxins of industrialization and mainstream society. Many people now accept that some individuals are sensitive to chemicals and that they may suffer varying degrees of illness. In fact, one survey found that up to 30 percent of the population think they are somewhat sensitive to chemicals; severe problems are reported by 2 percent of these people.

Even segments of the federal government seem to be several steps ahead of the scientific community in their willingness to accept chemical sensitivity. In 1990, the Americans with Disabilities Act included MCS as a recognized condition, and by mid-1992, the Department of Housing and Urban Development established disability status for the disorder. Congress has even held hearings on whether the chemicals in carpets cause sick-building syndrome which is thought to be caused by chemicals and inadequate ventilation systems in workplaces. Some people who suffer from sick building syndrome go on to develop MCS.

Organized support groups for MCS victims have sprung up in the last decade, and some have succeeded in pushing research money through Congress. Mary Lamiella, founder and president of the National Center for Environmental Health Strategies, says that she sees new signs of acceptance of MCS everywhere but in the lawsuits that chemical companies are fighting and in the medical and scientific mainstream establishment.

"Things have changed. A lot of industry groups, such as those that make pesticides or perfumes, no longer deny that there is a problem. They are jumping on a bandwagon in a sense, because they fear consequences if they don't respond," says Lamiella.

Arousing Interest

Lamiella admits that the economic stakes are high in whether MCS is ever recognized as a medical condition—insurers, government agencies that provide medical care and compensation, the chemical industry, and others are already being hit with claims and lawsuits, and more would surely follow. But she also claims that "it is only the established medical research community that is comfortable saying that there isn't a problem, and that they don't have any money [for research] anyway."

Indeed, MCS is not recognized by the Centers for Disease Control; it has no diagnostic criteria or tests, nor is a case definition expected soon. The list of symptoms and chemical culprits changes from patient to patient, but common complaints can include fatigue, concentration or memory difficulties, irritability, nervous tension, depression, daytime drowsiness, food cravings, insomnia, headaches, nasal congestion, muscle and joint aches, ringing in the ears, gastrointestinal distress, and palpitations.

No one knows how many people are sensitive to chemicals. And some physicians who don't believe in MCS call others who do quacks. There is, as Lamiella said, surprisingly little money to research the phenomenon; the few studies undertaken are done using "found" funds-monies borrowed from other research studies.

Government officials say publicly that they are neutral about the issue; some privately add that they are protecting themselves against a political backlash. They also note that numerous symposia convened around MCS, such as the National Research Council's 1991 meeting, have gone nowhere. But despite the skepticism, new views of the interactions between brain and body have caused some regulators and a handful of scientists to take note.

The group taking the lead on MCS is the CDC's sister, the Agency for Toxic Substances and Disease Registry (ATSDR), which is trying to put together an interagency working group to study the issue. Participants will include government agencies such as the National

Institute of Occupational Safety and Health, several branches of Health and Human Services, including the National Institutes of Health and the National Institute of Environmental Health Sciences, the EPA, and the Departments of Agriculture, Defense, Veterans Affairs, and Justice.

The working group is an effort to get the dialogue on MCS underway, said Barry Johnson, assistant administrator for ATSDR. "There are serious questions that remain in terms of researching the clinical expression and symptoms of MCS," said Johnson. "But what is not, in my mind at least, in question is that some people are in health distress."

Johnson continued, "This is an issue that the ATSDR has chosen to take seriously, and we want to bring light to a dim subject. But there is no simple path to getting on with scientific and clinical issues. I cannot guarantee that even when we all come together, there will be agreement that there is a need for coordinated activity."

A New Name for an Old Problem?

Chemical sensitivity may not be new. The reclusive, asthmatic French novelist Marcel Proust (1871-1922) spent the last years of his life in a cork-lined bedroom in Paris. He warned visitors not to wear perfume.

A medical syndrome of chemical sensitivity was first described in 1951 by Chicago allergist Theron Randolph, who noted that several of his patients had a "petrochemical problem" in that they became ill when passing through the heavily industrialized areas of northwest Indiana and South Chicago. He advised patients to avoid a wide range of everyday chemical exposures and food to see whether they improved.

His followers, who became known as "clinical ecologists," began to treat self-reporting patients who could find no relief with mainstream medicine. They used a variety of practices, including sauna therapy, vitamin and mineral supplementation, and sublingual or intradermal administration of chemicals to diagnose and treat the condition.

These practices and diagnoses have resulted in an ongoing acrimonious debate. Allergists have called clinical ecologists "pseudoscientists," convincing many in medicine that the diagnoses and treatment used by clinical ecologists are unproven and ineffective. "I have seen nothing to demonstrate that [MCS] exists," William Waddell, chair of pharmacology and toxicology at the University of

Louisville School of Medicine, told the journal *Science*. He blamed the syndrome on an "irrational fear of man-made chemicals." Others go further, accusing clinical ecologists of brainwashing their patients, who did not know what was wrong with them, into believing their illness springs from chemicals.

A stinging rebuke of clinical ecology was published in a July 1989 position paper in *Annals of Internal Medicine*:

> Clinical ecology lacks scientific validation, and the practice of "environmental medicine" cannot be considered harmless. Severe restraints are placed on patients' lives and in many cases, invalidism is reinforced as patients develop increasingly iatrogenic disability. Treatment by clinical ecologists frequently creates a severe financial burden for patients and imposes significant costs on heath insurers and worker's compensation issues.

Fueling this dissent was a spate of reports that suggested clinical significance to the disorder. Specifically, support for MCS sufferers carne in 1989 when a study commissioned by the New Jersey Department of Health was issued. The study was conducted by Nicholas Ashford, a chemist and lawyer who is an associate professor of technology and policy at the Massachusetts Institute of Technology, and Claudia Miller, an allergist and immunologist at the University of Texas Health Science Center in San Antonio. Their study concluded that chemical sensitivity is "widespread in nature and is not limited to what some observers would describe as malingering workers, hysterical housewives, and workers experiencing psychogenic illness." Ashford and Miller found evidence of chemical sensitivity in industrial workers, occupants of "tight buildings" with no air flow to the outside, people who live in communities where the water and air are contaminated by toxic chemicals, and other people exposed to chemicals in consumer products, drugs, and pesticides. The researchers said that while no definitive conclusions were possible, "chemical sensitivity does exist as a serious health and environmental problem, and public and private sector action is warranted at both the state and federal levels."

In 1991, Ashford and Miller wrote a book, *Clinical Exposures Low Levels and High Stakes*, that reviewed MCS literature and proposed biological motels of the disorder. Those who considered the syndrome to be due to psychological factors began their own studies. For example, John Selner, an allergist and respiratory specialist at the University of Colorado Health Sciences Center in Denver, claims he can cure most of his MCS patients by systematically deprogramming them to eliminate their "false beliefs" about chemicals. One of the most vocal critics of MCS, Abba Terr, a professor of medicine at Stanford University, thinks chemophobia is at the root of these patients' illness, although he has said that no form of psychotherapy will help many of them.

After a controlled study, reported in the 15 July 1993 issue of the *Annals of Internal Medicine*, found no physiologic differences between MCS patients and controls, except that MCS patients had more depression, Terr wrote an editorial that suggested physicians treat MCS patients with behavior modification therapy. "Seasoned internists, other primary care physicians, and specialists recognize in these patients an all-too-familiar pattern of over-utilization of medical diagnostic facilities because of longstanding unexplained symptoms," he wrote. "The only thing that distinguishes environmental illness or multiple chemical sensitivity from this pattern is the attribution of symptoms to environmental exposures." Other journals weighed in. In 1992, the *Journal of the American Medical Association* published a report from its Council on Scientific Affairs, concluding that MCS "should not be considered a recognized clinical syndrome."

Stories and Studies

At the same time, a handful of researchers pursued physiological mechanisms that could explain MCS. What they have to work with is, in large part, anecdotal evidence that paints a common picture. "Anecdotal stories are just that, but they become very powerful when they come from so many different people across the country," says Lamiella.

Generally, many patients can identify specific circumstances that initiated their illnesses. Some say it began after an overwhelming exposure to chemicals, such as a spill on their job or exposure to pesticides; an informal survey of almost 7,000 self-reported chemically sensitive people say their illness started with a pesticide exposure. Or MCS can come on after a new, chronic, medium-level exposure, such as moving into a new house with significant emissions of volatile organic compounds from the building materials or the carpet. After the initial event, symptoms seem to wax and wane with low-level chemical exposure.

When patients think they know the source of the irritant and remove it, symptoms disappear.

Once the syndrome has been initiated, a "spreading phenomenon" reportedly occurs, in which sensitivity generalizes from the original trigger to low doses of multiple, chemically unrelated substances, such as perfume, tobacco smoke, auto exhaust, and newsprint. A majority of patients also report new sensitivities to common foods, alcoholic beverages, and drugs they have taken for years.

To explain this spreading of sensitivity, some clinical ecologists theorize that initial high-level exposure, or chronic low-level exposure to chemicals causes the immune system to overreact to subsequent exposures or to lose some of its ability to protect the body against harmful substances. The immune system, they point out, also carries out precise regulatory interactions between itself and the endocrine and nervous systems, so a dysfunctional immune system could possibly lead to a multitude of symptoms.

One study, conducted by Alan Levin, professor of immunology at the University of California at San Francisco, found that some components of immunity can be abnormal in MCS patients. He found that T-cell and B-cell counts and the ratio of helper T- to suppressor T-lymphocytes are altered in these patients. Similarly, William Rea, a clinical ecologist in Dallas, Texas, reported abnormal levels of complement, T-lymphocytes, red blood cells, and immunoglobulin G in his patients.

But research findings on immune systems of MCS patients have not been consistent; to date, no single, consistently abnormal immunological parameter has been found in these patients. Terr, for example, found normal levels of immunoglobulins, complement components, and lymphocyte subsets in a review of the medical records of 50 patients diagnosed with the disorder. Many allergists point out that formation of IgE, the immunoglobulin associated with allergy, is very specific for particular substances, such as ragweed or bee venom, and that it cannot be spread to chemically unrelated substances.

All in the Head

Now research into MCS has delved into other physiologic pathways, many of which center on nervous system interactions. One scientist, William Meggs, of the Department of Emergency Medicine at East Carolina University School of Medicine, believes that volatile organic chemicals irritate fibers in the airway, leading to inflammation, and then to systemic symptoms. The inducing exposure may alter the regulation of respiratory mucosa in such ways that subsequent chemical exposure would result in a heightened inflammatory response.

Other scientists, including two leading MCS researchers, Miller and Iris Bell of the Department of Psychiatry at the University of Arizona Health Sciences Center, are postulating an "integrated" MCS hypothesis that ties the biological and psychiatric elements of MCS together. The key, they say, is the rich neural connections that lie between the olfactory system and the limbic and temporal regions in the brain's cerebral hemispheres, which, in part, regulate mood and autonomic functioning. They argue that many environmental chemicals gain access to the central nervous system via the olfactory and limbic pathways, inducing lasting changes in limbic neuronal activity and overall cortical arousal levels, altering a broad spectrum of behavioral and physiological functions to produce clinical MCS syndromes.

The limbic system is adjacent to the olfactory bulb, which contains nerves that are the brain's most direct contact with the external environment; there is no protective blood-brain barrier. Each olfactory nerve consists of bipolar neurons with one end in the upper part of the nose and the other in the brain's olfactory bulb. Odors can elicit electrical activity in the amygdala and hippocampal areas of the limbic system via this pathway. And subsensory exposure to chemicals can cause protracted, if not permanent, alterations in the electrical activity of the limbic region, beginning first with the most sensitive structures, such as the part of the amygdala that analyzes odor, says Miller.

The amygdala, the most sensitive portion of the brain to chemical stimuli, has been dubbed "emotion central," according to Miller. It is involved in feelings and activities related to self-preservation, such as hunger and the fight-or-flight response, and it is important in regulating mood states.

Furthermore, the hippocampus, important in learning and memory, is seen by some researchers as a prime target for toxins. Damage to the hippocampus may affect the synthesis, storage, release, or inactivation of excitatory and inhibitory amino acids that serve as neurotransmitters in this area of the brain. The hippocampus also regulates body temperature, eating, drinking, digestive and metabolic activities, aggressive behavior, and physical manifestations of emotion such as increased heart rate and elevated blood pressure. The hippocampus is also the area where the sympathetic and parasympathetic nervous systems converge. Says Miller, "Many symptoms that patients experience with food and chemical activities could be related to the autonomic nervous system."

Bell has taken the model a step further to postulate that these systems are so intertwined that dysfunction in either can produce emotional problems or chemical sensitivity, and vice versa. "The olfactory system, hypothalamus, and limbic system pathways would provide the neural circuitry by which adverse food and chemical reactions could trigger certain neural, psychologic, and psychiatric abnormalities," said Bell, adding that patients with chemical sensitivities have reported food cravings, binges, violence, or hypersexual activity following chemical exposure.

Bell also thinks that traumatic psychosocial events, like childhood abuse, could trigger changes in limbic activities, such as a heightened sensitivity to chemicals, that can result in MCS. She said that there is no question that the majority of MCS patients have a history of depression—many studies profiling MCS patients have pointed that out. Her own studies of college students and the retired elderly in Tucson who have reported some sensitivity to chemical exposure have found elevated rates of "generalized distress and negative affectivity, including depression, anxiety, and irritability." This relationship between depression and physiological symptoms is, of course, the old chicken-and-egg question. Many MCS detractors say that the depression influences the degree to which a patient rates symptoms of their malaise.

To back her theory, Bell cites interesting, albeit divergent, lines of evidence. In her surveys, she found that a self-reporting of shyness correlated most often with chemical sensitivity. And in animal models of shyness, if the amygdala is stimulated, the animal increases avoidance behavior.

Psychologists have long thought of the amygdala and limbic systems as regulators of social interaction and emotional tone, says Bell. That area of the brain is also the first place that gets information about noxious smells. If a patient acquired a vulnerability in the limbic system different from a "normal" person, he or she may be more prone to olfactory stimuli. Removal of the olfactory bulb in laboratory animals serves as a model for depression that researchers have used to test the effectiveness of antidepressant drugs, Miller says.

One study may underscore Miller and Bell's hypothesis. To understand what symptoms MCS patients share in common, researchers at the Robert Wood Johnson Medical School in New Jersey comprehensively analyzed 11 patients considered "pure"—they had no previous physical or psychiatric conditions to explain their symptoms, nor were they under the care of a clinical ecologist or part of an MCS support group. "Therefore, they were not simply repeating patterns that had been suggested to them," says Howard Kipen, associate professor at the medical school and at the Environmental and Occupational Health Sciences Institute (EOSHI).

What Kipen and colleagues found is that none of the subjects showed medical, allergic, or immunologic abnormalities, or premorbid psychiatric conditions, but that all had an increased sensitivity to odors, and six of them had poor memory performance on functional tests which were consistent with some form of central nervous system dysfunction. What was not clear, however, was how the patient's psychological disposition (some of them were depressed and anxious) interacted with the CNS symptoms, mediated through smell. "The psyche sits on the CNS," said Kipen.

To help answer this question, Kipen will use a facility built at EOSHI for testing air pollutants to conduct studies in which MCS patients will be exposed to chemicals at such a low threshold that patients won't be able to smell them. Any symptoms patients report will be followed by physiological tests, said Kipen.

Integral to Bell's model are the processes by which the limbic system is sensitized, which she calls "time-dependent sensitization" (TDS) and "kindling." A TDS model "predicts that finding that either a chemical exposure event or a stressful life event at the initiation point of illness in an MCS patient increases, not decreases, the likelihood of future amplified reactivity to both chemicals and stress," said Bell. Kindling, a very specific type of TDS, is best seen when animals are given enough low levels of electrical stimuli to induce a seizure, even though the stimuli is not enough to produce a seizure on its own. Subsequently, the process becomes permanent—seizures are always produced on low voltage. An analogous phenomenon is seen in psychiatry; an important psychosocial event triggers a first episode, and the disorder then begins to be repeated with smaller and smaller events.

Bell says that animal experiments have found such cross-overs in that stress to an animal can set off neuronal sensitivity. She added that female animals have shown greater susceptibility to TDS, accounting, perhaps, for the large percentage of MCS patients who are women. Bell said that, in her view, MCS has more in common with post-traumatic stress disorder than with sick-building syndrome, to which it is usually and erroneously, compared.

Johnson of the ATSDR calls Bell's hypothesis "fascinating, a neat theory that ties a lot of observations together." But he noted, as does Bell herself, that no specific evidence exists to support that view. "There's no animal model for MCS, and there's no federal money to create one. The few of us that work on MCS find a little money in other budgets," she said.

Johnson agrees, saying that MCS research may continue to suffer from medicine's worst vicious circle: "There are clearly people who are in distress, but in order to derive a case definition for MCS to be used by physicians to derive a diagnosis, we need to bring some science to bear on the debate, but it has been difficult to mobilize funding, because, in part, there's no case definition, nor any belief that there will be one in the near future."

Gulf War Veterans

The health problems of thousands of Gulf War veterans may be a mystery to military officials, but Claudia Miller thinks she has a good clue. "Many of these veterans are suffering from the same kind of symptoms seen in people with multiple chemical sensitivity," she said. "We have to look to MCS as a working hypothesis."

An estimated 4,000 Persian Gulf veterans returned from the war complaining of widespread health problems such as fatigue, depression, irritability, memory and concentration difficulties, muscle aches, shortness of breath, diarrhea, and a host of other problems which they attribute to exposures in the Gulf. Such exposures include combustion products from oil-well fires, paints, fuels, pesticides, and solvents. Some legislators and veterans have also raised the specter of possible chemical or biological warfare.

Miller became involved in the Gulf War mystery in 1992, when she was hired as a consultant by the Department of Veterans Affairs to examine Gulf War patients and diagnose them. An allergist and immunologist at the Texas Health Science Center at San Antonio, Miller is nationally known for her research on chemical exposure and its relationship to human illness.

In 1993, after Miller was appointed to the VA's scientific panel on Gulf War illness, she pressed for clinical research on MCS in general, because she felt sure MCS was at the root of these veterans' problems. Now the government is going to help Miller test her theory. Earlier this year the Department of Defense and Department of Veterans Affairs came up with more than $900,000 to supplement $300,000 that Congress had already approved last year to build an environmental chamber that would allow researchers to test the effects of chemicals, one by one, on MCS patients. It will be the first such federal research project devoted to MCS research.

The environmental medical unit, which several universities are vying for, will have eight beds in four rooms. The unit will be super clean—the air will be filtered, the walls will be porcelain, and furniture will not be made of synthetic materials, which can release a constant low-level stream of chemicals.

After participants "detoxify" in the chamber for several days, they will be given very low levels of a variety of chemicals. Participants will be blinded to these chemical challenges; concentrations will be so low that the subjects will not be able to smell them or taste them. The reaction of the subjects to each substance will be measured and analyzed, and if a subject does react, a battery of physical and neurological tests will follow, such as tests of pulmonary function and cerebral blood flow. Participants will stay in the chamber for about six weeks.

"The environmental unit is critical to ending the debate about whether MCS is real or imagined," said Miller.

Major General Ronald Blanck, commander of Walter Reed Army Medical Center in Bethesda, has gone on record in support of the environmental medical unit tests. Miller's work has great potential importance to determine the etiology of Gulf War disease, Blanck said. "More significantly," he said, 'it has tremendous potential benefit to society, which is increasingly being exposed to low levels of a variety of chemicals in the environment

—by Renee Twombly

Renee Twombly is a freelance writer in Durham, North Carolina.

Part Seven

Radiation and Noise Pollution

Chapter 40

Noise: A Health Problem

Introduction

"Health is a state of complete physical, mental and social well-being. Governments have a responsibility for the health of their people which can be fulfilled only by the provision of adequate health and social measures."

World Health Organization

Racket, din, clamor, noise. Whatever you want to call it, unwanted sound is America's most widespread nuisance. But noise is more than just a nuisance. It constitutes a real and present danger to people's health. Day and night, at home, at work, and at play, noise can produce serious physical and psychological stress. No one is immune to this stress. Though we seem to adjust to noise by ignoring it, the ear, in fact, never closes and the body still responds, sometimes with extreme tension, as to a strange sound in the night.

The annoyance we feel when faced with noise is the most common outward symptom of the stress building up inside us. Indeed, because irritability is so apparent, legislators have made public annoyance the basis of many noise abatement programs. The more subtle and more serious health hazards associated with stress caused by noise traditionally have been given much less attention. Nonetheless, when we are annoyed or made irritable by noise, we should consider these

---

EPA. Office of Noise Abatement. August 1978.

symptoms fair warning that other things may be happening to us, some of which may be damaging to our health.

Of the many health hazards related to noise, hearing loss is the most clearly observable and measurable by health professionals. The other hazards are harder to pin down. For many of us, there may be a risk that exposure to the stress of noise increases susceptibility to disease and infection. The more susceptible among us may experience noise as a complicating factor in heart problems and other diseases. Noise that causes annoyance and irritability in healthy persons may have serious consequences for those already ill in mind or body.

Noise affects us throughout our lives. For example, there are indications of effects on the unborn child when mothers are exposed to industrial and environmental noise. During infancy and childhood, youngsters exposed to high noise levels may experience learning difficulties and generally suffer poorer health. Later in life, the elderly may have trouble falling asleep and obtaining necessary amounts of rest.

Why, then, is there not greater alarm about these dangers? Perhaps it is because the link between noise and many disabilities or diseases has not yet been conclusively demonstrated. Perhaps it is because we tend to dismiss annoyance as a price to pay for living in the modern world. It may also be because we still think of hearing loss as only an occupational hazard.

The effects of noise on health are often misunderstood or unrecognized. Well-documented studies to clarify the role of noise as a public health hazard are still required, but we at least know from existing evidence that the danger is real. In the following nine sections, this chapter describes the ways that noise endangers our health and well-being:

Hearing Loss
Heart Disease
The Body's Other Reactions
Noise and the Unborn
Special Effects on Children
Intrusion at Home and Work
Sleep Disruption
Mental and Social Well-Being
Danger to Life and Limb

Hearing Loss

"Deafness, like poverty, stunts and deadens its victims."

Helen Keller

Noise loud enough to cause hearing loss is virtually everywhere today. Our jobs, our entertainment and recreation, and our neighborhoods and homes are filled with potentially harmful levels of noise. It is no wonder then that 20 million or more Americans are estimated to be exposed daily to noise that is permanently damaging to their hearing.

Noise Can Cause Permanent Hearing Damage

When hearing loss occurs, it is in most cases gradual, becoming worse with time. The first awareness of the damage usually begins with the loss of occasional words in general conversation and with difficulty understanding speech heard on the telephone. Unfortunately, this recognition comes too late to recover what is lost. By then, the ability to hear the high frequency sounds of, for example, a flute or piccolo or even the soft rustling of leaves will have been permanently diminished. As hearing damage continues, it can become quite significant and handicapping. And there is no cure. Hearing aids do not restore noise-damaged hearing, although they can be of limited help to some people.

People with partial deafness from exposure to noise do not necessarily live in a quieter world. The many sounds still audible to them are distorted in loudness, pitch, apparent location, or clarity. Consonants of speech, especially high frequency sounds such as "s" and "ch," are often lost or indistinguishable from other sounds. Speech frequently seems garbled, sounding as it the speaker has his or her "head in a barrel." When exposed to a very loud noise, people with partial hearing loss may experience discomfort and pain. They also frequently suffer from tinnitus—irritating ringing or roaring in the head.

People with Hearing Loss Suffer Discomfort and Social Isolation

There is even further pain the hard-of-hearing person faces: the emotional anguish caused, perhaps unintentionally, by friends and associates who become less willing to be partners in conversation or companions in other activities. Indeed, the inability to converse normally makes it difficult for partially deaf people to participate in lectures, meetings, parties, and other public gatherings. For a person with hearing loss, listening to TV, radio, and the telephone—important activities of our lives—is difficult, if not impossible.

As hearing diminishes, a severe sense of isolation can set in. The greater the hearing loss, the stronger the sense of being cut off from the rest of the world. What eventually may be lost is the ability to hear enough of the incidental—sounds that maintain our feeling of being part of a living world. The emotional depression following such hearing loss is much the same, whether the impairment has been sudden or gradual.

Hearing Loss is Not Solely an Occupational Hazard

The idea that hearing loss is solely the result of industrial noise is dangerously erroneous. Noise levels in many places and in some of the transportation vehicles we use are well above the levels believed to cause hearing damage over prolonged periods. As a rule, whenever we need to raise our voices to be heard, the background noise may be too loud and should be avoided.

Heart Disease

"We now have millions with heart disease, high blood pressure, and emotional illness who need protection from the additional stress of noise."
Dr. Samuel Rosen, Mt. Sinai Hospital

While no one has yet shown that noise inflicts any measurable damage to the heart itself, a growing body of evidence strongly suggests a link between exposure to noise and the development and aggravation of a number of heart disease problems. The explanation? Noise causes stress and the body reacts with increased adrenaline, changes in heart rate, and elevated blood pressure.

Noise, however, is only one of several environmental causes of stress. For this reason, researchers cannot say with confidence that noise alone caused the heart and circulatory problems they have observed. What they can point to is a statistical relationship apparent in several field and laboratory studies.

The best available studies are those that have been conducted in industrial settings. For example, steel workers and machine shop operators laboring under the stress of high noise levels had a higher incidence of circulatory problems than did workers in quiet industries. A German study has documented a higher rate of heart disease in noisy industries. In Sweden, several researchers have noted more cases of high blood pressure among workers exposed to high levels of noise.

Some laboratory tests have produced observable physical changes. In one instance, rabbits exposed for 10 weeks to noise levels common to very noisy industries developed a much higher level of blood cholesterol than did unexposed rabbits on the same diet.

Similarly, a monkey subjected to a day-long tape recording of the normal street noises outside a hospital developed higher blood pressure and an increased heart rate. In a test on humans, people subjected to moderately loud noise during different states of sleep exhibited constriction of the outer blood vessels.

Among the more serious recent findings in settings other than the laboratory or industry is the preliminary conclusion that grade school children exposed to aircraft noise in school and at home had higher blood pressures than children in quieter areas. The exact implications for these children's health are not known, but certainly this finding is cause for serious concern.

Because the danger of stress from noise is greater for those already suffering from heart disease, physicians frequently take measures to reduce the noise exposure of their patients. For instance, a town in New Jersey moved a firehouse siren away from the home of a boy with congenital heart disease when his doctor warned that the sound of the siren could cause the boy to have a fatal spasm. Another doctor ordered a silencing device for the phone of a recuperating heart patient.

As William Stewart, former Surgeon General of the United States, has pointed out, there are many incidents of heart disease occurring daily in the U.S. for which "the noise of twentieth century living is a major contributory cause." While the precise role of noise in causing or aggravating heart disease remains unclear, the illness is such a problem in our society that even a small increase in the percentage of heart problems caused by noise could prove debilitating to many thousands of Americans.

- Noise may produce high blood pressure, faster heart rates, and increased adrenaline.

- Noise may contribute to heart and circulatory disease.

"Loud noises once in a while probably cause no harm. But chronic noise situations must be pathological. Constant exposure to noise is negative to your health."
                                    Dr. Gerd Jansen, Ruhr University

The Body's Other Reactions

In readiness for dangerous and harmful situations, our bodies make automatic and unconscious responses to sudden or loud sounds. Of course, most noise in our modern society does not signify such danger. However, our bodies still react as if these sounds were always a threat or warning.

In effect, the body shifts gears. Blood pressure rises, heart rate and breathing speed up, muscles tense, hormones are released into the bloodstream, and perspiration appears. These changes occur even during sleep.

The idea that people get used to noise is a myth. Even when we think we have become accustomed to noise, biological changes still take place inside us, preparing us for physical activity if necessary.

Noise does not have to be loud to bring on these responses. Noise below the levels usually associated with hearing damage can cause regular and predictable changes in the body.

What happens to the human body when confronted with ever-present noise? In a world where steady bombardment of noise is the rule rather than the exception, the cumulative effects of noise on our bodies may be quite extensive. It may be that our bodies are kept in a near constant condition of agitation. Researchers debate whether the body's automatic responses build on each other, leading to what are called the "diseases of adaptation." These diseases of stress include ulcers, asthma, high blood pressure, headaches, and colitis.

In studies dating back to the 1930s, researchers noted that workers chronically exposed to noise developed marked digestive changes which were thought to lead to ulcers. Cases of ulcers in certain noisy industries have been found to be up to five times as numerous as what normally would be expected.

Similar research has identified more clearly the contribution of noise to other physical disorders. A five-year study of two manufacturing firms in the United States found that workers in noisy plant areas showed greater numbers of diagnosed medical problems, including respiratory ailments, than did workers in quieter areas of the plants.

From a study done with animals, researchers concluded that noise may be a risk factor in lowering people's resistance to disease and infection.

To prevent aggravation of existing disease, doctors and health researchers agree that there is an absolute requirement for rest and relaxation at regular intervals to maintain adequate mental and physical health. Constant exposure to stress from noise frustrates this requirement. In doing so, it has a potentially harmful effect on our health and well-being.

- Noise can cause regular and predictable stress in the human body.
- People do not get used to noise— the body continues to react.
- Noise may aggravate existing disease.

"There is ample evidence that environment has a role in shaping the physique, behavior and function of animals, including man, from conception and not merely from birth. The fetus is capable of perceiving sounds and responding to them by motor activity and cardiac rate change."
Lester W. Sontag, The Fels Research Institute

Noise and the Unborn

While still in its mother's womb, the developing child is responsive to sounds in the mother's environment. Particularly loud noises have been shown to stimulate the fetus directly, causing changes in heart rate. Related work also has demonstrated that, late in pregnancy, the fetus can respond to noise with bodily movements such as kicking.

Just as the fetus is not completely protected from environmental noise. The fetus is not fully protected from its mother's response to stress, whether it is caused by noise or other factors. When her body reacts to noise, the physical changes she experiences may be transmitted to the fetus. And it is known that the fetus is capable of responding to some changes in the mother's body of the type produced by emotion, noise, or other forms of stress.

In contrast to the more direct risk, this indirect fetal response may threaten fetal development if it occurs early in pregnancy. The most important period is about 14 to 60 days after conception. During this time, important developments in the central nervous system and vital organs are taking place. Unfortunately, women are often unaware that they are pregnant for much of this period, and are thus unlikely to take extra precautions.

While very little research has addressed these questions, due to the difficulties of studying humans in this respect, certain suggestive human research has been done.

A Japanese study of over 1,000 births produced evidence of a high proportion of low-weight babies in noisy areas. These birth weights were under 5 1/2 pounds, the World Health Organization's definition of prematurity. Low birth weights and noise were also associated with lower levels of certain hormones thought to affect fetal growth and to be a good indicator of protein production. The difference between the hormone levels of pregnant mothers in noisy versus quiet areas increased as birth approached.

Studies have also shown that stress causes constriction of the uterine blood vessels which supply nutrients and oxygen to the developing baby. Additional links between noise and birth defects have been noted in a recent preliminary study on people living near a major airport. The abnormalities suggested included harelips, cleft palates, and defects in the spine.

Taken together, this information points to the possibility of serious effects of noise on the growth and development of the unborn child. While it cannot be said at what level maternal exposures to industrial and environmental noise are dangerous to the fetus, these findings do create some concern. It is known that extreme stress of any type will certainly take a toll on the fetus, but, in the case of noise, it is not known how much is required to have an effect. Whatever the effect, the risk of even a slight increase in birth defects is considerably disturbing.

- The fetus is not fully protected from noise.
- Noise may threaten fetal development.
- Noise has been linked to low birth weights.

Special Effects on Children

"Levels of noise which do not interfere with the perception of speech by adults may interfere significantly with the perception

of speech by children as well as with the acquisition of speech, language, and language-related skills."
National Academy of Sciences Report

Good health includes the ability to function mentally as well as physically. This is especially true during growth and development.

Adults have worried about the effects of noise on children ever since the early 1900s when "quiet zones" were established around many of the nation's schools. These protective areas were intended to increase educational efficiency by reducing the various levels of noise that were believed to interfere with children's learning and even hamper their thinking ability.

Today's worries are little changed from those of the past. Researchers looking into the consequences of bringing up children in this less-than-quiet world have discovered that learning difficulties are likely by-products of the noisy schools, play areas, and homes in which our children grow up. Two primary concerns are with language development and reading ability.

Because they are just learning, children have more difficulty understanding language in the presence of noise than adults do. As a result, if children learn to speak and listen in a noisy environment, they may have great difficulty in developing such essential skills as distinguishing the sounds of speech. For example, against a background of noise, a child may confuse the sound of "v" in "very" with the "b" in "berry" and may not learn to tell them apart. Another symptom of this problem is the tendency to distort speech by dropping parts of words, especially their endings.

Reading ability also may be seriously impaired by noise. A study of reading scores of 54 youngsters, grades two through five, indicated that the noise levels in their four adjacent apartment buildings were detrimental to the children's reading development. The influence of noise in the home was found to be more important than even the parents' educational background, the number of children in the family, and the grades the youngsters were in. The longer the children had lived in the noisy environment, the more pronounced the reading impairment.

Assuming a child arrives at school with language skills underdeveloped because of a noisy home, will he or she fare any better at school? Again, the answer may depend on how noisy the classroom is. In a school located next to an elevated railway, students whose classrooms faced the track did significantly worse on reading tests than did similar students whose classrooms were farther away. In Inglewood, California, the effects of aircraft noise on learning were so severe that several new and quieter schools had to be built. As a school official explained, the disruption of learning went beyond the time wasted waiting for noisy aircraft to pass over. Considerable time had to be spent after each flyover re-focusing students' attention on what was being done before the interruption.

But the problem may be well beyond the capacity of the schools to correct. Children who live in noisy homes and play in noisy areas may never develop the ability to listen well enough to learn once they are of school age. To avoid this prospect, our concern for the health and welfare of the nation's children must be broadened to address the total environment in which they grow up.

- Noise may hinder the development of language skills in children.
- Noise disrupts the educational process.

Intrusion at Home and Work

"Interference with speech communication by noise is among the most significant adverse effects of noise on people. Free and easy speech communication is probably essential for full development of individuals and social relations, and freedom of speech is but an empty phrase if one cannot be heard or understood because of noise."

EPA Report

If there is one common denominator degrading the quality of all our lives, it may well be the almost constant intrusion of noise: in the home, at work, and in public areas. One of the most bothersome aspects of this intrusion is its interference with conversation. We may not always be aware of it, but we frequently must speak up to be heard. Others must often do the same to be understood by us.

Loss of the ability to speak at a normal level and be heard may be far more damaging than we realize. People who live in noisy places tend to adopt a lifestyle devoid of communication and social interaction. They stop talking, they change the content of the conversation, they talk only when absolutely necessary, and they frequently must repeat themselves. These reactions are probably familiar to all of us.

Interference with indoor conversation represents only a small part of the intrusion problem. Outdoors, the combination of continuous daytime noise caused by street traffic, construction equipment, and aircraft interrupts speech and can discourage conversation there as well. For millions of Americans residing in noisy urban areas, the use of outdoor areas for relaxed conversation is virtually impossible.

Noise not only makes conversation difficult, indoors or out, it also seems to hinder work efficiency. In general, noise is more likely to reduce the accuracy of work rather than the total quantity. And it takes a greater toll on complex compared to simpler tasks. When noise is particularly loud or unpredictable, errors in people's observation tend to increase, perception of time may be distorted, and greater effort is required to remain alert. Loud noise also can increase the variability of work, leading to breaks in concentration sometimes followed by changes in work rate.

Even when noise does not interfere with the work at hand, work quality may suffer after the noise stops. Studies and reports from individuals also suggest that people who work in the midst of high noise levels during the day are more, rather than less, susceptible to frustration and aggravation after work. Relaxing at home after a noisy workday may not be an easy thing to do. When the home is noisy itself, the tired and irritated worker may never be able to work out the day's accumulated stress during the course of the evening.

Noise in industrial settings may have the most pronounced effects on human performance and employee health. A coal industry study indicated that intermittent noise conditions during mining have a great likelihood for causing distraction leading to poorer work. Other studies have confirmed additional effects of noise exposure, including exhaustion, absentmindedness, mental strain, and absenteeism—all of which affect worker efficiency. In the words of Leonard Woodcock, former president of the United Auto Workers, "They (auto workers) find themselves unusually fatigued at the end of the day compared to their fellow workers who are not exposed to much noise. They complain of headaches and inability to sleep and they suffer from anxiety . . . Our members tell us that the continuous exposure to high levels of noise makes them tense, irritable, and upset."

- Noise interferes with conversation and social interaction.
- Noise hampers work efficiency.

Sleep Disruption

> *"The din of the modern city [includes] noises far above levels for*
> *optimum sleeping. Result: insomnia and instability."*
>
> Dr. Edward F. Crippen,
> *Former Deputy Health Commissioner of Detroit*

Sleep is a restorative time of life, and a good night's sleep is probably crucial to good health. But everyday experience suggests that noise interferes with our sleep—in a number of ways. Noise can make it difficult to fall asleep, it can wake us, and it can cause shifts from deeper to lighter sleep stages. If the noise interference with sleep becomes a chronic problem, it may take its toll on health.

Human response to noise before and during sleep varies widely among age groups. The elderly and the sick are particularly sensitive to disruptive noise. Compared to young people, the elderly are more easily awakened by noise and, once awake, have more difficulty returning to sleep. As a group, the elderly require special protection from the noises that interfere with their sleep.

Other age groups seem to be less affected by noise at bedtime and while asleep. But their apparent adjustment may simply be the result of failing to remember having awakened during the night. Sleep researchers have observed that their subjects often forget and underestimate the number of times they awaken during sleep. It may be that loud noises during the night continue to wake or rouse us when we sleep, but that as we become familiar with the sounds, we return to sleep more rapidly.

Factors other than age can influence our sleep. Studies suggest that the more frequent noise is, the less likely a sleeper is to respond. Certain kinds of noises can cause almost certain responses, however. A mother may wake immediately at the sound of a crying baby, but may tune out much louder traffic noise outside.

Disruption of sleep does not necessarily include awakening. Shifting in depths of sleep may be more frequent than awakening. For instance, recent studies have shown that shifts from deep to light sleep were more numerous because of noise, and that light sleep became lengthened at the expense of deep sleep.

Studies have also been made of noise complaints and what kinds of annoyance led people to file them. Surveys taken in communities significantly affected by noise indicated that the interruption of rest, relaxation, and sleep was the underlying cause of many people's complaints.

When noise interferes with our sleep—whether by waking us or changing the depth of sleep—it makes demands on our bodies to adapt. The implications of these demands for our general health and performance are not well understood. Nonetheless, we need restful sleep and many of us are not getting it. As a result, for millions of Americans, trying to get a good night's sleep still means reaching for sleeping pills.

- Noise affects the quantity and quality of sleep.
- The elderly and sick are more sensitive to disruptive noise.
- When sleep is disturbed by noise, work efficiency and health may suffer.

Mental and Social Well-being

"The Noise, The Noise. I just couldn't stand the Noise."
Suicide note left by a desperate homeowner.

The most obvious price we pay for living in an overly noisy world is the annoyance we frequently experience. Perhaps because annoyance is so commonplace, we tend to take our daily doses of it for granted, not realizing that the irritability that sometimes surfaces can be a symptom of potentially more serious distress inside us. When noise becomes sufficiently loud or unpredictable, or if the stress imposed is great enough, our initial annoyance can become transformed into more extreme emotional responses and behavior. When this happens, our tempers flare and we may "fly off the handle" at the slightest provocation.

Newspaper files and police records contain reports of incidents that point to noise as a trigger of extreme behavior. For instance, a night clerical worker, upset about noise outside his apartment, shot one of the boys causing the disturbance after he had shouted at them, to no avail, to "Stop the noise." As other examples, sanitation workers have been assaulted, construction foremen threatened, and motorboat operators shot at, all because of the noise they were producing.

Such extreme actions are not the usual responses to noise and stress. Some people cope with loud noise by directing their anger and frustration inward, by blaming themselves for being upset, and by suffering in silence. Others resort to a denial of the problem altogether, considering themselves so tough that noise does not bother them. Still, others deal with noise in a more direct manner: they take sleeping pills and wear ear plugs, increase their visits to doctors and keep their windows closed, rearrange their sleeping quarters and spend less time outdoors, and write letters of complaint to government officials.

Most of the time these ways of contending with noise are not likely to eliminate the noise or any underlying annoyance. Short of taking extreme action—which is unlikely to solve the problem either—most people who cannot cope with noise in these ways typically direct their anger and frustration at others and become more argumentative and moody, though not necessarily violent. This noise-induced, anti-social behavior may be far more prevalent than we realize.

Indeed, noise can strain relations between individuals, cause people to be less tolerant of frustration and ambiguity, and make people less willing to help others. One recent study, for example, found that, while a lawn mower was running nearby, people were less willing to help a person with a broken arm pick up a dropped armload of books. Another study of two groups of people playing a game found that the subjects playing under noisier conditions perceived their fellow players as more disagreeable, disorganized, and threatening. Several industrial studies indicate that noise can heighten social conflicts both at work and at home. And reports from individuals suggest that noise increases tensions between workers and their supervisors, resulting in additional grievances against the employer.

Although no one would say that noise by itself brings on mental illness, there is evidence that noise-related stress can aggravate already existing emotional disorders. Research in the United States and England points to higher rates of admission to psychiatric hospitals among people living close to airports. And studies of several industries show that prolonged noise exposure may lead to a larger number of psychological problems among workers.

- Noise can cause extreme emotions and behavior.

- Anti-social behavior caused by noise may be more prevalent than is realized.

Danger to Life and Limb

"Inability to hear auditory warning signals or shouts of caution because of noise has also been implicated in industrial accidents."
Alexander Cohen,
National Institute for Occupational Safety and Health

Two people were killed when Senator Robert Kennedy's funeral train passed through Elizabeth, New Jersey. Because of the noise from Secret Service and news media helicopters, they did not hear the warning blasts from the train that hit them.

Although the evidence is scanty, the inability to hear warning signals because of high background noise is thought to be the cause of many accidents each year. For example, traffic accidents occur and lives are lost because drivers are unable to hear the sirens from nearby or passing emergency vehicles. One study has estimated that when a fire truck or ambulance is in the process of passing a truck, the truck driver is able to detect the siren for only a very short time—three seconds or less. The rest of the time the truck's noise drowns out the siren, and the warning is undetected.

Nowhere is the concern over preventable accidents greater than in industrial settings, where noise levels not only can interfere with concentration and can cause hearing loss, but can hinder communication between employees as well—particularly in times of emergency. A study of medical and accident records of workers in several industries found that a significantly higher number of reported accidents occurred in noisier plant areas. The Federal Railroad Administration is aware of this hazard and has identified "high noise-level conditions" as a possible contributor in 19 accidents causing deaths of 25 railroad employees in a 22-month period.

Reports from industrial officials also indicate that the effectiveness of warning signals and shouts in noisy areas is considerably diminished and that accidents and injuries are more frequent. The effects of masking and speech interference can be dramatic, as in the case of an accident in an auto glass manufacturing plant. Noise levels were so high that a worker whose hand was caught in manufacturing equipment received no aid since no one heard the screams. As a result, the hand was lost. As additional examples, two pressroom auto workers in Ohio were permanently disabled when they failed to hear approaching panel racks or warning shouts.

Thus it is an unfortunate result of high background noise levels that people cannot respond in life and death situations when they are unable to hear approaching hazards or shouts of alarm.

- Noise can obscure warning signals, causing accidents to occur.

- Noise can interfere with shouts for help, preventing rescue attempts.

A Final Word

"It is truly a serious problem to escape from noise."
William Dean Howells, American Author

When unwanted sounds intrude into our environment, noise exists. We have all experienced to varying degrees the annoyance and irritation caused by noise. Sometimes this annoyance is brought about by disruption of our sleep or difficulty in falling asleep. At other times, it may be because we have to raise our voices over background noise to be heard or because we are distracted from our activities.

Except for the serious problem of hearing loss, there is no human illness known to be directly caused by noise. But throughout dozens of studies, noise has been clearly identified as an important cause of physical and psychological stress, and stress has been directly linked with many of our most common health problems. Thus, noise can be associated with many of these disabilities and diseases, which include heart disease, high blood pressure, headaches, fatigue and irritability.

Noise is also suspected to interfere with children's learning and with normal development of the unborn child. Noise is reported to have triggered extremely hostile behavior among persons presumably suffering from emotional illness. It is suspected to lower our resistance, in some cases, to the onset of infection and disease.

However, most Americans are largely unaware that noise poses such significant dangers to their health and welfare. The reasons for this lack of awareness are clear. Noise is one of many environmental causes of stress and cannot easily be identified as the source of a particular physical or mental ailment by the layman. Another reason is that biomedical and behavioral research is only now at the point where health hazards stemming from noise can actually be named, even though some specific links have yet to be found.

Dr. William H. Stewart, former Surgeon General, in his keynote address to the 1969 Conference on Noise as a Public Health Hazard, made the following point: "Must we wait until we prove every link in the chain of causation? I stand firmly with (Surgeon General) Burney's statement of 10 years ago. In protecting health, absolute proof comes late. To wait for it is to invite disaster or to prolong suffering unnecessarily. I submit that those things within man's power to control which impact upon the individual in a negative way, which infringe upon his sense of integrity, and interrupt his pursuit of fulfillment, are hazards to public health."

It is finally clear that noise is a significant hazard to public health. Truly, noise is more than just an annoyance.

> *"Calling noise a nuisance is like calling smog an inconvenience. Noise must be considered a hazard to the health of people everywhere."*
>
> *Dr. William H. Stewart, former U.S. Surgeon General*

Chapter 41

Electromagnetic Field Exposure and Cancer Studies

For the past few years, public concern has been growing over the possible health effects of low-frequency electromagnetic fields (EMF) produced by power transmission and distribution lines located near residential areas, as well as from electrical devices used in the home.

Electromagnetic fields are electric and magnetic fields created by electric charges; electric fields result from the strength of the charge, and magnetic fields arise from the charge motion. They are characterized as non-ionizing radiation when they lack sufficient energy to remove electrons from atoms. In contrast, the energy in ionizing radiation, such as x-rays and gamma rays can break atomic bonds and cause chromosomal changes. Electromagnetic fields are emitted from devices that produce, transmit, or use electric power. These include power lines, transmitters, and common household items, such as electric clocks, shavers, computers, televisions, electric blankets, heated waterbeds, microwave ovens, "Ham" radios, and cellular telephones. The intensity of the field drops off as distance from the source increases.

Over the past 15 years, there have been 11 studies of children and five of adults evaluating residential exposures to magnetic fields and proximity to power lines in relation to the risk of cancer. The findings have been mixed for children and generally negative for adults, although correlations have not been observed between directly measured residential EMF exposures and risk.

Before 1993, there were reports linking possible EMF exposure in the workplace with increased risks of leukemia and brain tumors

National Cancer Institute. *Cancer Facts*, April 25, 1995.

among adults. Since 1993, there have been four major studies that included EMF measurements. All looked at occupational EMF exposure (two published in 1993 by U.S. and Swedish researchers, one in 1994 by a Canadian and French research team, and one in 1995 by American researchers.)

Nonetheless, all the evidence pointing toward the likelihood that EMFs cause cancer has thus far proved "inconsistent," said Martha Linet, M.D., an epidemiologist with the National Cancer Institute's (NCI) Epidemiology and Biostatistics Program, Division of Cancer Etiology.

To evaluate possible human health effects of EMFs, scientists rely on epidemiological studies. However, these studies are often difficult to conduct due to the large number of subjects and variety of different exposures to be assessed, the need to obtain high participation rates, the effort to minimize the number of surrogate or next-of-kin respondents, and the necessity for considering potential confounding variables, including other workplace exposures.

The following summarizes research being conducted on or supported by NCI.

A Study of Extremely Low-frequency EMF Exposure and Childhood Leukemia

NCI and the Children's Cancer Group (CCG) are collaborating on a large-scale investigation to determine whether exposures to extremely low-frequency EMFs contribute to the development of acute lymphocytic leukemia (ALL) in children under age 15. ALL comprises 85 percent of all childhood leukemias in the Unites States.

The CCG is an NCI-supported, multicenter network of pediatric oncologists, epidemiologists, and other cancer researchers from 38 institutions and affiliated hospitals throughout the United States. The CCG is headquartered at the University of Southern California in Pasadena.

The study, directed by Dr. Martha Linet, was initiated in September 1989 because of public concern and a need for more precise epidemiologic data. It is part of a larger CCG investigation evaluating the risk of ALL associated with a wide range of factors, such as prenatal X-rays, childhood and maternal diseases, maternal drug use, maternal smoking, parental occupations, household chemical exposures, and familial cancer and related disorders.

For the EMF evaluation, 638 children with ALL and 613 matched controls were selected from the 1,900 cases and 1,900 controls (the latter identified by random-digit telephone dialing) who are participating in the comprehensive CCG study. The subjects, all under age 15, include residents of nine states: Illinois, Indiana, Iowa, Michigan, Minnesota, New Jersey, Ohio, Pennsylvania, and Wisconsin. A dosimetry study was conducted to determine the best way to estimate children's EMF exposure levels. Children under age 9 wore monitors that recorded all EMF exposures during a 24-hour period. When results were compared with EMF measurements made in homes, schools, and day-care centers, the home measurements were found to correlate closely with actual cumulative EMF exposures, while school and day-care center measurements contributed little to the overall EMF exposure history. Based on these finding, several types of home measurements were selected for use in the main EMF study to characterize exposures for all cases and controls.

The relationship between EMF radiation (from both household sources and electric power lines) and ALL is being examined by:

- measuring EMF levels in four rooms within current and former homes of children with leukemia and matched controls,

- interviewing parents about their children's EMF exposures (including prenatal exposures) from electrical appliances,

- diagramming the location, type, and size of external power lines near residences,

- measuring the earth's magnetic field in two rooms in order to determine is possible influence on EMF measurements,

- examining seasonal variability in EMF levels within selected homes over a one-year period,

- determining if electric meter readings and utility company records can be used to approximate within-home EMF measurements, and

- replicating the personal EMF dosimetry study on selected control subjects in both younger (0-8 years) and older (9-14 years) age groups.

Data on individual subjects will be used to estimate the amount of prenatal and lifetime EMF exposure. Estimates will be made both for the children who developed ALL and their matched controls. It will then be determined whether EMF exposure is correlated with increased risk of childhood ALL. This study will provide one of the first comprehensive and complete measures of EMF exposures in children's residences. Results from the study should be available in 1996.

Brain Cancer Studies

The causes of tumors of the brain and nervous system tumors are largely unknown, but genetic factors and a variety of environmental exposures have been implicated to varying degrees, said Peter Inskip, Sc.D., of NCI's Division of Cancer Etiology. Certain heritable syndromes, such as neurofibromatosis, predispose persons to developing tumors of the nervous system, but such syndromes are rare. Parents and sibling of children with brain cancer appear to have a slightly increased risk of developing brain tumors.

Epidemiological studies have linked central nervous system cancers with a variety of environmental exposures, including physical, chemical, and biological agents, according to Dr. Inskip. Public concern recently surfaced over the possibility that hand-help cellular telephones, as well as other sources of EMFs, may cause brain cancer. While there is strong evidence that high doses of ionizing radiation, such as from radiotherapy, can increase the risk of tumors of the central nervous system, the picture is less clear concerning possible risks posed by low doses of ionizing radiation or EMFs. Most studies of groups occupationally exposed to low doses of ionizing radiation have not found an increased risk of brain cancer.

The few studies of EMFs and cancer of the nervous system have focused on low-frequency (50-60 Hz) fields, such as those associated with electric power lines and household appliances. There is very little information available concerning possible risks associated with microwave frequencies, such as from hand-held cellular telephones (800-900 MHz). While the possible health hazards of EMF exposure remain an active area of research, expert panels that have reviewed the existing evidence have judged that available data are insufficient to support the conclusion that EMFs cause cancer.

Dr. Inskip is heading a comprehensive study of malignant and benign adult brain tumors to identify environmental and genetic causes for these serious but poorly understood diseases. NCI and extramural researchers will examine numerous factors that may affect brain cancer incidence, including cellular telephone use, occupational exposures, residential appliances, diet, vitamin supplements, reproductive and medical history, inherited susceptibility, and other factors, The NCI case-control study is being conducted at hospitals in Phoenix, Pittsburgh, and Boston, and will include 800 newly diagnosed brain tumor cases and an equal number of matched controls. The controls will be patients admitted to the same hospitals, with any of a variety of non-cancer diseases or conditions.

Researchers plan to gather information about possible risk factors through in-person interviews, self-administered questionnaires, and biochemical and molecular genetic analyses of blood samples. The occupational component of the study will improve on previous efforts to evaluate occupational risk factors for brain cancer by asking job-specific questions about tasks performed, specific chemicals and equipment used, and whether or not protective gear was worn. The early identification of brain tumor cases will provide the opportunity to interview brain cancer patients directly, rather than having to depend on a family member for the needed information.

A distinction will be made between cordless phones, which are commonly used in homes, and cellular phones, which operate at a higher frequency (800-900 MHz) and power. Information to be obtained about use of cellular telephones will include the types of phones used (hand-held, car, transportable cellular phones or cordless phones), duration of use, and frequency of use.

Researchers will also look at family histories of brain tumors and other cancers; consumption of vitamins, fruits, and vegetables; consumption of foods and beverages containing N-nitroso compounds or their precursors; medical and dental exposures to ionizing radiation; reproductive histories; exposure to viruses; and pre-existing medical conditions. Data collection began in June 1994 and will finish in 1997. Separate analyses will be conducted for the different types of brain tumor.

Radar Exposure and Cancer

In 1980, the National Academy of Sciences conducted a 20-year follow-up study of 20,000 U.S. Navy personnel to determine whether sailors exposed to high intensity microwave radiation (radar) were more likely to get cancer than 20,000 sailors with no or minimal radar exposure. The study, which was published in the July 1980 issue of the *American Journal of Epidemiology*, found no association between radar exposure and cancer. Currently NCI and the National

Academy of Sciences are conducting a 40-year follow-up study on the 20,000 U.S. naval personnel exposed to EMFs from radar equipment used during the Korean War versus the 20,000 receiving no or minimal radar exposure. The results of this study will be available in 1998.

NCI Grants

In addition, the NCI supports a number of grants to determine whether EMFs are associated with cancer risk. These projects will be funded for four more years.

Brain Cancer

The University of California, San, Francisco, is enrolling approximately 15 percent of the projected 450 newly diagnosed cases of brain cancer patients and 450 controls needed for a large-scale study of brain cancer. Patients from the San Francisco area will participate int his study, which is jointly funded by NCI and the National Institute of Environmental Health Sciences (NIEHS).

NCI is also supporting several studies by the American Health Foundation in New York. A case-control study of brain cancer is identifying over 150 cases and controls in five collaborating hospitals in New York, Rhode Island, and Ohio. Information on EMF exposures, cellular telephone use, and other potential risk factors will be examined.

The American Health Foundation also is conducting a study to see how many New York state cellular phone subscribers were diagnosed with cancer from 1990 through 1993, as recorded by the New York State Cancer Registry.

NCI is funding two epidemiologic case-control studies, including 500 children with brain tumors at the University of Southern California, Los Angeles, and 300 children in Israel, assessing whether exposure to EMFs or radio frequency radiation, among other possible risk factors, is associated with an increased risk of brain tumors.

Leukemias and Lymphomas

Exposures to EMFs have been suggested as risk factors for leukemia. An NCI grant to the University of Torino, Italy, is supporting a case-control study of 3,400 Italians with leukemia or lymphoma to assess EMF exposures, as well as exposure to solvents and pesticides.

Breast Cancer

An NCI-supported case-control study of breast cancer (800 cases) is in progress as the Fred Hutchinson Cancer Research Center in Seattle, and another case-control study of breast cancer, supported by NCI and NIEHS, is being conducted by the University Medical Center at Stony Brook, New York. This study is part of NCI's Long Island Cancer Study, which is investigating environmental factors and breast cancer. Both studies will measure in-home EMF exposures and proximity to power lines as possible risk factors.

Through a grant to the University of North Carolina at Chapel Hill, NCI will support the development of a new program of research on the environment and breast cancer, including a national conference on EMFs and breast cancer. (EMF exposure may lower melatonin, a hormone found in the pineal gland. Melatonin may be protective against breast cancer.)

A project at Brigham and Women's Hospital, Boston, is evaluating whether electric blankets are associated with breast cancer in a group of 121,700 nurses studied since 1976. These projects, together with research being conducted by intramural researchers at NCI, and grants supported by NIEHS, should provide us with a comprehensive evaluation of cancer risks from EMF exposures.

The Cancer Information Service (CIS)

The Cancer Information Service (CIS), a program of the National Cancer Institute, provides a nationwide telephone service for cancer patients and their families, the public, and health care professionals. CIS information specialists have extensive training in providing up-to-date and understandable information about cancer and cancer research. They can answer questions in English and Spanish and can send free printed material. In addition, CIS offices serve specific geographic areas and have information about cancer-related services and resources in their region. The toll-free number of the CIS is 1-800-4-CANCER (1-800-422-6237).

Chapter 42

Keeping Medical Devices Safe from Electromagnetic Interference

How could a nurse work without a beeper? An ambulance without a two-way radio? A doctor without a cellular phone?

Today's medical professionals rely heavily on wireless communication devices to help them do their jobs efficiently. And yet the proliferation of such gadgetry is not without its problems. Increasingly, medical and communications devices may be at odds with each other.

The problem is electromagnetic interference (EMI), and it's becoming a growing concern among hospital staffs, electronics manufacturers, and the Food and Drug Administration. Every electrical device emits electromagnetic energy. This energy can interfere with other devices the way a hair dryer creates "snow" on a nearby television.

Most of the time the problem is merely annoying. For example, EMI could cause static on the screen of a hospital computer. But whenever anything interferes with a lifesaving medical device like a pacemaker or an apnea monitor, the results can affect the patient.

Between 1979 and 1993, FDA received reports of more than 100 suspected incidents of EMI with medical devices. Because the interference was almost always fleeting and difficult to reproduce, most of those reports have not been verified or duplicated in laboratory settings. Nevertheless, FDA suspects EMI caused most of them, including the following:

- A pacemaker failed during an ambulance ride while the two-way radio was in use.

FDA Consumer, May 1995.

- A man in a powered wheelchair was seriously injured when his chair rode off a cliff at high speed. He was several miles from a radio tower and three blocks from a busy road, where mobile radios were likely in use.

- A pulse oximeter machine displayed a pulse rate and oxygen level on a dead body when a telemetry receiver that was part of the system was placed too close to the body.

- A fetal heartbeat detector picked up local radio and CB broadcasts instead of the baby's heartbeat.

As wireless technologies proliferate and the airways become more crowded, EMI is bound to increase. However, FDA, the medical device manufacturers, and members of the electronics industry are taking steps to minimize the danger it poses.

It will not be easy to make all medical devices immune to unwanted electromagnetic waves. The exposure, frequency, location, orientation, and design of a device all influence whether it will experience EMI.

"It's a complex phenomenon, and we don't yet know how it occurs in some cases," says Don Witters, an FDA physicist and chairman of an agency working group examining the problem.

"There are large uncertainties here. You can make a device immune to a certain level, but it really depends on several complex things interacting."

Clutter on the Airways

Sources of possible electromagnetic interference increase every year. Citizens Band radios, cellular telephones, wireless computer links, microwave signals, radio and television broadcast transmitters, pagers, and many other machines emit electromagnetic waves that could interfere with other devices.

For practical purposes, it's impossible to stop electromagnetic waves completely at their source. Modern society has become much too dependent on the convenience of instant communication. And since medical devices themselves often emit electromagnetic waves, using several machines at once in a hospital room can cause problems.

It is much more feasible to build electromagnetic compatibility (EMC) into new medical devices, so they can operate accurately in an environment flooded with electromagnetic waves, and so they don't give off any more waves than necessary.

"There's really no place to get away from electromagnetic waves. They're in the room, they're in the air," says Witters. "Even the body itself is electrical and acts as a transmitter for energy. Your body can generate electrostatic energy by walking across a wool rug on a winter day."

In an effort to investigate EMI problems with medical devices, FDA has already examined a few devices that are especially sensitive to electromagnetic waves.

Apnea monitors, for example, can be very sensitive. Used on premature babies and adults with sleeping disorders, the monitors are supposed to sound an alarm if the patient stops breathing while asleep.

In 1987, a physician in Nebraska reported to FDA that monitors in some neighborhoods of Omaha would not work properly. FDA tested monitors both at the site and in the laboratory and found that certain models are, indeed, very sensitive to electromagnetic waves.

The monitors can mistake low levels of modulated electromagnetic waves for breaths, therefore failing to sound the alarm if the patient stops breathing. Some monitors were so sensitive that a person walking across the room changed the waves in the room enough to fool the monitor.

FDA asked the manufacturer of the most sensitive monitor to recall the device. This machine malfunctioned when the monitor or the cables were touched or when an electrostatically charged fabric was waved over it.

While not as sensitive as the apnea monitors, powered wheelchairs may also encounter EMI-related problems. FDA has tested these and powered scooters in its laboratories after receiving a number of reports of the machines malfunctioning.

FDA engineers found that the wheelchairs' brakes would release and the wheels would begin turning in relatively low-strength electromagnetic fields. A police radio held about a meter away (3 feet, 4 inches) could cause some wheelchairs to move.

In response to this problem, in May 1994 FDA asked wheelchair manufacturers to ensure that all new chairs be at least reasonably immune to EMI (FDA recommends an immunity of 20 volts per meter), that they be labeled with the immunity level, and that purchasers be warned about the possibility of EMI and how to avoid it. FDA has also been working with the Rehabilitation Engineering Society of North America to develop EMC standards for wheelchairs. The goal is to increase the amount of electromagnetic waves the chairs can withstand without malfunctioning (that is, increase the immunity to EMI).

Today, FDA requires all new powered wheelchairs, respiratory devices, and implanted pacemakers to meet rigorous FDA guidelines for EMC before they can be approved. FDA plans to develop guidelines for other medical devices as needed.

It will probably be easier to design and build new devices that are electromagnetically compatible than to retrofit old ones. Some devices can be protected more easily than others. A large x-ray machine or MRI machine, for example, can be placed in a shielded room to protect it from interference and limit its emissions from affecting other devices. A pacemaker, on the other hand, travels with the patient. It must be able to sense tiny electrical impulses from the patient's body without interference from other energy waves in the area.

What Consumers Can Do

Consumers and health professionals who use sensitive medical devices can take steps on their own to protect themselves from unwanted interference. FDA recommends the following:

- Be aware that EMI can cause steady, momentary or intermittent disruption of the performance of many medical devices.

- Follow the recommendations of the device manufacturer for avoiding EMI.

- Purchase equipment that conforms to EMC standards. New apnea monitors, pacemakers, respiratory devices, and powered wheelchairs must meet certain EMI guidelines. Older equipment may not meet them. Not all products are labeled with immunity levels or whether they meet EMC standards. The user may need to contact the manufacturer for that information.

- As much as possible, try to keep known sources of interference (such as cellular phones and hand-held transceivers) from coming too close to patient monitors and other sensitive electronic medical devices.

- When an EMI problem is suspected, contact the manufacturer of the medical device for assistance. Local clinical engineers (often employed as equipment technicians in hospitals) may also be able to identify and correct the problem.

- Report the device problem to FDA's MedWatch Program (1-800-FDA-1088) and note if the problem is believed to be linked to interference from a recognizable source of electromagnetic energy in the vicinity.

"FDA certainly has made this a priority," says Witters. "We're beginning to address this across a whole range of devices and that will take some time to do."

In the meantime, he says, consumers should report any problems by calling FDA's MedWatch Program and should make a conscious effort to keep sensitive medical devices away from transmitters like cellular phones and walkie-talkies. Says Witters, "The key in dealing with this is awareness."

Cellular Phone Phobia?

The popular television series "ER" ran an episode last fall about a cellular phone wreaking havoc in a hospital emergency room. The electromagnetic waves radiating from someone's phone caused a powered wheelchair to spin out of control and a woman's implant cardiac defibrillator to fire without cause.

This fictional situation is based on a real life problem. Some European hospitals have already banned cellular phones from their buildings, and FDA has encouraged hospitals in the United States to take such action if warranted.

But that doesn't mean these phones should be outlawed everywhere. Though a popular target for blame, cellular phones are likely a small part of the problem, says Don Witters, an FDA physicist and chairman of an agency working group examining the problem.

Cellular phones generate a very small amount of the total electromagnetic waves in the atmosphere. But because of their mobility, these phones have the potential to get closer to most medical devices than, say, a radio station transmitter on top of a hill.

Patients and doctors who routinely use sensitive medical devices should be aware of the problem and consider keeping cellular phones away from their equipment.

The Cellular Telecommunications Industry Association, concerned about the problem electromagnetic interference poses for cellular phones, has given seed money to start a research center at the University of Oklahoma to explore the issue.

—by Rebecca D. Williams

Rebecca D. Williams is a writer in Oak Ridge, Tenn.

Part Eight

Environmental Pollutants and Food

Chapter 43

Is It Worth the Worry?
Determining Risk

Of the many health concerns challenging the public trust in recent years, food safety looms large. Pesticide use is the issue most familiar to many of us, but recent news stories reflect a multitude of other worries: dioxin leaching into milk from paperboard milk containers, lead in ceramic products leaching into food, *Salmonella* bacteria in eggs causing outbreaks of illness, color additives banned for possible carcinogenicity (cancer-causing ability), and possible risks from hormones given to cows to increase milk production. These are but a few issues raising the level of public concern and confusion.

Consumers are not alone in their frustration. "Scientists, managers and regulators who study risks for a living are constantly dismayed because the public seems to worry about the 'wrong' risks," says Robert Scheuplein, Ph.D., of FDA's Center for Food Safety and Applied Nutrition. He notes, for example, that "for several decades, food and color additives have topped the list of perceived consumer risks among the substances FDA regulates, despite the view of FDA and other professionally qualified groups that objectively they belong at the bottom."

What Is "Safe?"

Just what substances in foods do or do not pose a safety risk, how are the risks assessed, and how should they be managed? These are

FDA Consumer, June 1990.

Factor or Class of Factors	Percent of All Cancer Deaths	
	Best Estimate	Range of Acceptable Estimates
Tobacco	30	25-40
Alcohol	3	2-4
Diet	35	10-70
Food additives*	<1	-5-2
Reproductive and sexual behavior	7	1-13
Occupation	4	2-8
Pollution	2	<1-5
Industrial products	<1	<1-2
Medicines and medical procedures	1	0.5-3
Geophysical factors**	3	2-4
Infection	10 ?	1-?
Unknown	?	?

*Allowing for a possibly protective effect of antioxidants and other preservatives.
**Only about 1%, not 3%, could reasonably be described as "avoidable. " Geophysical factors also cause a much greater proportion of non-fatal cancers (up to 30% of all cancers, depending on ethnic mix and latitude) because of the importance of UV light in causing the relatively non-fatal basal cell and squamous cell carcinomas of sunlight-exposed skin.

After Doll, R. and Peto, R. The Causes of Cancer: Quantitative Estimates of Avoidable Risks of Cancer in the United States Today. Journal of the National Cancer Institute, June 1981, page 1256.

Table 43.1. *Proportions of Cancer Deaths Attributed to Various Different Factors*

the questions with which government agencies, special interest groups, and consumers continue to grapple.

Remarkable advances in scientific knowledge and technology over the past half century have heightened public expectations for a risk-free environment and quick solutions to public health problems. But these very same scientific advances have raised new questions that confound how we are to define what is "safe." (See "Weighing Food Safety Risks" in the September 1989 *FDA Consumer.*)

A 1949 FDA monograph stated: "A substance proposed for use in foods should show no chronic toxicity in animals in an amount equivalent to 100 times the proposed human use level, i.e., a safety factor of 100 should be present." Thus, the safety standard for a substance was set to be at least 100 times lower than the highest dose at which the chemical causes no ill effects in animals. Later, the Delaney Clause of the 1960 Color Additive Amendments to the Food, Drug, and Cosmetic Act prohibited approval of any product shown to have a cancer-causing effect, no matter how small.

New, highly sensitive chemical methods for detecting minuscule quantities of cancer-causing agents (in parts per billion or parts per trillion) have complicated decision-making about safety and placed new pressures on regulatory agencies. Also, highly sensitive methods of measuring toxic changes in animals have further complicated the interpretation of long-term study results. Scientists can now detect multiple subtle biochemical and physiological changes that had previously gone unobserved. However, the health significance to humans of these changes is often unclear, creating a regulatory dilemma.

How accurately can results from animal studies, the current standard for evaluating toxicity, be applied to humans? This question has perplexed scientists for a long time.

At the turn of the century, Harvey Wiley, father of the Food and Drugs Act of 1906, conducted food additive experiments with human volunteers. Then, as now, scientists were not certain how conclusively results of animal studies could be extrapolated to humans. Wiley's volunteers, dubbed the "poison squad," consumed graduated doses of suspect chemicals, such as borax, sodium benzoate, formaldehyde, and salicylic acid. Wiley's methods and conclusions were controversial, however, disputed both by the affected industries because of possible economic repercussions and among scientists who disagreed with his studies.

Testifying before the House Subcommittee on Interstate and Foreign Commerce in 1906, Wiley had the following exchange with Congressman James D. Mann concerning the use of borax as a preservative:

> Mr. Mann: Does your report show that in your opinion the use of borax has a deleterious effect upon the organs of the body?

> Dr. Wiley: Of course, you understand, Mr. Mann, the tests that we have made are not the same as those made upon animals fed for pharmacological experiments because after a given time the animals are killed and their organs are examined, and the changes in the cells are studied by the microscope. We were precluded from doing that.

> Mr. Mann: Is that your conclusion?

Dr. Wiley: My conclusion is that the cells must have been injured, but I had no demonstration of it, because I would not kill the young men and examine the kidneys.

Today, nearly a century later, scientists are still trying to refine methods of assessing risk to humans without endangering human life.

Adding to the confusion is frequent disagreement among experts. In his book *News and Numbers*, medical reporter Victor Cohn quotes Tim Hammonds of the Food Marketing Institute: "The public has become used to conflicting opinion . . . Many have come to feel that for every Ph.D., there is an equal and opposite Ph.D."

On the Other Hand

In EPA's publication "Explaining Environmental Risk," Peter Sandman, Ph.D., director of Rutgers University's Environmental Communications Research Program, points to another source of frustration, the qualifications, conditions and limitations that seem always to accompany experts'statements. He explains that everyone outside his or her own field prefers simplicity, precision and certainty to complexity, approximation and tentativeness. Sandman tells about Senator Edmund Muskie's complaint about experts who kept qualifying their testimony with the phrase, "on the other hand . . . " "Find me an expert with one hand," Muskie said.

"The dichotomization of risk," says Sandman, "distorts the reality that nothing is absolutely safe or absolutely dangerous, and polarizes 'more-or-less' disagreements into 'yes-or-no' conflicts."

The complexity of assessing and managing risk can be illustrated by last year's Alar scare. Alar is a growth-regulating chemical that was used on apples. The environmental group Natural Resources Defense Council charged that children exposed to Alar were at increased risk for cancer. After much media attention, the chemical was pulled from the market. Its manufacturer stopped selling it, and the Environmental Protection Agency proposed to phase out all allowable residue levels. Yet, according to Bruce Ames, chairman of biochemistry and director of the Department of Environmental Health Sciences at the University of California at Berkeley, the human cancer risk from Alar is about the same as that from tap water (which contains the carcinogen, chloroform) and about 30 times lower than from peanut butter (which can contain aflatoxin, a natural carcinogen).

A bill sponsored by Representative Henry Waxman (D-Calif.) and Senator Edward Kennedy (D-Mass.) would allow the use of additives and permit pesticide residues that present no more than a risk of one cancer case in a million over a lifetime of exposure. This "negligible risk" standard would replace the much debated Delaney Clause, whose "zero-risk" standard is no longer practical.

When FDA assesses a cancer risk at less than one in a million, it means that at most, there will be one cancer in a million. The risk, in fact, may be closer to zero, causing no additional cancers. "The upper bound nature of these risk estimates are generally misperceived by the public, however," says Scheuplein. "For example, if I say I have less than $1 million in my pocket, people will generally assume that I have closer to about $5 than to $999,000. But with risk, it's different—people generally assume the worst."

Also, risk estimates are averages for a population; they are not tailored to individuals. Rather, an individual's entire exposure history and genetic background probably affect susceptibility to any single carcinogenic chemical.

Natural Versus Man-made

Scheuplein stresses that the primary threat of cancer from food is the food itself, not pesticides and other contaminants: "The nation's food supply contains a lot of natural carcinogens that dwarf all the synthetic sources."

Carcinogens are found naturally in many spices, in smoked or salted fish, pickled vegetables, corn, peanuts, and broiled or fried protein-rich foods such as beef, pork, eggs and chicken, for example. On the other hand, many foods contain substances such as vitamins A, C and E that seem to have a protective effect against cancer.

In 1981, British investigators Richard Doll and Richard Peto published a 117-page report in the *Journal of the National Cancer Institute* on "The Causes of Cancer: Quantitative Estimates of Avoidable Risks of Cancer in the United States Today." In their report, commissioned by the U.S. Congress, the researchers attributed 35 percent of cancer deaths at least in part to diet.

Dietary guidelines issued by the National Cancer Institute, the American Cancer Society, the federal government (U.S. Departments of Agriculture and Health and Human Services), and the American Heart Association are all similar in their conclusions about the roles of various foods in promoting or helping to prevent cancer. Emphasis is on reducing fat intake, increasing fiber intake, avoiding obesity, and limiting consumption of alcoholic beverages and of salt-cured, salt-pickled, and smoked fish.

Based on the Doll and Peto numbers and an analysis of the quantity of cancer-causing agents in the diet, Scheuplein concluded that the risk of dying of cancer from dietary exposure to both natural and man-made carcinogens was approximately 7.7 percent. Even this figure reflects a combined effect of the carcinogenic substances in the food and the diet itself, that is, the cancer-causing effect of fats, smoked foods, alcohol, and other substances. The risk from naturally occurring carcinogens alone was at least 7.6 percent, and probably much closer to 7.7 percent.

"Most of the dietary risks are people's personal choices," Scheuplein noted. "They are not imposed on people by corporations. Apparently that's a hard lesson. People want to blame somebody." He added, "I think we should be doing more about diet and less about specific chemical residues. The notion that you can ban one or two of the carcinogens in ordinary food and improve your health doesn't make sense."

This is not to dismiss all concerns about food contaminants, but rather to put these risks in perspective and to examine how public perception of risk differs from scientific assessment of risk. For example, as mentioned earlier, the lifetime risk of death from natural carcinogens in the diet is at least 7.6 percent. Yet people are overwhelmingly more willing to accept these dietary risks than the much smaller risk of cancer from Alar.

Outrage Factors

Risk perception scholars have identified more than 20 "outrage factors" that, according to Rutgers University's Peter Sandman, risk managers cannot ignore in making policy decisions about managing environmental risks. Sandman defined the following nine in the November 1987 *EPA Journal*:

- Voluntariness: A voluntary risk is much more acceptable to people than a coerced risk, because it generates no outrage. Consider the difference between getting pushed down a mountain on slippery sticks and deciding to go skiing.

- Control: Almost everybody feels safer driving than riding shotgun. When prevention and mitigation are in the individual's hands, the risk (though not the hazard) is much lower than when they are in the hands of a government agency.

- Fairness: People who must endure greater risks than their neighbors, without access to greater benefits, are naturally out-raged—especially if the rationale for so burdening them looks more like politics than science. Greater outrage, of course, means greater risk.

- Process: Does the agency come across as trustworthy or dishon-est, concerned or arrogant? Does it tell the community what's going on before the real decisions are made? Does it listen and respond to community concerns?

- Morality: American society has decided over the last two de-cades that pollution isn't just harmful, it's evil. But talking about cost-risk trade-offs sounds very callous when the risk is morally relevant. Imagine a police chief insisting that an occa-sional child molester is an 'acceptable risk.'

- Familiarity: Exotic, high-tech facilities provoke more outrage than familiar risks (your home, your car, your jar of peanut but-ter).

- Memorability: A memorable accident (Love Canal, Bhopal, Times Beach) makes the risk easier to imagine, and thus (as we have defined the term) more risky. A potent symbol, the 55-gallon drum, can do the same thing.

- Dread: Some illnesses are more dreaded than others; compare AIDS and cancer with, say, emphysema. The long latency of most cancers and the undetectability of most carcinogens add to the dread.

- Diffusion in time and space: Hazard A kills 50 anonymous people a year across the country. Hazard B has one chance in 10 of wiping out its neighborhood of 5,000 people sometime in the next decade. Risk assessment tells us the two have the same ex-pected annual mortality: 50. 'Outrage assessment' tells us A is probably acceptable and B is certainly not.

Hazard + Outrage = Risk

Why is that? Rutgers' Sandman attributes this seeming paradox to a disparity in what scientists define as "hazardous" and what the public perceives as risk. The environmental risks that will kill us often don't match up with those that most anger and frighten us, he writes in a November 1987 article in the *EPA Journal.*

"To the experts," Sandman explains, "risk means expected annual mortality. But to the public (and even the experts when they go home at night), risk means much more than that." The "much more" is what Sandman calls "outrage." He maintains that the public pays too little attention to "hazard" or death rate, and the experts pay absolutely no attention to outrage. Not surprisingly, he says, they rank risks differently.

People's concerns are often more a function of outrage than hazard. The risks associated with a high-fat, low-fiber diet are more acceptable in the public's mind than the risk posed by Alar. For one thing, there is no "villain," no one to blame. Second, food choices are voluntary, not forced, so that people can, quite literally, "pick their own poison."

Third, the issue of chemicals in food has been transformed into a "moral" issue. It is no longer a simple matter of harmful versus innocuous, but of good versus evil. Things "natural" are persistently viewed as "good," whereas chemicals added to foods are seen as "bad"— this despite the fact that, taken together, natural carcinogens overwhelm synthetic ones in their harmful effects.

Sandman emphasizes that outrage factors are not "distortions in the public's perception of risk [but rather] intrinsic parts of what we mean by risk," and must be considered in forming policy about risk management. He contends that when a risk manager continues to ignore these factors, and continues to be surprised by the public's response of outrage, "It is worth asking just whose behavior is irrational."

Medical reporter Victor Cohn echoes this belief: "The public is not entirely illogical," he says. "It is easier to cope with the known than the unknown and mysteriously threatening. We decide for ourselves whether to accept the risks of driving, drinking, smoking, or hang gliding. We may feel very different about a risk someone imposes on us, or a risk that could decimate a population if the worst happens."

Sandman examines the role of the media in contributing to the confusion concerning risk. An analysis of news stories on environmental risk submitted by newspaper editors in New Jersey showed that reporters focused on the politics of risk rather than the science of risk, politics being more newsworthy.

"Only a handful of the articles told readers what standard [if any] existed for the hazard in question, much less the status of research and technical debate surrounding the standard," Sandman points out. "Yet the public needs to understand abstractions like the uncertainty of risk assessments, the impossibility of zero risk, the debatable assumptions underlying dose-response curves and animal tests." Sandman advises journalists not to assert that the issue is "risky or not," but "how risky" it is.

Managing Risk

Health protection agencies have a responsibility to carry out risk assessments and use them judiciously to protect the public on the basis of the data available. Therefore, agencies sometimes must act before there is much more than even a "glimmer of certainty," as Scheuplein puts it, about the scientific accuracy of their conclusions. It is important to remember that the published risk estimates are inherently protective and not predictive.

Former FDA toxicologist W. Gary Flamm, Ph.D., in a chapter in *Risk and Reason: Risk Assessment in Relation to Environmental Mutagens and Carcinogens*, notes that there are few places outside of the United States where quantitative risk assessment is used for determining safe levels of carcinogenic substances. Flamm, who is now with Science Regulatory Services, International, in Washington, D.C., writes, "We could ask ourselves, is that because the United States is ahead of everyone else . . . or is it that the rest of the world knows something that we do not know and that ultimately we will come to realize that there are better ways of controlling risks to carcinogenic substances than the methods we are currently developing and using?"

The answer to this question may be a long time coming. In the meantime, Sandman proposes that "First, we need to teach people about hazard, to help them understand what the serious risks are. That's the long-term solution. Second, we have to do everything we can to make serious hazards outrageous; the furor over second-hand smoke, for example, has probably saved thousands of smokers' lives. And third, we have to stop goosing the outrage of insignificant hazards—environmentalists have to stop doing it on purpose, and government has to stop doing it by mistake."

For More Information

For more information about risk assessment in foods, see these *FDA Consumer* articles:

- "An Unwanted Souvenir: Lead in Ceramic Ware," December 1989-January 1990.
- "Deciding About Dioxins," February 1990
- "Perspectives on Food Biotechnology," March 1990
- "EBDCs: Becoming a Household Word," March 1990
- "Keeping Up with the Microwave Revolution," March 1990
- "Bovine Growth Hormone: Harmless for Humans," April 1990
- "Salmonella Enteritidis: From the Chicken to the Egg," April 1990
- "Red No. 3 and Other Colorful Controversies," June 1990

— by Marian Segal

Marian Segal is a member of FDA's public affairs staff.

Chapter 44

What's Eating Us about What We're Eating?

Most people know the old adage: an apple a day keeps the doctor away. Increasingly, Americans are paying heed to the adage and taking it many steps further, eating their greens and downing their multivitamins in the hope of staving off all types of cancer. But the daily bombardment of conflicting advice about what to eat to stay healthy is enough to kill your appetite.

The connection between nutrition and cancer prevention is still controversial. The Food and Drug Administration will not allow labeling to the effect that food, food supplements, and vitamins prevent disease because it hasn't been proven. Almost all cancers of epithelial origin, such as prostate, colon, breast, and lung, are believed to be affected by diet, however, and scientists are struggling to pinpoint exactly how diet contributes to the development and progression of these cancers. In particular, researchers are investigating the contribution of fat and calories to a variety of cancers, including those outside the digestive tract, and the roles of fiber, nutrients, and antioxidant vitamins in cancer development. People are eager to hear the results of such research, hoping for a dietary prescription to prevent cancer.

The growth of the National Cancer Institute's diet and cancer budget is evidence of the increasing interest in the diet-disease connection. Diet and cancer research began at NCI in 1974 with less than $3 million and grew by 1990 to more than $67 million. This funding was boosted by a series of scientific review reports, such as the one

Environmental Health Perspectives Volume 103, Number 6, June 1995.

in 1980 by the National Research Council that suggested that many common human cancers, including cancers of the esophagus, stomach, liver, colon/rectum, lung, breast, and prostate are influenced by dietary patterns.

Follow-up reports by the U.S. Public Health Service and the National Research Council emphasized that further basic and applied nutritional research is needed, including clinical prevention trials. According to Peter Greenwald, director of the Division of Cancer Prevention and Control at NCI, the challenge that the agency and investigators face is huge: "to effectively translate diet and cancer information into a significant reduction of cancer incidence and mortality."

There is conflicting information about the precise role of dietary factors, and cause-and-effect relationships have not been established: for every confirmatory finding, another study finds no association. And many of the research questions are still fundamental; for example, when studying the contribution of fat in diet, should researchers really be looking at calories, since fat is so laden with calories? Most disturbing to some researchers is that in most cases the mechanisms behind diet and cancer have not been detailed. And the preliminary models that exist have been disputed.

Furthermore, there has been a reluctance to base recommendations for the modification of human diets on observations in experimental animals. Too often, some researchers say, laboratory animals are obese, so the contribution of nutrients to their health cannot be separated out.

"Teasing apart nutrition is a long row to hoe, and we have only just gotten started," said Bernard Weinstein, director of the Comprehensive Cancer Center at Columbia-Presbyterian Cancer Center. "With the thousands of compounds people put in their mouths, the study of diet is unbelievably complex."

After years of study costing millions of dollars, NCI's Greenwald says that the knowledge at hand can suggest only general advice on how to cut your chances of getting cancer. "There is enough strong evidence to say that eating patterns affect your risk, not only of cancer, but of heart disease and diabetes, and that you should cut your fat and stay trim," he said. "Although we have no answers yet on how specific constituents of food contribute to cancer, there are no studies that show you can be worse off by eating more vegetables and fruits."

Contradictory Evidence

Critical dietary factors implicated in the development of breast, colon, and other epithelial cancers consist of macronutrients such as

474

fat and fiber; micronutrients, such as vitamins and minerals; and the hundreds of non-nutritive constituents in vegetables and fruits. For example, a diet rich in micronutrients found in fruits and vegetables appears to be protective for several types of cancer, including cancers of the lung, colon, rectum, bladder, oral cavity, stomach, cervix, and esophagus. Increased body weight is associated with postmenopausal breast and endometrial cancer. But the most vocal debates swirl around the contribution of fat in the diet for colon, rectum, breast, and prostate cancer.

This debate centers on the relative value of diet-disease associations depending on what type of study is done—epidemiologic reviews, case-control studies, or randomized clinical trials. A major problem with most epidemiological studies is that they rely on the recall of the eater. Few randomized trials are conducted because they are expensive and difficult to manage. Problematic in all of these studies, researchers say the question of what other lifestyle factors may play a role. For example, a person who doesn't eat much fat is likely to eat more fruits and vegetables and be committed to other health measures such as exercise and reduced alcohol consumption. So the question remains: how can the separate effects of these variables be determined?

Cancer researcher Cheryl Ritenbaugh of the University of Arizona says that in general such studies need to be more structured. Speaking at the Fourth International conference on Prevention of Human Cancer, held in Tucson, Arizona, in June 1992, Ritenbaugh said: "There is a need for prospective, placebo-controlled clinical trials to rest the low-fat, high-fiber, and increased numbers of fruit and vegetable servings hypothesis in specific high-risk populations, for breast, colon, lung, and prostrate cancer."

Breast cancer. Breast cancer research may be the most contentious area of research and illustrates the difficulties in drawing connections between nutrition and malignancies. Greenwald summarizes the state of research on nutrition and breast cancer this way: "[Regarding] fat, there is a fair amount of agreement, but strong views the other way. Antioxidants are less clear, but need to be studied. Estrogen contribution is a hypothesis, but it is important. There are contradictory studies on pesticides. The contribution of exercise is debated. More study is needed on alcohol as a contributing factor."

The primary support for the proposed link between dietary fat and cancer is based on studies comparing countries such as Japan and China which have low fat intake and low rates of breast cancer, as well as cancers of the colon and prostrate, with countries such as the United States where fat intake is high and there are high rates of breast cancer. Similar correlations have also been observed in regions within countries, like Italy, in which the fat-consuming north has higher levels of breast cancer than the south, where the diet is leaner. But results of such epidemiological studies have different implications to researchers who question whether other variables may be responsible.

For example, scientists question whether low breast cancer rates in women in some countries are due not to eating less fat and its associated calories, which can trigger cell division, but due to having less body fat, a genetic factor contributing to cancer. Other researchers hypothesize that less fat consumption in childhood delays the onset of menstruation, and thus exposure to estrogen (prolonged estrogen exposure is considered a risk factor in breast cancer). Also, short stature has been positively correlated with low cancer rates in developing countries. Another factor to consider is that many rural populations have low breast cancer rates, where foods are often grown without harmful pesticides and residents may not be exposed to industrial contaminants or electromagnetic fields. Researchers are also studying the beneficial effects of fresh air and exercise in these populations, as well as lower alcohol consumption.

Some studies do seem to confirm the connection between fat and breast cancer. A 1990 meta-analysis of 12 case-control studies among postmenopausal women by the National Cancer Institute of Canada showed a 50 percent relative increase in breast cancer among women ingesting high intakes of saturated fat. Another analysis of postmenopausal women in Hawaii, by the Cancer Research Center of Hawaii, estimated that 10-20 percent of breast cancer could be prevented by significantly decreasing saturated fat intake.

Then a study appeared in October 1992 that rattled the accepted theories. The largest study of its kind, it offered convincing evidence that dietary fat and fiber do not play a role in breast cancer. Walter Willett and his colleagues at Brigham and Women's Hospital in Boston studied 89,494 women for 8 years, asking detailed questions about their diets and health. During the study period, 1,439 women developed breast cancer. But the researchers reported that no matter how they analyzed their data, they could not find any relationship between what the women ate and their chances of getting breast cancer. The fifth of the women who ate the least fat, those for whom fat accounted for less than 25 percent of total calories, were just as likely to get cancer as the fifth of the women who ate the most fat, for whom fat accounted for more than 49 percent of their calories.

Criticism of Willett's study was intense and continues today because he claims no large study, epidemiological or randomized, will find any different result. Greenwald says Willett's study relied on the recall of participants, and there were "methodological and design problems," said Ernst Wynder, director of the American Health Foundation. "The totality of evidence, including a half century of animal model data, ecological data, the meta-analysis of 12 case-control studies, and plausible biological mechanisms which support the fat hypothesis" should be considered before drawing conclusions from this single study, said Wynder.

The NCI has launched a large trial to reconcile the positive correlations from international studies with the lack of positive findings from Willett's study and other case-control and cohort studies. But the $140-million, 15-year Women's Health Trial has provoked a storm of controversy because of concerns about the study's statistical power to detect an effect. Ross Prentice, head of the division of Public Health Sciences at the Fred Hutchinson Cancer Research Center in Seattle which is leading the Women's Health Trial, countered that the study is meant to answer "the public health question." Said Prentice, "The purpose is to identify a practical strategy for women to reduce their risk of cancer and other common diseases through dietary modifications that the general public can adhere to. . . . It is much less important to know exactly which change caused what degree of risk reduction, although it is of intellectual interest."

What about the contribution of food nutrients, particularly antioxidant vitamins E and C and beta-carotene (vitamin A) in reducing the risk of developing breast cancer, and indeed any cancer? Results from a 1993 study in China showed that people who took vitamins A and E had a 13 percent lower risk of dying from cancer and raised hopes that disease prevention was as close as a multivitamin. But, that same year, Willett reported that large intakes of vitamin C or E didn't protect against breast cancer. He did, however, observe a significant inverse association of vitamin A intake and breast cancer risk.

Colon cancer. There is perhaps a less ambiguous association between dietary fat and colon cancer, which, along with rectal cancer, is the most common form of cancer in the United States. Positive associations between animal (but not vegetable) fat consumption and colon cancer rates have been seen in many, but not all, studies. The question here has largely been which kind of fat is implicated. In the 1992 Harvard study of 89,000 nurses, those whose diets were high in red meat and animal fat were more likely to develop colon cancer than those who ate poultry and seafood. Another study of 49,000 men, published in 1992 by the Harvard School of Public Health, showed that those who ate a high-fat, low-fiber diet quadrupled their risk of developing precancerous colon polyps. But in this study, the risk was said to be due to the consumption of saturated fat (corn oil or corn/ safflower oil), rather than polyunsaturated or monounsaturated fat intake (coconut oil, olive oil, marine fish oil). A further analysis of the same data earlier this year found that men with a high alcohol intake and a diet low in fruits, vegetables, and whole-grain foods are particularly vulnerable to colon cancer.

A review of the epidemiological literature concerning the contribution of fat, fiber, and calories in colon cancer by Bandaru Reddy, a researcher in the division of nutritional carcinogenesis at the American Health Foundation, found that most epidemiological models suggest that fat intake may be even more important than calorie intake in colon carcinogenesis. "However, the literature remains confusing, although the majority of these researchers agree that diets low in fat, high in dietary fibers, and high in fruits, vegetables, and calcium content are inversely associated with colon cancer risk," Reddy wrote in the journal *Preventive Medicine* in 1993.

Because many studies of fiber have shown a protective effect against colon cancer, the question arises whether it is fiber or fat that is a primary risk factor for colon cancer. Johanna Dwyer, a Tufts University cancer researcher, says. "I think it is both fat and fiber, but researchers generally fall into one camp or another."

To answer the question, the NCI is undertaking the Multisite Polyp Prevention Study to study the effect of decreasing dietary fat intake and increasing dietary fiber intake, both of which can be achieved through eating more fruits and vegetables. The randomized, controlled study is based on the assumption that because there is a strong association between colon polyps and the development of colon cancer, an intervention that reduces the recurrence of large-bowel polyps has a strong likelihood of reducing the incidence of large-bowel cancer. The study is being conducted at 10 academic medical centers across the United States and is enrolling 2,000 male and female colon cancer patients over the age of 35. Half of the patients will be randomized to a control group with no intervention except for information on basic nutrition, and the other half will be assigned to the diet intervention group with target goals of eating 20 percent of calories from fat, 18 grams of fiber per 1,000 calories and 5-8 servings of fruits and vegetables daily. The recurrence of polyps in both groups at the end of years one and four will determine the effectiveness of dietary intervention. Initial results from an Australian Polyp Prevention Project of 400 colon cancer patients show no difference in the incidence of new cancers in a group randomized to a low-fat diet, but do show a trend for reduction of cancer spread in the group randomized to a high-fiber diet, according to Reddy.

Meaningful Mechanisms

If human studies can't answer the question, can laboratory experiments? Some researchers believe the mechanisms by which fat affects cancer risk have been neatly worked out, while some argue that most, animal nutritional experiments have no relevance to humans because the animals are generally obese, thus skewing the contribution of calories to carcinogenesis.

David Rose, associate director of the American Health Foundation, has conducted numerous animal studies that he says, show fat can be associated with cancer in two ways. According to one theory, fat intake can change specific fatty acids on the cell membrane, altering their function and the production of prostaglandins, which can then suppress the functioning of the immune system. High-fat diets and omega-6 polyunsaturated fatty acids, such as corn oils, have these effects, but omega-3 fatty acids, such as fish oil, do not, Rose says.

The second mechanism involves the way the body handles estrogen. One of the least controversial notions about breast cancer is "that estrogen plays some sort of promotional role," Rose asserts. Dietary fat can alter the production, metabolism, and excretion of estrogen. High-fat diets alter the type of bacteria and enzymes found in the intestinal tract, leading to an increased capacity to break down estrogen, allowing more estrogen to be reabsorbed into the body. "It [estrogen] may not initiate the tumor, although some people think that's possible, but it helps the cancer develop," says Rose. "High fiber in a diet has the reverse effect by decreasing the ability of estrogen to be reabsorbed."

This "gut story" may play a role in many cancers, including colon and prostate cancer, Rose says. While estrogen may not be involved in these other cancers, the ability of the intestinal tract to eliminate potential carcinogens is.

479

Willett believes estrogen may be important, but not specifically for the reasons Rose cites. He believes elevated levels of estrogen cause women to menstruate earlier, and therefore heightens the degree to which estrogen is active. Observational studies have shown that early menarche is associated with earlier onset of breast cancer. Willett also postulates that "energy restrictions" or low caloric intake in early life could confer a protective effect on breast cancer, whether or not the energy is derived from fat or calories. He notes a high association between tall women and breast cancer, saying that rapid growth in youth may set in motion the wheels of uncontrolled cancerous cell division. "Energy restriction during growth has emerged as a promising hypothesis which may explain much of the international variability—but it doesn't suggest a feasible intervention," Willett says.

Studies on the role of calories in breast cancer have centered on body mass because caloric intake contributes to obesity. But study findings have been puzzling, according to Louise Brinton, of the NCI's Environmental Epidemiology Branch. Although increased body mass has now been fairly consistently shown to increase the risk of the development of postmenopausal breast cancer, "there has been a surprising lack of attention on weight loss as an intervention for lowering breast cancer risk," she says.

But here animal studies may provide some insights. Like a growing number of scientists who study diet and cancer in laboratory animals, Angelo Turturo of the Division of Biometry and Risk Assessment at the FDA's National Center for Toxicological Research believes control of calories is the key to many types of cancer. "Just as an effect of calorie restriction, live tumor incidence in lab animals can go from zero to 70 percent. You can shut it off with low calorie intake." When baby mice are given doses of a carcinogen and high calories, "they can get a liver tumor at one year," Turturo says. "But calorie-restrict other mice at four months who are also receiving the same carcinogen and they won't get cancer."

According to Turturo, tumorigenesis is often the result of a promotional effect on endogenous hormones and the stimulation of growth factors. The job of the endocrine system is to regulate growth and the development of organs based on available energy and physiology. "The question is not if calories promote cancer, but why wouldn't they promote cancer?" he says. "Some people have the bizarre notion that normal growth and carcinogenesis are not related. Calorie restriction can affect physiological, cellular, biochemical, and such molecular processes as endocrine homeostasis, promotion, oncogene expression, progression and the immune response, which affect all steps in the induction of toxicity." Turturo says that most epidemiological studies are "useless" and all interventional studies have failed because they rarely control for calorie intake. "We've known since the 1930s that calorie intake can significantly affect life span and that the most efficient modulator of cancer is total calories."

Animal experimentation can answer questions about cancer risk, but not if the animals are obese—as most are, maintains Frank Kari, a nutritionist at the NIEHS. Kari has found that some chemicals shown to be carcinogenic in these overweight animals do not produce cancer in calorie-restricted animals. "I noticed over the last decade that the average weight of rats and mice was increasing. Most of these animals eat and drink as much as they want and consequently are obese. I also noticed a relationship between lesions and weight and found that the heavier animals tend to die spontaneously of a lot of different chronic diseases," said Kari.

Kari designed a set of experiments, the results of which will be presented later this summer, that show that certain chemicals now regulated as carcinogens are not carcinogenic in rats and mice that are just 5-7 percent lighter than most laboratory animals. These chemicals include two commonly used pharmaceuticals, a food additive, and an industrial pollutant. "I found I could turn a carcinogen into a non-carcinogen just depending on how heavy the host is," said Kari. "What this means to me is that it calls into question how we now regulate chemicals. The big picture that we do not look at is the wide range of outcomes available in the host. It may mean we can set ourselves up nutritionally to be at risk to potential carcinogens."

Animal studies by the Health Protection Branch of National Health and Welfare in Ottawa, Canada, looked at the effects of dietary modifications on cell proliferation. They found that diet- and calorie-restricted mice showed less cell division in seven tissues, including the mammary gland, which was the most affected in non-restricted animals. "If a cell doesn't proliferate, it doesn't produce a tumor," says biologist Eric Lok. On the other hand, Lok adds, when a cell divides at a high rate given excess calories and energy, there may be a greater chance a somatic mutation will occur, possibly as a result of environmental chemicals, and will become fixed in the genome.

But Lois Gold, a biochemist at the University of California-Berkeley, maintains that animal studies such as those by Lok cannot answer the specific question of which dietary nutrients promote which cancer. "In rodents, we never get more than a 50 percent chance that a tumor will occur in the same site twice in these studies," she said. "All we are finding is that obese rats have more cell division." Weinstein disagrees with Gold's assertion that animal studies have little value. "Gold underrates the predictive value of the assays. There is a unity of biology across rats and humans that tells us valuable things. Dose responses may be a problem, but if you abandon them, you are left with nothing." What the field needs now is "more objective markers of the action in the body of what we eat. We have made too many inferences and associations," Weinstein says. "We need to take our cue from cardiovascular disease studies that routinely measure serum cholesterol, HDL, LDL, and other markers. We just cannot stay in the old rut of dietary history. We need to know what is happening in tissues, in DNA." Weinstein says that although such biomarkers will be expensive to develop, widespread use of them in interventional studies will reduce costs.

"We are at an exciting point where the revolution in our knowledge of the cellular and molecular basis of cancer can start to be applied with nutritional studies," Weinstein continues. "And we need to double our efforts because the public is already deciding what to do, in the absence of proof from us."

— by Renee Twombly

Renee Twombly is a freelance journalist in Durham, North Carolina.

Chapter 45

High-Tech Tools for Food Safety Sleuths

A geneticist couples two DNA strands, one natural from bacteria and one synthetic, and forms a hybrid that positively identifies a species of food-borne bacteria responsible for causing severe illness and death. In another laboratory, a chemist, using mass spectrometry, tracks the amount of an unwanted chemical in fermented products to parts per billion.

Both are FDA food scientists working on the persistent problems caused by contaminants that sometimes creep into what we eat and drink. Often the problem is bacterial, causing rapid development of illness. Other times it's chemical, with illness occurring immediately or at some future time because of cumulative effects.

Health problems from contaminants in foods are well documented. For example, a particularly virulent species of *Listeria* bacteria causes listeriosis, a disease the national Centers for Disease Control estimates results in 1,850 illnesses and 425 deaths annually in the United States. An example of a chemical problem is the presence of ethyl carbamate, a byproduct of fermentation, in alcoholic beverages and other fermented products. This chemical has been known to cause cancer in laboratory animals.

Up-to-the-minute technology helps food scientists lessen the dangers from these and other food contaminants.

FDA Consumer, November 1992.

The Need for Speed

Listeria monocytogenes, the species that causes listeriosis, was the culprit in one of the United States' most tragic food-borne illness outbreaks. In 1985, 48 people from the Los Angeles area who had eaten soft cheese contaminated with the bacteria died, and 94 others became ill.

More recently, last July food and agriculture ministries in France reported an outbreak of listeriosis that had started four months earlier. At the time of the report, there were 108 cases from all regions in France, including 21 deaths of newborn or elderly persons and five spontaneous abortions. The source of the outbreak had not yet been identified.

Serious complications of listeriosis include meningitis (brain infections) and septicemia (bacteria in the bloodstream). For pregnant women, the disease can be transmitted to the fetus, resulting in similar complications in the newborn, or miscarriage or stillbirth.

At the time of the Los Angeles outbreak, the deadly potential of the bacteria made quick identification imperative so that whatever food was causing the illness could be removed from grocery shelves immediately. But it took nearly a month using traditional laboratory methods to positively determine that *L. monocytogenes* had caused the illness.

Recognizing the need for a speedier laboratory technique to identify the bacterial species without sacrificing accuracy, Atin R. Datta, Ph.D., a geneticist with FDA's division of microbiology, and his FDA associates went to work on the problem. Datta's team developed a synthetic gene probe to positively identify *L. monocytogenes*, and today, food scientists can identify *L. monocytogenes* in only two to four days.

FDA's DNA probe has been accepted worldwide. After researchers in France find the source of the recent listeriosis outbreak there, it is expected that they will use the DNA probe to save time in positively identifying the bacteria.

How the DNA Probe Works

All food, unless it has been sterilized and packaged in a sterile container, contains many types of bacteria. Most are harmless to healthy people, but some, like *L .monocytogenes*, are capable of causing serious problems. In this procedure, the *Listeria* class of bacteria is isolated and if *L. monocytogenes* is present, it can be identified and counted in the first part of the DNA probe procedure, Datta spreads a diluted sample of food suspected of containing *Listeria* on the surface of a selective agar medium (a gelatinous substance). This allows *Listeria* bacteria to multiply by suppressing the growth of most other bacteria normally present in many foods. Within two days, the *Listeria* forms colonies on the agar.

When the colonies are formed, Datta presses membrane filter paper onto the agar plates containing the bacterial colonies. This transfers the bacterial colonies to the filter paper, giving the colonies a firm support base for the next step-colony hybridization.

In hybridization, bacterial colonies on the filter paper are treated with microwaves and strong alkaline solutions to break open the cells and release the DNA, uncoupling the natural double-stranded DNA into single strands. Next, synthetically produced, radioactive-labeled, single strands of *L. monocytogenes* DNA (called gene probes) are added to the bacterial colonies on the filter paper.

If *L. monocytogenes* is present, the synthetic gene probe finds it among the natural single strands of DNA and binds with it, forming a hybrid DNA molecule. The probe has been designed in such a way that only *L. monocytogenes* DNA will form the hybrid molecule; other bacterial colonies will not bond to this probe.

In the last step of the DNA probe procedure, Datta places a sheet of x-ray film on the filter paper holding the hybrid DNA molecules. Each colony containing hybrid molecules leaves a dark spot on the film. Because each colony has grown from a single cell, the number of dark spots tells Datta how many *L. monocytogenes* cells were in the original sample.

Other types of DNA probes are used in FDA labs for problems with Shigella, *Escherichia coli*, and other bacteria that cause food-borne illnesses. They're all labeled with radioactive material.

Handling radioactive material is a health hazard, and disposal is a costly environmental problem. (Currently, only three locations in the United States have appropriate disposal facilities for low-level radioactive waste.) So Datta and his associates are developing and testing a method that labels DNA probes with a non-radioactive material-horseradish peroxidase.

DNA probes labeled with horseradish peroxidase could be used to detect *L. monocytogenes* in foods in the same way as radioactive-labeled probes. Once this technique is standardized, Datta believes it will replace radioactive probes, not only for *Listeria* but also for other food-borne pathogens.

A Look at Mass Spectrometry

In other FDA food laboratories, chemists use mass spectrometry (MS) to do different types of analyses. MS enables chemists to identify organic chemicals such as dioxins, pesticides, and naturally occurring toxins. Combining the sophisticated technology of mass spectrometry with chromatographic techniques such as gas, super critical fluid, or high pressure liquid chromatography, FDA chemists can identify and count chemical contaminants in food.

They do it by introducing a small amount of an extract of a food sample into a chromatograph, where chemical contaminants or pesticide residues are separated into individual compounds. Then, in the mass spectrometer, an electronic beam bombards the separated chemicals, ionizing the molecules (giving them an electric charge) and fragmenting them.

The unique fragmentation pattern of individual ionized compounds allows the computer attached to the mass spectrometer to chart information about each and to identify the unknown chemical by comparing its spectrum, or "molecular fingerprint," to a known substance. The system also may allow chemists to accurately measure the amount of a chemical contaminant in a sample of food to parts per trillion levels and smaller.

FDA food chemists have developed laboratory procedures using MS to identify and count many kinds of food contaminants. For example, in an MS procedure using a technique called positive ion fast atom bombardment, chemists have characterized 12 of the neurotoxins in "red tide"—algae that bloom and produce toxins. These toxins can concentrate in fish and shellfish that feed on algae blooms. If eaten, the toxin—contaminated fish can cause serious illness and death. State authorities monitor waters and close the areas to fishing immediately when red tide appears.

FDA field laboratories around the country regularly apply MS and other laboratory procedures to identify and measure chemical contaminants in food. The Chicago district, for example, uses MS procedures to test milk and paper milk cartons for dioxin, a chemical contaminant that could migrate into milk from the paper containers (see "Deciding about Dioxins" in the February 1990 *FDA Consumer* and reprinted earlier in this sourcebook).

FDA and other government agencies have used MS research results to make decisions about food problems. In a food-related crisis in 1989, for example, FDA chemists, working with food scientists from the Centers for Disease Control, needed to identify an unknown impurity in L-tryptophan, a widely used dietary supplement

More than 1,500 persons who had taken the supplement had become ill and 39 died of eosinophilia-myalgia syndrome, a painful muscle and blood disorder. James Sphon, Ph.D., of FDA's Office of Physical Sciences, says that before starting the isolation and identification process, the mass spectrometrists had very little information about what the substance could be.

An FDA/CDC team developed a chromatographic procedure to show trace organic components in L-tryptophan. Using this procedure, along with epidemiologic data, FDA and researchers from medical centers and industry solved part of the mystery by identifying one impurity, 1,1'-ethylidene-bis-L-tryptophan (EBT), that could have been associated with the illness. Several other chemicals have been identified and through ongoing research, scientists will try to find out if these cause or contribute to eosinophilia-myalgia syndrome.

Flaws in Fermentation

FDA has also used mass spectrometry to measure the amount of ethyl carbamate (EC) in fermented products such as soy sauce, wines, or bakery products. EC, a chemical that sometimes forms as a byproduct of, the fermentation process, is a suspected human carcinogen (cancer-causing agent).

The problem of carcinogens in fermented products got international attention in 1985 when Health and Welfare Canada reported that its scientists had detected EC in certain alcoholic products at levels that exceeded newly established Canadian guidelines. FDA and the U.S. Bureau of Alcohol, Tobacco, and Firearms (ATF) immediately began sampling wines and whiskeys from domestic and foreign producers to determine the levels of EC. (FDA and ATF share responsibility for regulating alcoholic beverages—FDA regulates their safety and cleanliness; ATF regulates the manufacture, composition specifications, labeling, and advertising.)

As with the *Listeria* situation, there was a problem of time spent in the laboratory searching for the presence of EC. Before a sample of distilled spirits could be run through the mass spectrometer, chemists had to "clean up" the sample in an unusually extensive, time-consuming procedure.

So William Brumley Ph.D., formerly with FDA and now with the U.S. Environmental Protection Agency, developed a procedure using a more sophisticated mass spectrometer to shorten the analysis time. Brumley's procedure not only identifies and measures EC, it also does part of the sample cleanup.

In Brumley's approach, the MS analysis is carried a step further through an instrument called MS/MS. In this extended step, selected ions are collided with an inert gas. The impact breaks them into smaller, or "daughter" ions. This breakdown allows a more specific identification of the EC.

This year, John Roach, an FDA mass spectrometrist, began collaborating with scientists from 20 laboratories worldwide to evaluate Brumley's approach. The collaborative study will determine if the procedure is acceptable for common use within the scientific community.

FDA food scientists continually adapt DNA probes, mass spectrometry, and other procedures to fit the numerous types of food contaminant problems they encounter. (See "A Day in the Life of FDA's Food Safety Team," in the September 1988 *FDA Consumer*.)

Analytical methods used by FDA have been accepted in courts of law, and studies of most have been published in peer review journals. As FDA geneticist Datta and mass spectrometrist Brumley have shown, if new approaches are needed to solve a contaminant problem, FDA scientists can be called upon to develop them.

A Peek in the Toolbox

FDA food scientists use a number of analytical techniques. Grouped into categories according to their function, these tools and some of their applications are:

Chromatography (thin-layer, gas and liquid)

- separates complex mixtures (food extracts of various types) of similar components by measuring migration rates of component molecules through columns and through coatings on chromatography plates.

- analyzes food extracts for pesticide residues, chemical contaminants, and natural toxins; analyzes alcoholic beverages, fats, oils, and direct and indirect food additives.

Spectrometry (mass spectrometry, nuclear magnetic resonance and electron spin resonance, and infrared and ultraviolet spectroscopy)

- measures molecules or atoms of food components as they are ionized and fragmented in a magnetic field, as they are polarized in a magnetic field, or as they undergo absorption and emission of energy in irradiation.

- analyzes food additives, food contaminants, metals, fats, and oils; confirms the identity of pesticides, natural toxins and other chemical contaminants, and food additives and flavors; assists in identifying unknown complex organic structures.

Radiotracers

- measure isotopes that undergo radioactive decay but that, in all other respects, are identical to atoms normally found in chemicals.

- study food additives, food processing, animal metabolism, and biosynthesis of natural toxins; analyze foods for radioactivity.

Gene probes, enzyme catalysis, antibody-antigen interaction, and immunoassays

- depend on specific properties and interactions of substances being analyzed with antibodies, DNA fragments, and other components.

- analyze foods for amino acids, sugars, microbial toxins, other natural toxins (e.g., aflatoxins), and pesticides.

Analyzers (thermal energy analyzer, amino acid analyzer, and others)

- are specialized instruments, often automatic, that react to specific components or contaminants in food samples.

- analyze contaminants in foods (e.g., nitrosamines) and food packaging; assay vitamins, nutrients, and other food substances.

Electrochemistry (polargraphy, electrophoresis, anodic stripping, voltammetry)

- separates complex mixtures of components in a food product by use of an electric force field.

- analyzes food extracts for metals and pesticide residues; identifies preservatives, color additives, and species of fish.

Bioassays

- measure responses of living organisms (from viruses to bacteria, animal cells in culture to primates) to substances being analyzed.

- analyze food extracts for natural toxins, pesticides, nutrients, and hormones.

Computer-assisted analytical workstations

- control analytical instruments by use of highly sophisticated computers.

- monitor programs; calibrate, record and store information; maintain diagnostic control over analytical and data-gathering systems.

— by Judith Foulke

Judith Foulke is a staff writer for FDA Consumer.

Chapter 46

Chemicals We'd Rather Dine Without

A person's diet can never be entirely free of potentially harmful chemicals. Mother Nature has seen to that, having armed her bounty with an arsenal of poisons against molds, bacteria, insects and other predators.

And though people are responsible for such toxins in the diet as synthetic pesticides and industrial chemicals, nature's poisons are often more potent—certainly more prevalent. "We are ingesting in our diet at least 10,000 times more by weight of natural pesticides than of man-made pesticide residues," reported Bruce Ames, Ph. D., and other Berkeley, Calif, researchers in the April 17, 1987, issue of *Science*.

What turns the effects of a toxin from harmless to harmful, though, are the toxin's potency and the extent of a person's exposure to it. Fortunately, FDA has something to say about exposure. "As public health gatekeeper for most foods, FDA monitors the food supply for pesticide residues and contaminants, and agency data show that the amounts our bodies are exposed to are safe," said Richard Ronk, acting director of FDA's Center for Food Safety and Applied Nutrition (CFSAN).

The Federal Food, Drug, and Cosmetic Act has various provisions both to regulate the presence of contaminants in foods and to remove foods with unsafe contamination from the market. Imported foods with illegal residues can be refused entry into the country. In the case of domestic foods, FDA can impose the sanctions of seizure, injunction and prosecution.

FDA Consumer, September 1988.

Accents on Imports

During 1984 and 1985, FDA took a special look at ethnic foods on the U.S. market. Random sampling revealed an array of problems, such as vermin-infested dry foods and swollen and rusty cans. As a result, imported foods are getting extra FDA attention nowadays. (See "Imported Ethnic Foods: Exotic Fare but Buyer Beware" in the December 1986-January 1987 *FDA Consumer*.) The agency began a special ethnic foods program that includes not only stepping up its own import monitoring, but also urging state and local agencies to intensify their surveillance.

Soon, FDA will improve its tracking of imported foods—and contaminants they may have been found to contain—with a highly sophisticated and versatile computerized system called ISIS (for Import Support and Information System). According to Dennis Linsley, of FDA's Buffalo district office, "ISIS will do profiling for us—firms, products and countries—to give us a better idea of where the problems are. On the basis of this profiling, its artificial intelligence will in the future. actually be able to alert us to look at certain products."

Automated import records in the fully functioning ISIS will help FDA rapidly shift enforcement strategies—to keep importers from moving problem products from port to port—"port shopping"—to avoid detection, for instance. FDA will be able to detect trends more readily. And trends, in turn, can be used to help earmark future monitoring resources.

Smarter Sampling

To monitor foods for contaminants, FDA routinely samples items that are of dietary importance, such as produce. Foods suspected of illegal residues receive more intense watching.

An important part of FDA's safety sampling is a "market basket" or total diet study of foods that, according to government surveys, typify the American diet. Four times a year, identical purchases of 234 foods, including imports and processed foods, are made in three cities in a given region. The foods are shipped to FDA's Kansas City, Mo., laboratory, where they are peeled, cooked, baked, or otherwise made table-ready, and then analyzed for (among other things) pesticide residues, radioactive elements, and toxic metals. The results are used to determine actual dietary intakes of these chemicals by eight population groups, based on age and gender.

492

The concern with most chemical contaminants in foods is not over any immediate harm, but over the possibility of an increase in a health risk; due to long term exposure. Following is a look at some individual contaminants, along with steps FDA has taken to keep risks as low as possible for consumers. These contaminants are targets of the agency's ongoing surveillance. Some involve contamination problems that are currently being assessed to determine potential risks. (Also see "Invisible Villains" in the July-August 1988 *FDA Consumer* for information about bacterial contaminants.)

Mycotoxins

Mycotoxins are a group of naturally formed food toxins produced by molds growing on foods or feeds that have the potential to cause illness.

Best known are the aflatoxins. The highly potent aflatoxin B_1 has caused cancer in certain test animals. The exact extent of the risk that aflatoxins pose for people is yet unknown, but FDA believes it is in the best interest of consumers that dietary exposure be kept to minimal levels. FDA monitors foods to ensure this is the case. Aflatoxins can't be completely destroyed by heat or effectively removed by many types of food processing, so they may remain intact in finished products. The foods most often contaminated with aflatoxins are tree nuts, peanuts, and oil-seeds such as cottonseed. Animal feed ingredients, though are the primary source of aflatoxins.

When aflatoxins are found, levels typically are so low as to compare with finding a single copper slug in $10 million worth of pennies. Scientists at CFSAN have developed methods to detect aflatoxin levels as low as parts per billion in foods.

The ideal growth condition for most molds depends on an optimal combination of temperature, humidity, and the proper nutrients. Mycotoxins are most likely to be produced when plants are stressed, such as through drought, insect damage, or other adverse conditions. Cooling and freezing halt mold growth but don't eliminate mycotoxins already produced. Moldy food or feed shouldn't be fed to pets or farm animals. When in doubt, throw it out!

Lead in Ceramic Products

Most ceramic dinnerware is coated with a glaze containing lead or cadmium. Lead gives a shiny, smooth look; cadmium gives shades of yellow, orange and red. Both are toxic. If such a glaze is properly formulated, applied and fired, the final product is almost impervious to food and beverage interaction. But if any steps are improperly performed, the poisonous metal may leach into food. Most problems come from storing high-acid foods for long periods in improperly made ceramic containers. High levels of lead in the diet will go into bones and organs, where it can reside for as long as 30 years.

Since 1971, FDA has limited how much lead may leach from ceramic products. FDA tightened its limits in 1980 and is reassessing them again to see whether they should be even stricter. This reevaluation was prompted by research data that heightened concerns about lead from all sources and agency concern over certain food-ware, especially imports. "Fortunately, domestically manufactured dinnerware seldom exceeds the limits established by FDA," said Edward Steele, who directs the division of program operations, CFSAN.

Agency investigators routinely sample ceramic products, pewter, enamelware, and other household items for lead and cadmium. FDA exempts from its limits display-only products, provided they carry permanent warnings that they may cause food to become toxic and that they are not intended for storing or serving food or beverages.

The only sure way to know whether a ceramic piece is safe is to have it tested, but you can reduce the chances of lead poisoning by not using antiques or collectibles for food or beverages and by being wary of items bought in other countries or made by amateurs. (See also "Pretty Poison: Lead and Ceramic Ware" in the July-August 1987 *FDA Consumer*.)

Another significant man-made source of lead in food is lead-soldered cans. Efforts by FDA and the food industry have resulted in markedly decreased lead levels in canned foods in recent years. Many firms (including the entire soft drink industry) now use cans that don't require any lead solder.

FDA does not recommend storing acidic foods, such as tomatoes, in lead-soldered cans that have been opened. The lead dissolves and leaches into these foods rapidly due to the presence of acid and oxygen.

Because the very young are more vulnerable to the effects of lead, FDA has been especially concerned with the diets of infants and children. Now, all infant formula comes in cans without lead solder, and infant juices and foods are packaged in glass.

Lead also may be present in certain calcium supplements, so FDA periodically samples them. FDA surveys first centered on bonemeal supplements. Recently, however, the agency assigned its district offices to conduct a survey that included samples from other calcium sources, such as oyster shell and dolomite. "The results haven't been completely analyzed yet," said CFSAN consumer safety officer John Thomas, "but we have found no reason to be alarmed."

Paralytic Shellfish Poisoning

Toxins that cause potentially fatal paralytic shellfish poisoning (PSP) are produced by microscopic algae called dinoflagellates. PSP is frequently associated with a "red tide" (an explosive growth of the dinoflagellates turns the water reddish), though not all red tides are produced by poison-producing dinoflagellate species.

FDA coordinates regulation of shell fish safety through the Interstate Shellfish Sanitation Conference, a group composed of FDA, state agencies, and industry representatives. Ensuring that shellfish are harvested from clean waters falls to the states, which prohibit harvesting in areas contaminated by sewage, industrial wastes, or high levels of toxic dinoflagellates. FDA provides scientific expertise, evaluates the states' programs, recommends corrective measures states should take to ensure safe interstate shellfish shipments, and reports any deficient state programs to the interstate conference.

FDA conducts research on fish-related public health problems through its facilities in Washington, D.C.; Cincinnati; Seattle; Davisville, R.I.; and Dauphin Island, Ala. Studies cover such areas as decomposition of seafood, aquaculture, ciguatera toxins (which can occur in such coral reef fish as barracuda, grouper, and red snapper), the safety of surimi (ground fish formed to imitate shellfish), and improving detection of marine toxins and environmental contaminants.

Mercury in Fish and Shellfish

FDA first set limits for mercury in foods in 1969, after 120 people in Niigata, Japan, had fallen ill from eating fish contaminated with high amounts of mercury. Birth defects in offspring of some mothers in the group affected also were ascribed to mercury poisoning.

Between July 1 and Dec. 31, 1986, FDA checked 127 swordfish shipments from 15 countries for mercury. Samples from over 70 percent of the countries had illegal levels. Currently, swordfish imports are automatically detained until they are shown to meet FDA's requirements. Shipments are admitted only after the importer provides FDA with a certificate of analysis from a qualified independent laboratory to show the fish do not contain mercury levels of potential health concert. "Sixteen shippers have been taken off detention after having up to 20 consecutive legal shipments," said John Browne of FDA's import operations branch. "But we'll still monitor their swordfish and, if we find excessive mercury levels, that shipper's exemption from detention will be cancelled," he said.

Polychlorinated Biphenyls (PCBs)

Widely used for years in a variety of products, PCBs—a class of industrial chemicals—are no longer produced, because of their health risks. PCBs are linked to liver tumors and reproductive problems in test animals, so FDA has banned their use in machinery used to process food and animal feed. "FDA has seen no evidence that acute PCB exposure, which may occur from consumption of foods, causes adverse effects in people," said Michael Bolger, Ph.D., a CFSAN toxicologist. "Long-term effects from chronic exposure via foods are unknown," he said.

Because PCBs persist in soil and sediment in water, occasional contamination of food may be unavoidable. Further, they can't be eliminated from food by processing. To limit consumers' exposure, FDA has established tolerances for PCBs in susceptible foods and in paper food-packaging material. The most significant food source for PCB residues is fish, primarily freshwater fish such as coho and Chinook salmon from the Great Lakes, and bottom-feeding freshwater species from waters near other industrial areas—although coastal marine species also may contain PCBs. Any food found to contain levels exceeding the tolerances are subject to seizure and other legal remedies by FDA or the states. The state of New York, for instance, applied FDA's tolerances for PCBs to close some highly contaminated areas of the Hudson River to commercial fishing of striped bass. "Fish in interstate traffic are highly unlikely to contain unsafe levels of PCBs," said Bolger.

Dioxin

Though the chemical 2,3,7,8-tetrachlorodibenzo-p-dioxin has a scientific name that begins something like a football cheer, it is generally known by its blessedly shortened name, dioxin. It forms during the manufacture of chemicals such as certain pesticides and during the chlorine bleaching process applied to paper, including paper products used with some foods, such as coffee filters and paper plates.

Dioxin is believed to produce cancer and other harmful effects in some animals, even in small doses. The American Council on Science and Health, however, reported in a 1984 publication that studies of people occupationally exposed to dioxin "have not shown a relationship between dioxin and cancer and this offers us considerable assurance that traces in the environment do not cause a cancer hazard."

A major food source of dioxin for Americans is bottom fish from the Great Lakes, an area of the country with a great deal of industrial activity and chemical production. Several years ago, states in that area found they had a dioxin problem and, so, asked FDA about whether to issue advice on eating certain fish from certain waters and whether to restrict fishing. "Our advice was that, for a fishery whose fish average less than 25 parts per trillion (ppt) of dioxin, you probably don't need to control consumption," said Elizabeth Campbell of FDA. "But if the fish average more than 50 ppt," she said, "you probably shouldn't eat them. Between those levels, consumption should be restricted— probably once a week for the seasonal folks and no more than twice a month for people eating the fish there year-round."

Because dioxin contamination is a localized problem, it is unlikely that the fish sold in interstate commerce contain unsafe levels. "People who eat commercial fish normally eat a variety," Campbell said, "and even those who stick to one type of fish don't usually have a problem, because fish in interstate commerce generally come from different waters, only a few of which may contain any dioxin." Such occasional exposures aren't harmful, she said.

There also has been some concern about possible leaching of dioxin into foods from Kraft paper food-use production such as paper plates and coffee filters. The American Paper Institute, in a 1988 summary of a study it conducted, reported. "Even using assumptions that likely overstate the risk, consumption of coffee brewed using bleached paper filters does not present a significant, health risk—that is, the coffee is safe to drink." At the behest of the Environmental Protection Agency, paper manufacturers themselves are examining the processes used at their mills to try to prevent further environmental contamination with dioxin. Ronald Lorentzen, Ph.D. a carcinogen expert at FDA, said that FDA is working with EPA, industry, and other groups to determine what, if any, risks to people dioxin from paper products may pose.

Urethane in Alcoholic Beverages

Urethane (ethyl carbamate) is a chemical that forms during fermentation of alcoholic beverages. If the fermented product is heated, as in "baking" sherry and distilling bourbon, urethane levels increase. Urethane causes cancer in animals, but the extent of its risk to people is at present unclear. Legal responsibility for alcoholic beverages is shared by FDA and the Bureau of Alcohol, Tobacco, and Firearms (ATF). FDA ensures safety under the Federal Food, Drug, and Cosmetic Act; ATF regulates manufacture, composition, labeling and advertising under the Federal Alcohol Administration Act.

In November 1985, news reports from Canada stated that authorities there had found urethane in certain wines and distilled spirits. U.S. concern led FDA, ATF and industry to look for ways to assess and deal with the problem. Sampling revealed that, among distilled spirits, bourbons generally contained the highest urethane levels: up to several hundred parts per billion (ppb). Levels in some brandies were also high: from 200 to 12,000 ppb.

Since then, FDA has accepted two plans by industry to reduce urethane in alcoholic beverages. And FDA Commissioner Frank E. Young, M.D., Ph.D., has asked 27 foreign governments that levels in their countries' alcoholic beverages intended for export to the United States be "as low as technologically feasible—at least comparable to those of similar alcoholic beverages" produced here. At FDA's request, the National Toxicology Program, a federally funded research group, is giving urethane its highest research priority in 1988. Results of that research should provide the information FDA needs to better assess the significance of urethane in alcoholic beverages. (See also "Too Many Drinks Spiked with Urethane" in the April 1988 *FDA Consumer.*)

Priorities

FDA repeatedly reevaluates its food safety priorities so that resources go where the big concerns are. This does not mean, however, that safety in one area is sacrificed for safety somewhere else. As Commissioner Young noted during recent Congressional hearings, while microbial and other natural food contaminants may pose greater risks than do synthetic pesticides, "we must continue... to carry out a strong program to police, and thus minimize, illegal pesticide residues in the food supply so that the risks presented by dietary exposure... will remain low."

—by Dixie Farley

Dixie Farley is a member of FDA's public affairs staff.

Chapter 47

Perspectives on Food Biotechnology

The "new biotechnology" is in the news so much these days that it now goes by the handy nickname "biotech." In medicine, it has assumed heroic proportions, with *Science* magazine hailing it as the last great technical innovation of the 20th century—the progenitor of genetic probes, synthetic hormones, and other life-saving marvels.

In food production, however, it has not been so warmly welcomed:

- The European Economic Community has banned use of a genetically engineered hormone to increase milk production in dairy cows.

- American grocery chains have refused milk from such cattle.

- Activists fearing agricultural experimentation have sued to prevent field testing even of genetically engineered petunias.

What's Going on with Our Food Supply?

The short answer is "the new biotechnology," a scientific revolution less than 20 years old that's already changing the foods we eat.

The jargon of the "new biotech" may sound pretty ominous to the average consumer. "Cloning," "genetic manipulation," "cell fusion," and "mutation" may seem more like fantasies out of "Star Trek" than the results of processes we want to contemplate at the supermarket. Nonetheless,

FDA Consumer, March 1990.

these scientific processes are soon likely to be applied to more and more of our foods.

It's important to understand what food biotechnology is before forming our opinions about it. Although the jargon may sound unnatural, the science is the reverse. In fact, it can be viewed as a method of organizing nature to bring out the best in nature. It's essentially a refinement of what we've known—and done—for a very long time.

"Biotech" Old and New

Biotechnology is the use of biological systems—living things—to create or modify products.

Traditional biotechnology is almost as old as agriculture itself. The first farmer who bred the best bull with the best cow in the herd to improve the stock, rather than allowing the animals to breed randomly, was implementing biotechnology in a simple sense. The first baker who used yeast enzymes to make bread rise was likewise using a living thing to produce an improved product. Indeed, one anthropologist argues that a desire to raise grain for brewing beer—a classic biotechnology product—was the impetus for the first systematic farming 10,000 years ago.

The "old biotech" that produced these changes is obviously not a single process but a number of different methods. The one feature common to these traditional biotechnologies is use of natural processes to introduce changes in foods. The "new biotechnology" is likewise a number of methods of using organisms to make or modify products. It differs from traditional methods by modifying the genetic material of organisms directly and precisely. It enables the transfer of genes between diverse organisms, allowing combinations unlikely to occur by conventional means.

Unlike their predecessors, who progressed by trial and error, today's farmers can exploit the subtleties of genetics. Science has found ways for them to introduce quickly and directly specific crop and animal improvements that formerly took generations. The result may be the same, but the new precision multiplies the possibilities available for achieving specific practical results.

It was not always thus. Mark Twain spins the tongue-in-cheek yarn of an agricultural experimenter named William Beazeley who pined away because of his obsessive, but futile, desire to grow turnips on vines. Nineteenth-century readers scoffed at this absurd idea, but that satire of the 1860s could become a technical possibility in the 1990s if there were any point to achieving it. Fortunately, the new biotech projects in view have more practical goals than Beazeley's.

New biotech springs from our ability to rearrange or recombine DNA, the basic genetic material of living things, a feat made possible in 1974, when American scientists first cloned (isolated and duplicated) a specific gene. From that beginning, the new biotechnology has developed as wide a range of applications as traditional methods. In food production, it is revolutionizing old processes like fermentation and cross-breeding. Both in the field and in the food-processing plant, it is joining in the age-old quest for a healthy, abundant and nutritious food supply.

Evolution or Revolution?

In the 1860s, Gregor Mendel, an Austrian priest (who, ironically, had flunked biology in his teacher's examination), deduced the laws of heredity. Working with pea plants in his monastery garden, Mendel discovered he could predict the characteristics of plants bred from specific types of parents. From there it was just a short step to producing at will such characteristics as color, height, and pod position or appearance. Although published in the 1860s, his findings were ignored until researchers rediscovered and confirmed them in 1900.

Mendel's work ultimately made possible scientific farming based on genetics. By the 1930s, organ culture techniques made it possible to isolate plant embryos as a basis for breeding more successful hybrids. Corn production in the United States quickly doubled as a result. Through such methods, agricultural wheat was crossed with wild grasses in order to acquire such properties as greater yield, increased resistance to mildew and bacterial diseases, and tolerance for salt or adverse climate conditions.

Similar progress with many foodstuffs enabled China and India, threatened with famine in the mid-1970s, to invigorate their agriculture to the point that today they are net exporters of grain. Although much of this achievement came from ambitious applications of traditional biotechnology, the new biotech now sustains it, notably in work on rice and the other grains on which so many people worldwide subsist. Today, the new biotech strives to develop drought-tolerant crops that, in turn, could alleviate the famines devastating Africa.

New biotech continues its quest for fruitful harvests only under protest. In one case in Maryland, opponents long delayed field testing of corn engineered to resist the European corn borer, a caterpillar that annually spoils $400 million in American crops unless deterred by heavy treatments with pesticides. In Wisconsin, where farmers forfeit $800,000 yearly in crops and pesticide expenses in their losing battle against brown spot disease in green beans, university researchers had to curb their hunt for a new-biotech alternative because of difficulties getting approval for field tests.

One current focus of research is a tomato genetically engineered not to go soft for far longer than ordinary products. Its developer claims that it looks the same, feels the same, and tastes the same as other tomatoes; its nutritional value is identical. The only difference researchers found—a difference achieved by isolating and counteracting a single gene that makes tomatoes rot rapidly—is that this tomato keeps longer. The reversal of that one gene in the 10,000 making up the plant is all that was needed to make this biotech tomato significant.

Waiting in the wings is another tomato plant altered to contain a bacterial protein toxic to plant-attacking insects but not to other living things. The primary safety issues with both of these "new" tomatoes are whether their introduction of single new properties might mask other unforeseen changes as well, and whether the products of these new genes are safe to eat.

The Context of Controversy

Traditional biotechnology also continues to develop even as the new biotech comes into play. A recent triumph is the "beefalo," a hybrid animal whose meat combines the tenderness of domestic beef with the leanness of American buffalo. This development alarmed nobody and has won consumer acceptance.

Yet, when the traditional biotechnology of farmyard and field moves toward the "new biotech" of the laboratory, many people become alarmed at its very efficiency. As Margaret Mellon of the National Wildlife Federation put it, "I feel an affection for the natural world the way it is—the way four billion years of evolution have made it. I resist the notion of improving nature in the future, just as I lament the loss of nature as it was in the past." Refinements that once would have taken generations may now be induced deliberately and rapidly—too rapidly for such observers.

Perhaps our imaginations have been colored by gimmick picture postcards of gigantic foodstuffs, whether gondola-sized potatoes or enormous bass asserted to be typical of particular resorts. Perhaps films showing humanity beleaguered by Frankenstein monsters or mutant insects dispose us to envision enormities. More soberly, some critics make analogies to past introductions of novelties into our environment, such as kudzu plant, which became a troublesome weed, or the starlings whimsically imported into North America only to multiply and foul our cities. Others fear harm to consumers from new foodstuffs.

What is the individual to make of these fears? Is the new biotech following in the steps of the pioneer Mendel or the crackpot Beazeley? For example, bST (bovine somatotropin), a pituitary hormone produced in cattle, was recognized to increase milk production when injected into dairy cows as early as the 1930s. The recombinant technology of the 1980s allowed production of large amounts of pure bST, which could be used to increase milk yield and efficiency of production during part of the cow's lactation period.

Because it is a protein, bST is digested and inactivated when eaten. Furthermore, bST is inactive in humans. People produce human somatotropin, but it is considerably different in structure from bST.

Since cows produce bST naturally, it is and has always been present in their milk. Treating the animals with the proposed levels of bST doesn't increase the level of bST in milk above the levels occurring naturally. Nor does bST treatment alter the nutrient composition of milk. While FDA is still evaluating the animal and environmental safety of bST, the agency has determined that the milk from treated animals is safe for humans.

Recently, five U.S. supermarket chains publicized their refusal to buy dairy products from cows treated with bST. They curtailed purchases under pressure from a coalition of groups concerned with issues ranging from animal rights to an alleged current milk surplus and the survival of the small family farm. Uneasiness about the safety of consuming dairy products from "experimental animals" also apparently influenced the decision.

When it comes to farm crops, the U.S. National Academy of Sciences and its parent, the National Research Council (NRC), have not found any difference between the environmental safety of old and new biotech-derived plants. In 1989, NRC reported that "crops modified by molecular and cellular methods [i.e., the new biotechnology] pose risks no different from those modified by classical genetic methods for similar traits." It also noted that no adverse effects have developed from introductions of genetically modified organisms.

Moreover, some scientists argue that the precisely directed alterations of recombinant-DNA technology might in fact be far safer than the random shuffling of characteristics inevitable under more traditional techniques. As the NRC puts it, because "the new molecular methods are more specific, users of these methods will be more certain about the traits they introduce into plants" than those using traditional methods. Many projects now in the works to promote food safety (from displacing chemical pesticides or preservatives to improving food sanitation) are possible only through the new methods.

New Challenges for FDA

In insuring a safe, nutritious food supply, FDA can't be complacent about the implications of the new biotechnology or any technology. Old biotechnology occasionally posed regulatory puzzles, and FDA recognizes that the products of genetic technology give new twists to old regulatory questions.

Take the concept of food adulteration, for instance. The traditional idea of adulteration was that of impurities being added to a food—for instance, when milk might be exposed to *Salmonella* bacteria or in the case of fillers added to cereals. The new biotechnology, however, makes it possible to remove properties as well as to add them: the long-lasting tomato, for example. There are many exciting possibilities—like engineering cows or hens to eliminate the properties some people are allergic to in milk or eggs—but these undeniably raise questions about changes in quality.

The ultimate question may be how many properties can be changed in an organism before it becomes something else. A tomato improved in one specific way seems obviously to be still a tomato, but does it remain one if you alter it in 10 ways, or 20? When traditional methods crossed the tangerine with a grapefruit, the new genetic structure was clearly something else, now sold as a tangelo. The new biotech questions are far more subtle. FDA must grapple with concepts of this sort as it considers the many new biotech food applications now being developed.

Biotechnology on Your Table

Markedly different or even novel foods probably won't appear on the grocery shelves any time soon. In less spectacular form, however, the new biotechnology is already keeping its dinner date. For instance, Canadian salmon have been treated for most of this decade with a hormone that allows them to mature three times faster than normal, without changing the fish in any other way.

Most of the new biotech projects now in the works would do little to affect the taste or appearance of the food on the plate, although a few promise to improve the flavors and consistency of some vegetables or reduce the fat content of some meats. Most address foods in ways that can't readily be seen—by improving nutrition content, preventing spoilage, or even eliminating the need for chemical pesticides. Gene probes to detect rapidly the source of food-borne illnesses have already proven their worth to health authorities. For example, a synthetic DNA probe recently was used to detect a shellfish-related disease when other detection methods failed.

FDA recently surveyed more than 100 experts from government, business, and the universities to find out what sorts of developments in food biotechnology to expect in the near future. The survey made clear that the floodgates of innovation are opening. Nearly 800 different developments were reported as technically feasible, three-quarters of them potentially ready for commercial applications in a few years.

Prospects include meats with lower sodium and cholesterol content and longer shelf life, as well as weather-resistant crops with more abundant yield and nutritional content. Methods to better detect *Listeria* species or other food-borne germs are coming, to join the valuable gene probes already in use for detecting *Salmonella* and other bacteria. Plants engineered to do without chemical pesticides are beginning to sprout. Potatoes might some day be raised to last without preservatives. To the consumer's eye and palate, these first fruits of the new biotechnology will seem only subtly different, but the benefits should be substantial.

"Biotech Burgers" won't be available at the drive-in any time soon. Apples the size of pumpkins aren't right around the corner. And don't hold your breath waiting for Beazeley's turnip vines. But there may soon be the option of buying low-fat, low-cholesterol steaks, long-lasting, nutritionally superior vegetables, and pesticide-free fruits abundant because of an extended growing season, all courtesy of the new biotechnology.

—by Henry I. Miller, MD., and Stephen J. Ackerman

Henry I. Miller, M.D., is director of FDA's Office of Biotechnology.

Stephen J. Ackerman is a writer and consultant in Washington, D.C.

Chapter 48

Food Irradiation: Toxic to Bacteria, Safe for Humans

A measure FDA announced in the *Federal Register* this year may go unused because of consumer apprehension. On May 2, 1990, FDA issued a rule defining the use of irradiation as a safe and effective means to control a major source of food-borne illness—*Salmonella* and other food-borne bacteria in raw chicken, turkey, and other poultry. However. FDA has received written objections that it must evaluate before the rule can go into effect.

Experts believe that up to 60 percent of poultry sold in the United States is contaminated with *Salmonella*, according to Joseph Madden, Ph.D., acting director of FDA's division of microbiology. Madden adds that studies suggest that all chicken may be contaminated with the *Campylobacter* organism.

People often become ill after eating contaminated poultry. Symptoms may range from a simple stomachache to incapacitating stomach and intestinal disorders, occasionally resulting in death.

As equipment used to irradiate food is regulated as a food additive, the FDA rule is the first step in permitting irradiation of poultry. However, although the U.S. Department of Agriculture will soon propose a companion rule finalizing guidelines for commercial irradiation of poultry, industry groups cite consumer apprehension as a drawback to implementing the procedure. And reaction to FDA's new rule has elicited more questions than answers.

FDA Consumer, December 1992. Reprint of *FDA Consumer* November 1990. NIH publication no. 91-2241.

A Scary Word

Irradiating food to prevent illness from food-borne bacteria is not a new concept. Research on the technology began in earnest shortly after World War II, when the U.S. Army began a series of experiments irradiating fresh foods for troops in the field. Since 1963, FDA has passed rules permitting irradiation to curb insects in foods and microorganisms in spices, control parasite contamination in pork, and retard spoilage in fruits and vegetables.

But to many people, the word irradiation means danger. It is associated with atomic bomb explosions and nuclear reactor accidents such as those at Chernobyl and Three Mile Island. The idea of irradiating food signals a kind of "gamma alarm," according to one British broadcaster. (Gamma rays are forms of energy emitted from some radioactive materials.)

But when it comes to food irradiation, the only danger is to the bacteria that contaminate the food. The process damages their genetic material, so the organisms can no longer survive or multiply.

Irradiation does not make food radioactive and, therefore, does not increase human exposure to radiation. The specified exposure times and energy levels of radiation sources approved for foods are inadequate to induce radioactivity in the products, according to FDA's Laura Tarantino, Ph.D., an expert on food irradiation. The process involves exposing food to a source of radiation, such as to the gamma rays from radioactive cobalt or cesium or to x-rays. However, no radioactive material is ever added to the product. Manufacturers use the same technique to sterilize many disposable medical devices. Tarantino notes that in testing the safety of the process. Scientists used much higher levels of radiation than those approved for use in poultry. But even at these elevated levels, researchers round no toxic or cancer-causing effects in animals consuming irradiated poultry.

Beyond the Gamma Alarm

Market tests show that once consumers learn about irradiation, they will buy irradiated food. For example, Christine Brahn, Ph.D., of the University of California's Center for Consumer Research in Davis, Calif., reports that irradiated papayas outsold the nonirradiated product by more than 10 to 1 when in-store information was available. And Danny Terry, Ph.D.. a consumer researcher at Central Missouri State University in Warrensburg, Mo., says that a recent market test he conducted with irradiated strawberries showed that consumers who received written information about irradiation along with the fruit were slightly more interested in buying irradiated products in the future.

Nevertheless, concern about the process remains strong. Since 1989, three states (Maine, New York, and New Jersey) have either banned or issued a moratorium on the sale of irradiated foods. According to a U.S. General Accounting Office report prepared in May 1990 at the request of Rep. Douglas Bosco (D-Calif), "officials of these states told us that their states took the actions in response to public concern by citizen groups rather than as a result of scientific evidence questioning the safety of food irradiation."

Something quite aside from food safety appears to lie at the root of the entire controversy, which may explain why it continues to flourish in the face of all safety assurances," says Carolyn Lochhead in the August 1989 issue of *Food Technology* magazine. "Many opponents charge that the Food and Drug Administration, the World Health Organization. and the nuclear power industry are conspiring to promote the technique as a way to dispose of nuclear waste."

Lochhead discusses concerns that one source of radioactive material for food irradiation, cesium 137, is recovered from spent fuel rods in nuclear power plants. The conspiracy charge promotes unwarranted fear among consumers, says Lochhead.

"For economic, as well as other reasons," says Department of Energy of official Barbara Thomas, "the U.S. commercial nuclear power industry does not attempt to recover material, such as cesium 137, from spent fuel."

According to DOE, commercial irradiators in the United States choose their irradiation source (whether the gamma-emitting radioactive materials cesium 137 or cobalt 60 or accelerators that can produce electrons, x-rays or both) based on practical requirements, such as cost. The product to be irradiated also influences the choice. Many foods require low energy levels to kill harmful organisms, while medical supplies may need higher doses for sterilization.

However, the fallout from a falsely characterized cesium recovery plan has changed the legislative atmosphere. George Giddings. Ph.D. a consultant food constant scientist are expert in food irradiation matters, sees it as the "single most important issue in the food irradiation area." Giddings suggests that legislators are wary of supporting food irradiation measures some critics say are linked to increased nuclear activity, including the production of nuclear weapons.

A 1982 congressional amendment bars using spent commercial fuel for military purposes. The Department of Energy has no interest In changing this law.

Michael Colby, director of Food and Water, Inc., one of the more vocal groups lobbying against food irradiation, says the new poultry regulation will lead to nuclear hazards, "including the continued generation of radioactive wastes for which a secure isolation technology has yet to be developed." Colby submitted the comment during a 30-day objection period following publication of the final rule. In the case of food additives, FDA evaluates objections in order to determine whether any changes in the final rule are appropriate. Based on FDA's findings, those raising the objection may be entitled to a hearing before the commissioner.

FDA inspections of all irradiation plants conducted from 1986 to 1989 showed no violations of the food irradiation regulation.

Giddings contends that groups such as Food and Water play on the public fear of nuclear energy, misrepresent the safety questions surrounding food irradiation. They frame it as a populist issue to legislators and pressure them to introduce legislation banning food irradiation.

Consumer Uncertainty

Other consumer groups have taken more moderate positions. The Center for Science in the Public Interest, for instance, says that at a minimum, irradiated foods should be labeled—so that consumers know what they're buying.

Since 1966, FDA has required that irradiated foods be labeled as such. In 1986, a mandatory logo was added to this labeling requirement. The international logo, first used in the Netherlands, consists of a solid circle, representing an energy source, above two petals, which represent the food. Five breaks in the outer circle depict rays from the energy source.

Consumer surveys show mixed reactions. According to an article in the October 1989 issue of *Food Technology* magazine, which reviewed surveys conducted by various academic and consumer research groups. consumers are more concerned about chemical sprays and pesticide residues, preservatives, and food-borne illnesses than about food irradiation. A Louis Harris poll, conducted from 1984 through 1986, however, found that 76 percent of Americans consider irradiated food a hazard.

Product	Purpose of Irradiation	Dose Permitted (kGy)	Date of Rule
Wheat and wheat powder	Disinfest insects	0.2-0.5	8/21/63
White potatoes	Extend shelf life	0.05-0.15	11/1/65
Spices and dry vegetable seasoning (38 commodities)	Decontamination/ disinfest insects	30(max.)	7/5/83
Dry or dehydrated enzyme preparations	Control insects and microorganisms	10(max.)	6/10/85
Pork carcasses or fresh non-cut processed cuts	Control *Trichinella spiralis*	0.3(min.)- 1.0(max.)	7/22/85
Fresh fruits	Delay maturation	1	4/18/86
Dry or dehydrated enzyme preparations	Decontamination	10	4/18/86
Dry or dehydrated aromatic vegetable substances	Decontamination	30	4/18/86
Poultry	Control illness-causing microorganisms	3	5/2/90

Table 48.1. *U.S. Food Irradiation Rules*

"Consumer acceptance of irradiation as a treatment for foods is showing only minimal positive change, at best," said Fred Shank, Ph.D.. director of FDA's Center for Food Safety and Applied Nutrition, in a symposium on food irradiation at the 1990 annual meeting of the Institute of Food Technology. Shank said that the greatest concern about the process is its perceived association with radioactivity and nuclear power.

Another concern, raised often in comments to FDA when it proposed the use of radiation to kill microorganisms in spices and insects in fresh foods, is that irradiation may produce substances not known to be present in nonirradiated foods. These substances, described by scientists as "radiolytic products" sound more threatening than they actually are, says George Pauli, Ph.D., an FDA food irradiation expert and policy maker. For instance, Pauli says, when we heat food it often creates new substances that produce new tastes and smells. These substances could be called thermolytic products—an intimidating word for a harmless change.

In 1979, FDA established the Bureau of Foods Irradiated Food Committee (BFIFC) to review safety assessments of irradiated food. Experiments have shown that very few of these radiolytic products are unique to irradiated foods. In fact, the BFIFC estimated that approximately 9 percent of the substances identified as radiolytic products are found in foods that have not been irradiated—including raw, heated and stored foods. Moreover, many of these substances are not well known because the foods usually have not been studied at the minute (parts per million) levels scrutinized by chemists who analyzed the irradiated foods.

Proving the Absence of a Ghost

For 30 years, FDA has reviewed experiments attempting to show possible harmful effects of consuming irradiated food. But, just as we can't prove the absence of a ghost, scientists cannot point to some "thing" that proves the absence of risk." Pauli adds, "One can only search diligently.'"

The only relevant safety issue in food irradiation, BFIFC determined, would be the production of harmful substances. BFIFC examined all available data on such products obtained by the U.S. Army's high-protein food sterilization program. Only six substances (found in beef irradiated at 50 kiloGrays) of the 65 identified by Army researchers could not be verified in the literature as present in nonirradiated foods. These six substances were similar to natural food constituents.

The committee determined that even a diet consisting mainly of food irradiated at the one kiloGray level (see below) would not be likely to contain a significant amount of any of these products.

BFIFC concluded in 1980 that food irradiated at a dose not exceeding 1 kiloGray is safe for human consumption, and that animal tests are recommended only for foods irradiated above one kiloGray.

A second team of scientists then reviewed all animal feeding and other irradiated food toxicity studies—several hundred—from agency files and the scientific literature and reaffirmed the BFIFC recommendation.

Since then, FDA has set the use of food irradiation at levels higher than 1 kiloGray. The 1990 rule, for instance, would allow irradiation for poultry at levels up to 3 kiloGrays after animal data again revealed no hazardous effects.

In a separate review, the international community reached a similar conclusion. Representatives from the United Nations, the International Atomic Energy Agency, and the World Health Organization, making up the joint "Committee on the Wholesomeness of Irradiated Food," declared in 1980 that the irradiation of' any food up to an overall average dose of 10 kiloGrays causes no toxicological hazard and introduces no special nutritional or microbiological problems. The Codex Alimentarius Commission, a United Nations body responsible for developing international food standards, adopted the recommendation in 1983.

The Future of Food Irradiation

The World Health Organization believes irradiation can substantially reduce food poisonings. According to a 35-year WHO study, there has been a constant increase in the incidence of food-borne diseases, as well as emergence of new disease-causing organisms such as *Campylobacter* and *Listeria*.

Food irradiation would be another weapon in the arsenal against food-borne illness. FDA and WHO, however, emphasize that irradiation is not a substitute for careful handling, storage and cooking of food. Irradiated poultry can become recontaminated, for instance, if placed next to contaminated, nonirradiated poultry, or left unrefrigerated so that remaining organisms can grow.

To date, 35 countries have issued unconditional or provisional clearances allowing irradiation of commercial foods. Of the more than 140 industrial gamma irradiators in over 40 countries, 29 are used part-time to irradiate food items and conduct food-related research. (They are used mostly for sterilizing disposable medical supplies.) A 1989 Library of Congress report prepared for Congress estimates that by the early 1990s. Fifty-five facilities worldwide will be used for food irradiation and related food irradiation research.

However, as Tanya Roberts of USDAs Economic Research Service stresses, the future of irradiation depends upon consumer acceptance—based largely on proof that the process can produce safer foods at lower cost. Roberts estimates that the cost of medical treatment and lost productivity for five food-borne diseases trichinosis, toxoplasmosis, salmonellosis, campylobacteriosis, and beef tapeworm—totals more than $1 billion annually.

The last chapter in the story of food irradiation still remains to be written. Will the fear of nuclear energy prevent this technology from being used to its fullest potential? Or will education win acceptance for a procedure that can lower the incidence of food-borne illness? Only consumers can supply the answers.

Measuring Irradiation

Absorbed radiation is measured in units called "Grays." The amount of Grays refers to the level of energy absorbed by a food from ionizing radiation that passes through the food in processing.

1,000 Grays = 1 kiloGray (1 kGy)

In the past the term "rad" was commonly used. It stands for radiation absorbed dose.

100 rad = 1 Gy

Poultry Producers Respond

With one hand, poultry producers are giving a thumbs-up sign to FDA's rule permitting irradiation of poultry. With the other, they are putting its use on hold.

Stuart Proctor, executive vice president of the National Turkey Federation—which represents 95 percent of turkey growers and producers—says "we are encouraged by FDA's decision. The industry should be allowed to use any science available that makes food safe from food-borne illness and also is safe." He continues, "As soon as consumers are ready to accept the product, we'll use it."

As George Watts, president of the National Broiler Council says, "the U.S. poultry industry has always been a consumer-driven business. demonstrated by the variety of new products developed over the years to meet the American public's demand." He says that should consumers desire irradiated food products, "the industry will respond."

Perdue Farms, Inc., a large, East Coast chicken producer, says it has no plans to use the irradiation process. Steve McCauley, a company spokesman, said that the firm sees no need for decontaminating its poultry with irradiation because Perdue tests its products stringently. He claims this keeps them safe from contamination.

The need is for consumer education. Although poultry groups say they do not have the resources for the costly campaign needed, they believe that once consumers understand more about food irradiation, they will demand it.

Proctor compares reaction to food irradiation to earlier apprehension about microwave ovens. Once consumers recognized microwave cooking as safe, desire for fast and convenient food led to a microwave revolution. He said he could foresee the same demand for irradiated food, prompted by a desire to cut down on food-borne illness. Once consumers are no longer afraid of the process.

— by Dale Blumenthal

Dale Blumenthal is a staff writer for FDA Consumer.

Chapter 49

Artificial Sweeteners and Cancer: Cyclamate, Saccharine, and Aspartame

Data from population studies do not provide evidence of a clear association between artificial sweeteners and cancer in humans. Interest in such a possible association developed when early studies showed that cyclamate, one type of artificial sweetener caused bladder cancer in laboratory animals.

This finding in animals suggested that cyclamate may increase the risk of bladder cancer in humans; for this reason, the U.S. Food and Drug Administration (FDA) banned the use of cyclamate in 1969. However, results of studies conducted in more recent years have contradicted initial data on the sweetener. Currently, FDA is reviewing the data to evaluate cyclamate's safety for human consumption and to determine whether it should be approved for commercial use in restricted amounts.

Other scientific studies including one conducted in Canada several years ago, have linked saccharin with the development of bladder cancer in test animals. The FDA proposed a ban on that artificial sweetener in April 1977. The Saccharin Study and Labeling Act, passed by Congress in November 1977, placed an 18-month moratorium on any action against saccharin by FDA and required that all food containing the substance bear the following warning label: "Use of this product may be hazardous to your health. This product contains saccharin, which has been determined to cause cancer in laboratory animals." The moratorium has been extended to May 1997.

National Cancer Institute. *Cancer Facts*. May 1996.

During 1978 and 1979, the National Cancer Institute (NCI) and FDA conducted a population study on the possible role of saccharin in causing bladder cancer in humans. In general, people in the study who used an artificial sweetener had no greater risk of bladder cancer than people in the population as a whole. However, when only the data for heavy users were examined, there was some evidence of an increased risk, particularly in persons who consumed both diet drinks and sugar substitutes and who used at least one of these two forms heavily. (In the study, which included a large number of elderly people, heavy use was defined as six or more servings of sugar substitute or two or more 8-ounce servings of diet drink daily.) In addition, persons in the study who were heavy cigarette smokers and who also used artificial sweeteners had higher rates of bladder cancer than did heavy smokers who did not consume these products. It should be noted that heavy smoking itself increases the risk of bladder cancer.

The results of the NCI-FDA study, together with findings of previously conducted research with laboratory animals, suggest that consumption of saccharin and cyclamate is a weak potential risk factor for bladder cancer in humans. The FDA is reviewing this study and other ongoing research in an effort to assess possible health risks more accurately.

Another artificial sweetener, aspartame, contains a mixture of two amino acids (phenylalanine and aspartic acid). Under the trade name of Nutrasweet or Equal this sweetener was introduced to the market in July 1983 after tests showed that it did not cause cancer in laboratory animals.

For More Information

The Cancer Information Service (CIS), a program of the National Cancer Institute, is a nationwide telephone service for cancer patients and their families, the public, and health care professionals. CIS information specialists have extensive training in providing up-to-date and understandable information about cancer. They can answer questions in English and Spanish and can send free printed material. In addition, CIS offices serve specific geographic areas and have information about cancer-related services and resources in their region. The toll-free number of the CIS is 1-800-4-CANCER (1-800-422-6237).

Chapter 50

Bovine Growth Hormone: Harmless for Humans

Generations of Americans have been told that "Milk is nature's most perfect food," and the nutritional value of milk supports this claim. Milk sustains infants and is also beneficial to adults, including the elderly. Many people begin the day with it—by the glass, in cereal, coffee, and in baby's bottle. And because it is perceived as perfect and essential, some consumers and processors of milk products are highly uneasy about the decision of the Food and Drug Administration to allow marketing of milk from experimental herds injected with bovine growth hormone, also known as bovine somatotropin, or bST.

Some consumers suspect that this hormone, even if not harmful, at least detracts from the "purity" of milk. Such skepticism has many sources, ranging from a desire to protect children and an uneasiness about "nature-altering" biotechnology, to the underlying apprehension that life-sustaining gifts of agriculture are becoming polluted by chemistry. (See "Perspective on Food Biotechnology" in the March 1990 *FDA Consumer*.)

Writing not long ago about chemical firms that want to market bST, *Milwaukee Journal* columnist Joel McNally captured the public's wary state of mind: "Consumers," he wrote, "might have second thoughts about . . . milk enhanced by the same companies that gave us such taste treats as vinyl chloride and polystyrene."

Adverse publicity has made bST a hot political issue among dairy farmers, particularly in Wisconsin, Minnesota and Vermont, many of whom demand that the hormone be banned. At a meeting in

FDA Consumer, April 1990.

Washington, D.C., last summer, Jeremy Rifkin, president of the Foundation on Economic Trends and a frequent critic of biotechnology, launched a campaign (the second in three years) against bST as a potentially dangerous drug "with no redeeming social value." He was joined by consumer, animal welfare, and environmental groups, as well as 40 public officials. The grass-roots pressure resulted in a partial boycott of milk produced by experimental herds that receive injections of the growth hormone in clinical animal studies being performed by commercial sponsors of the drug.

Subsequently, the supermarket chains of Safeway, Kroger, Stop & Shop, and Vons last August said they had agreed to not market milk from the bST-supplemented cows, and Kraft USA, Borden's, and Ben & Jerry's Homemade (the Vermont ice cream maker) announced they would not use it in their products. The country's largest dairy cooperative, Associated Milk Producers Incorporated, issued a statement that its 21,000 members will not give the hormone to their cows.

"People are nervous about this substance," says Alan Parker, the Ben & Jerry spokesman. Coming on the heels of the widely publicized concerns about Alar—the growth regulator for apples whose cancer-causing metabolites resulted in the manufacturer withdrawing it from the market—the experiments with bST, in Parker's view, made many "consumers feel that they're losing contact with their food."

Unfounded Fears

BST is biologically inactive in humans. FDA concluded almost five years ago, based on extensive scientific investigation, that milk and meat from bST-supplemented experimental dairy cows may be used for human consumption without causing a risk to the public health. Fears about the growth hormone's effect on human health do not withstand close scrutiny.

Furthermore, talk about "natural" milk in the American marketplace is a piece of nostalgic fiction. Gone are the days when one consumed milk in the "natural" state in which it was drawn from the udder. Milk that is pasteurized to destroy bacteria, homogenized to evenly distribute fat, and fortified with vitamin D to improve nutritional qualities is the result of technological advances. Skim and low-fat milk are supermarket best sellers. Even the recent introduction of unrefrigerated ultra-long-life milk, yet another type of processed milk, represents the application of current technology to milk, and it has met little consumer resistance.

Some scientists believe that bST will ultimately benefit the dairy industry—as have the application of other technologies—by increasing the efficiency of milk production and controlling the retail prices of milk and dairy products to consumers.

BST is a natural product of the pituitary gland of cattle. It stimulates growth in immature cattle and, as a Russian scientist first noted in 1937, it increases milk yield in lactating cows. Research on the substance until the early '80s was stymied by shortages of bST, which could only be extracted from slaughtered animals and varied in purity. In recent years, however, newly perfected genetic engineering techniques have enabled scientists to produce the hormone in sufficient quantity and quality for intensive study. The early findings that bST increases milk production 10 to 25 percent gave the hormone such economic potential that four firms—Monsanto, American Cyanamid, Upjohn, and Elanco—applied to FDA for marketing approval for their brands of genetically produced bST.

Grounds for Decision

Before FDA allows the full-scale commercial marketing of bST, or any new animal drug, the manufacturer must provide sound scientific data showing that its bST product is effective for the proposed use (increasing milk production) and causes no safety concerns for human or animal health. The sponsor must also provide adequate data on the environmental impact of the drug's use. However, in the meantime, FDA has allowed the marketing of meat and milk from bST-supplemented cows in experimental herds because it has determined that these foods meet the requirement of federal law. Federal law permits the commercial sale of food products from animals in investigational studies only when the sponsor has demonstrated that they present no public health risk. Some of the main scientific grounds for FDA's decision are:

- Bovine somatotropin is a protein hormone, and this means that when a product containing bST is eaten, it breaks down during digestion in the gastrointestinal tract into inactive fragments without any effect on the person (or cow) who ate it. That is why cows must be injected with bST for it to be effective.

- Experiments with rats have shown that they are unaffected by oral administration of bST. Rats are an appropriate model because bST is biologically active in rats when injected. Thus, any bST escaping digestion in the rat would have biological effects, such as effects on growth.

- Studies indicate that bST is not effective in humans and other primates even if injected. In the 1950s, physicians tried to treat human dwarfism in children by injecting them with bovine somatotropin, but it had no effect because the amino acid structure of human somatotropin is 35 percent different from bST.

- BST is a natural constituent of milk. It is produced by the pituitary gland and has always been present in the meat and milk of cows. The bST injected to increase milk production merely increases the amount to which the cow is exposed.

- Supplementation with bST does not significantly affect the nutritional qualities of milk or interfere with milk processing. Subtle changes, primarily in the milk fat, occur in the first few weeks of bST supplementation due to metabolic adjustments in the cow. However, this is temporary, and because it occurs to some degree during early lactation in untreated cows the milk contains milk fat well within the normal composition range. Other studies have shown that bST has minimal, if any, effect on the remaining components and characteristics of milk, including protein, minerals, protein coagulation, cholesterol, starter cultures, and flavor. In fact, FDA scientists are not aware of any technology that can detect a difference between milk and dairy products from bST-supplemented cows and similar products from untreated cows.

Other Considerations

There is, however, at least one area of controversy concerning bST that, under the law, FDA may not consider in making its approval decision: the potential social and economic impact of the growth hormone on the nation's dairy farmers. According to the drug's opponents, the lower prices of a more plentiful milk supply will adversely affect thousands of small dairy farms in an already precarious economic situation.

Fear for the continued existence of family farms has fueled the opposition to the growth hormone in the dairy states and increased support for activist Rifkin's anti-bST campaign. Rifkin was back in Washington this past January once again to claim that bST is, among other things, bad for farmers, cows and taxpayers. In support of family farms, Ben and Jerry's Homemade, which buys milk from s.nall Vermont producers, last August placed on its ice cream containers a sign opposing the hormone and calling for the preservation of small farms. Since then, the firm has received more than 1,000 requests for more information on the issue.

On the other hand, many bST supporters realize that dairy farming has changed a great deal since the 1950s—largely as a result of technological innovation—and believe that further changes in the industry are inevitable due to emerging technologies.

It does appear that even after FDA answers all scientific questions about bST and reaches a decision about its approval for general use in the nation's dairy cattle, it may continue to be a controversial topic. However, one thing is certain. Bovine somatotropin will not be approved for commercial use unless, and until, FDA is completely satisfied that scientific data show that it meets all safety amid efficacy requirements for commercial marketing.

—by Beverly Corey

Beverly Corey is a member of FDA's speech-writing staff.

Chapter 51

Consuming Lead with Your Meal: Deadly Leaching from Dishes, Glasses and Mugs

Lead Threat Lessens, but Mugs Pose Problem

Throughout history, lead in food and drink has been synonymous with disaster. Historians suspect that some ancient empires tumbled when leaders became deranged or died of poisoning because they used lead to sweeten wine, drank from lead-lined aqueducts, and used utensils made with lead-based clays and paints.

These days, knowledge of the dangers of lead poisoning keeps manufacturers and governments vigilant about the amounts that get into food. Small amounts of lead leach from glazes and decorative paints on ceramic dinnerware, from lead crystal, and, less frequently, from pewter and silver-plated hollowware. Also, because lead is generally in the environment, it makes its way into food through soil and water.

The levels of lead in food and drink today are the lowest in history, 90 percent lower than 12 years ago. This is mostly due to the U.S. food industry's voluntary elimination of lead solder to seal the seams of food cans and the removal of lead from automobile gasoline that settled on crops and in water.

But concern remains about lead leaching into food from ceramic ware, especially mugs. While analyzing risks from dietary lead, FDA scientists found that about 80 percent of adult exposure to lead from food in contact with ceramic hollowware comes from frequent or daily use of mugs for hot beverages.

FDA Consumer, August 1993.

Risk to Fetus

In a February 1992 report to the Society of Toxicology, FDA scientists Clark D. Carrington, Ph.D., P. Michael Bolger, Ph.D., and Robert J. Scheuplein, Ph.D., said there can be a substantial incremental risk to a developing fetus from lead leaching into food from ceramic hollowware.

Hot acidic beverages such as coffee and tea, both caffeinated and decaffeinated, cause the greatest leaching. FDA toxicologists agree that pregnant women should avoid daily drinking of hot coffee or tea or other hot acidic beverages, such as tomato soup, from lead-glazed ceramic cups or mugs. However, the occasional use of these pieces is not a problem, even during pregnancy.

Consumers also need to be aware of the potential for lead to leach from ceramic plates, bowls and pitchers. Glaze, improperly formulated or fired, can leach large quantities of lead into food. Consumers who suspect a ceramic product has been improperly glazed or fired, should avoid using it for food, or should test the piece for excessive lead leaching before using it.

Responsible manufacturers of ceramic ware use all the proper precautions, but even with properly glazed pieces, low amounts of lead may migrate into food. FDA advises consumers to avoid storing acidic beverages, such as fruit juices and iced tea, in lead-glazed pitchers because, even cold, acidic beverages have a greater tendency than other foods to cause leaching of lead.

New Action Levels

Recent studies on the effects of lead on the fetus, infants, toddlers, and adults in amounts well below those previously believed harmful prompted FDA to reduce its action levels (guidelines telling industry at what point FDA may take regulatory action) for lead leaching from all ceramic hollowware. The action levels specify how much lead may leach from the ceramic piece into a special test solution during a 24-hour test at room temperature. This was the third reduction since action levels for lead leaching from ceramic ware were first set in 1971.

The new action levels are based primarily on how frequently a type of ceramic ware is used, the type of food it holds, the temperature of the food, and how long the food comes in contact with the ceramic ware. For example, a coffee mug is generally used every day to hold a hot acidic beverage, often several times a day, and a pitcher could be used to store fruit juice. Cups and mugs were put into a separate category, and they, along with pitchers, were given an action level of 0.5 parts per million, the lowest for all ceramic ware.

Manufacturers of materials used by ceramic hobbyists and handicrafters are aware of lead contamination problems, and label their products with special instructions. Public affairs specialists in FDA district offices work with state health officials and organizations to develop special education materials for handicraft and pottery associations to avoid potential sources of lead exposure that fall beyond FDA regulatory control.

In addition, FDA has notified embassies in Washington, D.C., of the new action levels so that foreign manufacturers and exporters will have the necessary information to meet the new levels. FDA samples and tests for lead leaching from imported and domestic ceramic ware sold in this country, but the agency cannot check it all. For example, products that enter the country through informal channels, such as those brought by travelers from abroad, are not monitored by FDA.

Because of its heightened focus on ceramic ware, in February 1992, FDA inspectors in every port in the country conducted a short-term intense surveillance of ceramic products used for food, ranging from fine bone china to inexpensive imported pottery. Assisted in many cases by state authorities, FDA inspectors examined more than 5,000 lots of ceramic ware from 29 countries. Nearly 700 lots of domestic ceramic ware from approximately 90 firms were also examined. The results were encouraging. Using the best screening methods available, FDA examiners found that only about 1 percent of imported and 3 percent of domestic ceramic ware exceeded the action levels. (See "New Initiatives for Import Safety," *FDA Consumer*, October 1992.)

FDA also has taken new regulatory steps to ensure that lead continues to stay at lowest possible levels in food. On Nov. 25, 1992, the agency published in the *Federal Register* a proposed regulation that would prohibit the use of tin-coated lead foil capsules (coverings for the cork and neck area) on wine bottles because lead from the capsule may get into the wine. Another proposal, published Jan. 5, 1993, would set a limit for lead in bottled water of no more than 5 parts per billion. And FDA intends to propose a regulation that would prohibit lead solder in food cans. The prohibition would also apply to imports—food in lead-soldered cans would not be allowed to enter the country.

On April 1, 1993, FDA published interim action levels for lead in food packaged in lead-soldered containers. Products that exceed these levels are subject to regulatory action, including recalls. The interim action levels will be in effect until FDA can permanently ban lead-soldered food cans.

Lead and Cans

Before the U.S. canning industry voluntarily eliminated the use of lead in solder to seal food cans, FDA estimates that from 14 to 45 percent of lead in food came from such seals. During the food packaging process, the can body, with its side seam mechanically crimped together, passed over a pot of molten solder, where a rotating roll transferred solder to the seam. The excess solder was then wiped from the can, and the can was cooled until the solder was set. Although solder was not applied to the inside of the can, some of it had to bleed through the ends of the side seam to make a strong, leak-proof can. The minute amount of solder that bled through the seam later leached into the food inside. Sometimes, more lead would contaminate the can's inner surface from the solder dust in the vicinity of the solder pot or splashes from the wiping station.

As more information on lead toxicity became available, the canned food industry consulted with FDA on ways to make a safer product. In response, industry voluntarily switched to unseamed cans and to sealing can seams with non-lead-solder techniques, such as forge and wire welding.

The industry voluntarily stopped packaging infant formula in lead-soldered cans in 1982, according to information submitted to FDA by the Infant Formula Council. As for all of the other canned foods, the Can Manufacturers Institute informed FDA that as of November 1991, lead-soldered cans were no longer produced in the United States. But lead-soldered cans are permitted in some countries that export canned food to us.

The interim action levels published this April primarily affect imported food. FDA estimates that up to 10 percent (some 230 million pounds) of food imported each year may be packaged in lead-soldered cans. Some ethnic groups use imported canned foods as staples in their diets. Also, food in lead-soldered cans may enter the United States through individual purchases outside the United States. A 1991 San Diego County screening program for lead in children's blood led to detection by the Board of Health of a dangerously high blood-lead level in a 1-year-old child whose parents had brought back fruit juice in lead-soldered cans from a grocery store across the Mexican border. Investigators found that the same product had entered the United States through import channels. The juice products were recalled nationwide (see "Toddler's Blood Test Leads to Juice Recall" in the Investigators' Reports section of the December 1992 *FDA Consumer*).

The upcoming FDA proposal to prohibit the use of lead-soldered food cans would prevent such incidents. As an additional measure, FDA has sent letters to more than 65 countries to inform them of FDA's concerns and to learn about their regulations on lead-soldered food cans. Many of the countries that responded are aware of the problems with lead solder in food cans and have established their own lead limits or have adopted those set by the World Health Organization. FDA urges exporters to stop manufacturing lead-soldered food cans, and has made its concerns known through these letters and other discussions at world forums over the last few years.

Foil Capsules on Wine Bottles

Many imported and domestic wines have lead foil capsules (coated on both sides with a thin layer of tin) covering the cork and neck of the bottle. The capsule is used to prevent insect infestation of the cork area and as an oxygen barrier. It's also used to impart an image and feel that are perceived as important to product differentiation and to the marketing of fine wines.

Data on the lead content in wine with lead foil seals were developed by the U.S. Bureau of Alcohol, Tobacco, and Firearms (ATF). Higher lead levels were found in samples of wines poured from the bottle than in unpoured samples. The ATF report concluded that "significant lead contamination" could result if the wine seeps between the cork and the wrap or capsule, causing the foil seal to corrode and leave lead salt deposits on the rim. Although the lead levels found do not pose a short-term health hazard, FDA's concern is with long-term exposure for individuals who regularly consume wine.

Based on these findings, FDA proposed a regulation to declare lead foil wraps for wines to be a food additive that is unsafe, and further to prohibit the use of such wraps on wine bottles. Many wine producers in the United States and Europe have already stopped using them.

FDA advises consumers to wipe the rim and top of the cork of wine bottles sealed with foil with a cloth dampened with water or lemon juice before removing the cork. Pregnant and lactating women have long been advised to avoid alcoholic beverages, including wine. Lead contamination is another good reason for pregnant women to refrain from drinking wine.

Crystal Ware

Recent studies have found that lead can leach into food from lead crystal hollowware. The International Crystal Federation has provided FDA a report of its research on lead leaching into food and alcoholic beverages, and the industry has started a program in which manufacturers share technological developments to reduce lead leaching. Also, FDA has initiated studies of its own on lead leaching from crystal ware.

Until FDA reviews all the data and determines what further actions, if any, need to be taken, the agency advises consumers not to store alcoholic beverages in lead crystal decanters, and pregnant women not to routinely drink from lead crystal glasses. Infants should not be fed with lead crystal baby bottles.

FDA tested 60 samples of crystal ware from 17 different countries for leachable lead content. In the experiments, FDA scientists used in the glassware an acetic acid solution similar in acidity to household vinegar. Results showed that over a 24-hour period, amounts of lead released into the solution ranged from non-detectable levels to 7.2 parts per million. One experiment shows that when acidic juices or warmed infant formula were poured into crystal baby bottles, lead levels in the beverages rose. FDA and the crystal ware industry are performing additional studies on the release of lead by crystal glassware.

FDA presently has no maximum allowable level for lead leached from crystal ware. But experts recognize that lead is hazardous to health. Because lead accumulates in the body, limiting exposure to it is essential.

FDA Consumer, May 1991.

Because lead is ubiquitous, FDA recognizes that no effort will totally eliminate lead from the food supply, however desirable that may be. But FDA and many other federal, state and local governments are working together through all available means to reduce exposure to lead. The initial focus is on the sources likely to result in the greatest exposure.

FDA uses as many sources as it can to get the story of lead to consumers, both of the harm it causes, and about how to prevent poisoning. Careful attention to consumer advisories can prevent unnecessary exposure to this age-old health problem.

Danger Even at Low Levels

Even at low levels, lead not excreted through the digestive system accumulates in the body and is absorbed directly into blood and soft tissues, including the kidney, bone marrow, liver, and brain. When lead leaves the bloodstream, it is stored in bone, along with other minerals, where it continues to build over a lifetime.

In average adults, 10 to 15 percent of lead that reaches the digestive tract is absorbed. Young children and pregnant women, however, absorb as much as 50 percent. The body cannot distinguish between calcium and lead. Once lead enters the body, it is assimilated in the bloodstream in the same manner as calcium, and, because young children and pregnant women absorb calcium more readily to meet their extra needs, they also absorb more lead. Those with calcium deficiencies absorb even more. And lead, even in small amounts, may become toxic wherever it settles. (See "Getting the Lead Out of Just About Everything," *FDA Consumer*, August 1991.)

Lead also gets into the blood of pregnant women from their own bone stores. During a period of physiological stress, such as in pregnancy or lactation, bone stores of minerals, including the normally inert lead, can be mobilized back into a woman's blood and increase her blood-lead level. As this blood circulates, it is picked up by the fetus.

FDA considers children and pregnant women at highest risk for lead poisoning. FDA toxicologists say that for pregnant women, lead exposure is an actual, rather than potential, problem. Besides potentially harming her own health, lead can damage the developing fetus because it crosses the placental barrier.

A 1987 report in the *New England Journal of Medicine* shows that as little as 10 micrograms of lead per deciliter of fetal blood could damage a fetus early in pregnancy during its most vulnerable period of nervous system development. It can also cause premature birth or lower birth weight. In adults, 30 micrograms of lead per deciliter of blood can cause high blood; pressure and damage nerves and red blood cells.

FDA toxicologists have set provisional total tolerable intake levels (PTTILs) of lead from all sources at 25 micrograms per day for pregnant women, and 6 micrograms per day for infants and children up to six years. For every microgram per day of lead intake, blood lead levels increase 0.16 micrograms per deciliter of blood in children and 0.04 micrograms per deciliter of blood in adults.

PTTILs represent the intake level FDA believes provides a reasonable margin of protection from the measurable toxic effects of lead from all food and non-food sources. Scientists have not found a no-effect level of toxicity from lead. If additional research shows that lower blood lead levels cause measurable adverse health effects, the PTTILs would be reduced even further.

Advice for Consumers

Consumers can guard against exposure to lead in food by observing the following guidelines:

- If you are pregnant, avoid the daily use of ceramic mugs when drinking hot beverages such as coffee or tea, and avoid the daily use of lead crystal ware.

- Do not feed babies from lead crystal bottles.

- Do not store acidic foods such as fruit juices in ceramic containers.

- Do not store beverages in lead crystal containers.

- Limit the use of antique or collectible housewares for food or beverages to special occasions.

- Stop using items that show a dusty or chalky gray residue on the glaze after they are washed.

- Follow label directions on any ornamental product with a warning such as, "Not for Food Use—Plate May Poison Food. For Decorative Purposes Only."

- If your wine is sealed with a foil capsule, wipe the rim of the bottle with a cloth dampened with water or lemon juice before removing the cork.

FDA is aware of three kits to test for lead leaching from ceramic ware that consumers can use at home. These kits are not always sensitive enough to detect lead at the new lower levels, but they can be valuable for identifying items that release larger amounts of lead. For information about these kits and other questions about lead, contact the local FDA office, listed in the blue pages of the phone directory, or call FDA headquarters at (301)443-4667.

The National Safety Council, under a grant from the federal government, maintains a National Lead Information Center with a toll-free number (1-800) LEAD-FYI, or (1-800)532-3394 — where callers may request a Spanish or English language information package. Also, most U.S. ceramic manufacturers maintain toll-free lines through which consumers may obtain information about lead levels in their products. Public affairs specialists in FDA district offices can provide consumers with these numbers.

—by Judith E. Foulke

Judith E. Foulke is a staff writer for *FDA Consumer*.

Chapter 52

Pesticides in Food

Pesticide residues on infant foods and adult foods that infants and children eat are almost always well below tolerances (the highest levels legally allowed) set by the Environmental Protection Agency. This was the conclusion of a recent Food and Drug Administration report based on the agency's monitoring of these types of foods over the last seven years.

The FDA report, "Monitoring of Pesticide Residues in Infant Foods and Adult Foods Eaten by Infants and Children," was published in the May-June 1993 issue of the *Journal of the Association of Official Analytical Chemists International*.

The authors, consumer safety officer Norma Yess and chemists Ellis Gunderson and Ronald Roy of the Center for Food Safety and Applied Nutrition, based their findings on food samples from the three approaches FDA uses to monitor pesticides: regulatory, incidence and level, and Total Diet Study.

Through the regulatory approach, FDA checks foods close to the point of production for levels of residues and, if they are violative, considers enforcement action. Incidence and level is a study approach that analyzes selected samples of certain foods. Total Diet Study is an approach that uses data from supermarket shopping.

Of more than 10,000 food samples reported from regulatory monitoring, fewer than 50 were violative. No residues over EPA or FDA action levels were found in samples from the incidence and

---

FDA Consumer, June 1993.

level studies. In the Total Diet Study, no residues were found in infant formulas, and no residues over FDA or EPA allowed levels were found.

Shared Responsibility

The responsibility for ensuring that residues of pesticides in foods are not present at levels that will pose a danger to health is shared by FDA, EPA, and the Food Safety and Inspection Service of the U.S. Department of Agriculture. Pesticides of concern include insecticides, fungicides, herbicides, and other agricultural chemicals.

EPA reviews the scientific data on all pesticide products before they can be registered (or licensed) for use. If a product is intended for use on food crops, EPA also establishes a tolerance.

FDA is responsible for enforcing these tolerances on all foods except meat, poultry, and certain egg products, which are monitored by USDA. In addition, FDA works with EPA to set "action levels"—enforcement guidelines for residues of pesticides, such as DDT, that may remain in the environment after their use is discontinued. The guidelines are set at levels that protect public health.

Regulatory Monitoring

In its regulatory monitoring to enforce EPA-set tolerances, FDA checks foods for pesticide residues as close to production of the commodity as possible at distributors, at food processors, or, if imported, at entry into the country. If illegal residues are found in domestic samples, FDA can take regulatory action, such as seizure or injunction. For imports, FDA can stop shipments at ports of entry.

The FDA report used data from FDA regulatory monitoring between 1985 and 1991. The authors chose eight foods that infants and children eat in relatively large quantities: apples, bananas, oranges, and pears; apple, grape and orange juices; and milk.

FDA found 50 violative samples, representing only 0.3 percent of domestic products and 0.6 percent of imports reported under the regulatory monitoring approach.

All foods sampled in regulatory monitoring are analyzed unwashed and unpeeled, even bananas. Yess explains that because food processors, and most consumers, wash or peel produce before eating or using it in food products, many of the violative samples reported in the

FDA study showed higher residues than the actual amount people are exposed to. Studies have shown that residues of many pesticides can be washed off fresh produce, a good practice for anyone fixing a salad or snacking on grapes.

Of the 50 violative samples, nearly all were pesticide residues for which there were no tolerances or EPA "approval for use" on the specific food sampled. Since pesticides are registered for specific crops, residues on crops for which the pesticide has not been registered are illegal.

A few samples had residues higher than EPA tolerances or FDA action levels in effect at the time; a number of tolerances were revised between 1985 and 1991. The revisions for daminozide (Alar), for example, reflect that it has not been used in agriculture since 1989.

Some domestic milk samples showed small amounts of chlorinated pesticide residues. The registration for food use for these compounds expired more than 20 years ago, but because they persist in the environment, residues are still found at low levels.

Incidence and Level Studies

When FDA wants to know more about specific pesticides, commodities, or pesticide-commodity combinations, the agency supplements its regulatory monitoring by analyzing selected samples of certain foods in incidence and level monitoring.

For the pesticide residue report, the authors used the results of two studies. One study targeted five specific commodity-pesticide combinations for infant foods and other foods commonly eaten by infants and children. The analyses for this study were directed by FDA and completed in 1990 through a cooperative agreement with a USDA laboratory in Gulfport, MS. The other study, also in 1990, analyzed whole pasteurized milk samples through an FDA-supported contract.

Both studies included results of analyses of several pesticides and pesticide-commodity combinations that have been the focus of public attention within the last five years. No residues over EPA tolerances or FDA action levels were found in samples from either of the two studies.

The first study involved five tasks. In the first, about 900 samples of commercially prepared infant foods and formulas were collected and analyzed for residues of the following pesticides:

- benomyl-thiabendazole (fungicides)

- daminozide (sprayed on apple trees to prevent premature drop, no longer used by growers)
- ethylenethiourea (ETU, a breakdown product of a fungicide)
- aldicarb (an insecticide, acaricide against snails, and nematocide against worms)
- the organochlorine group of pesticides (older, more persistent pesticides, including those no longer used in foods).

The other four tasks were analyses of adult foods eaten by infants and children:

- apples, bananas, oranges, and pears for benomyl-thiabendazole
- apple and grape juices, applesauce, and canned pears for daminozide
- grape juice for ETU
- bananas, oranges, and orange juice for aldicarb.

Three-quarters of the samples collected for all tasks were from large retail grocery stores in six states: Massachusetts, Illinois, Michigan, Wisconsin, Minnesota, and Washington. The remaining samples were collected in the Gulfport, MS, area (the home of USDA's National Monitoring and Residue Analysis Laboratory, where the FDA-directed study was done). The prepared infant foods and formula samples were selected mostly from the major manufacturers.

The second study showed the results of sampling for residues of the organochlorine group of pesticides in whole pasteurized milk. Organochlorine pesticide residues—mostly DDT, DDE and dieldrin—were found in 398 of the 806 milk samples, but all were well below EPA tolerances or FDA action levels.

Samples for the milk study came from monthly collections at 63 sampling stations that are a part of EPA's Environmental Radiation Ambient Monitoring System, located in large metropolitan areas throughout the United States. At each sampling station, milk from selected sources was combined to represent the milk routinely consumed in that area. Portions of the milk were sent to an FDA contract laboratory for analysis.

Total Diet Study

For its report, FDA also used data from the Total Diet Study, which is used to monitor a number of nutritional concerns, including pesticides.

As part of the Total Diet Study, FDA staffers shop in supermarkets or grocery stores four times a year, once in each of four geographical regions of the country. Shopping in three cities from each region, they buy the same 234 foods (including meat), selected from nationwide dietary survey data to typify the American diet. The purchased foods are called "market baskets."

Foods from the market baskets are then prepared as a consumer would prepare them. For example, beef and vegetable stew is made from the collected ingredients, using a standard recipe. The prepared foods are analyzed for pesticide residues, and the results, together with USDA consumption studies, are used to estimate the dietary intakes of pesticide residues for eight age-sex groups ranging from infants to senior citizens.

For their report, the FDA researchers included results from 27 market baskets collected and analyzed between 1985 and 1991. Included were 33 different infant foods (both strained and junior), 10 adult foods eaten by infants and children, and four types of milk. The infant foods included cereals, combination meat and poultry dinners, vegetables, desserts, fruits and fruit juices, and infant formulas. The adult foods included apples, oranges, pears, and bananas; apple, grape and orange juices; applesauce; grape jelly; and peanut butter. Milks were chocolate, evaporated, low-fat (2 percent), and whole.

No residues were found in the infant formulas, and no residues over EPA tolerances or FDA action levels were found in any of the Total Diet Study foods. Low levels of malathion were found in some cereals because malathion is widely used both before and after harvest on grains. Low levels of thiabendazole, a post-harvest fungicide used on many fruits, were found on some of the fruits and fruit products.

The low levels of pesticide residues found in the Total Diet Study and incidence-level monitoring samples show how processing foods or otherwise preparing them for consumption at the table can reduce residue levels. Washing at home removes much of the residues. But commercial food processing steps, such as peeling and blanching, can further reduce residues. For example, the highest finding of thiabendazole in raw apples was 2 parts per million (EPA tolerance is 10 ppm), 0.08 in apple juice, and 0.06 in applesauce.

Also, agricultural specialists from major infant food manufacturers work with their contract growers to minimize pesticide applications and to ensure that only those pesticides specified in the contract are applied. Therefore, when pesticide residues are found on infant foods, they are usually well below EPA tolerances.

Wash Before Eating

Washing fresh produce before eating is a healthful habit. You can reduce and often eliminate residues if they are present on fresh fruit and vegetables by following these simple tips:

- Wash produce with large amounts of cold or warm tap water, and scrub with a brush when appropriate; do not use soap.
- Throw away the outer leaves of leafy vegetables such as lettuce and cabbage.
- Trim fat from meat, and fat and skin from poultry and fish. Residues of some pesticides concentrate in animal fat.

Supermarkets, as a rule do not wash produce before putting it out, but many stores mist it while it's on display. Misting keeps the produce from drying, but surface residues drain off also, in much the same way as from a light wash under the kitchen faucet.

A 1990 report in the *EPA Journal* by three chemists from that agency, Joel Garbus, Susan Hummel, and Stephanie Willet, summarized four studies of fresh tomatoes treated with a fungicide, which were tested at harvest, at the packing house, and at point of sale to the consumer. The studies showed that more than 99 percent of the residues were washed off at the packing house by the food processor.

A 1989 study reported by Edgar Elkins in the *Journal of the Association of Official Analytical Chemists* showed the effects of peeling, blanching and processing on a number of fruits and vegetables. For example, in the case of benomyl, 83 percent of the residues found on fresh apples were removed during processing into applesauce, 98 percent of residues from oranges processed to juice were removed and 86 percent of residues from fresh tomatoes processed to juice were removed. Another study in 1991 by Gary Eilrich reported in an American Chemical Society Symposium, showed similar results.

NAS Evaluation Expected

The National Research Council of the National Academy of Sciences (NAS) is expected to issue a report this summer on its evaluation of the methods the government uses to estimate the health risks to infants and children from, dietary exposures to pesticide residues. At issue is whether federal pesticide risk assessments, on which Environmental Protection Agency tolerances are based, adequately protect special segments of the population, particularly infants and children.

Tolerance levels reflect both the toxicity of a chemical and anticipated dietary exposure. Risks are calculated from two types of exposure estimates:

- the potential risk from a one-time exposure
- a composite average lifetime risk, which includes a proportionately greater exposure in childhood.

FDA and U.S. Department of Agriculture monitoring for pesticide residues consistently show that levels rarely exceed or approach established tolerances. Estimated dietary intakes of pesticides by children and adults in the United States are also well below Acceptable Daily Intakes (ADI) established by the Food and Agriculture Organization and the World Health Organization, seldom exceeding 1 percent of the ADI.

In response to a request from Congress in 1988, NAS convened a 14-person committee representing academia, medicine, state governments, industry, USDA, and Canada's health agencies. EPA asked the committee to address:

- the ways in which children are more or less susceptible to the toxicity of pesticides in their diets
- diets of various age groups
- pesticide-use patterns on crops likely to contain residues that cause concern
- improvements EPA could make in its toxicological testing requirements and methods of estimating risk to improve protection for infants and children.

— by Judith E. Foulke

Judith E. Foulke is a staff writer for FDA Consumer.

Judith Levine Willis also contributed to this article.

Chapter 53

Human Breast Milk: As a Potential Biological Hazard

Human Breast Milk Is Contaminated

Editorial:
For a thorough scientific evaluation of the level of contamination of human breast milk, see "Chemical Contaminants in Human Milk" in Environmental Health Perspectives, Volume 103 Supplement 6.

If breast milk from American women were bottled and sold commercially, it would be subject to ban by the U.S. Food and Drug Administration (FDA) because it is contaminated with more than 100 industrial chemicals, including pesticides. FDA has set limits on contamination of commercial milk by pesticides, and human milk routinely exceeds those limits by a wide margin (see Table 53.1).

We do not want to discourage breast feeding. Breast feeding is a highly desirable practice, despite the presence of toxic chemicals in human milk. Breast feeding gives an infant immunity against gastrointestinal diseases and respiratory infections; it may also offer protection against food allergies. The emotional bonding that takes place between mother and child can be exceedingly important as well. Furthermore, the alternatives (prepared formulas) are all less healthy.

Still, it is important for Americans to recognize the consequences of allowing the chemical industry (and, more recently, the incineration industry) to expand unchecked, and contamination of breast milk

Rachel's Hazardous Waste News published by Environmental Research Foundation, number 193. "Human Breast Milk Is Contaminated." August 1990.

is one well-established consequence. The problem is not widely acknowledged or often discussed, perhaps because it forces us to ask ourselves, what kind of people allow their infant children to ingest low concentrations of a hundred industrial poisons with every mouthful of their mother's milk?

Scientists first discovered that human breast milk was contaminated with DDT in 1951. DDT, like many other chlorinated organic chemicals, is soluble in fat but not very soluble in water, so when it enters the body it is not easily excreted and it builds up in fatty (adipose) tissue. The main way that females excrete such chemicals is through their breast milk. Breast milk contains about 3 percent fat (average) and fat-soluble chemicals collect there. Unfortunately, this contaminates infant children who breast feed. *When examining data on milk contamination, be aware that concentrations are sometimes given as ppm [parts per million] for fat, or ppb [parts per billion] for whole milk; fat concentrations are about 30 times higher than whole milk concentrations, so, for example, 2.5 ppm in fat is approximately equivalent to 75 ppb whole milk.*

The most extensive survey of the milk of American women was conducted by U.S. Environmental Protection Agency in 1975. They took samples from more than 1,000 women, but analyzed them for only a few pesticides. They found DDT in 100 percent of samples, PCBs in 99 percent of samples, and dieldrin in 83 percent of samples. EPA says DDT, dieldrin and PCBs are all "probable carcinogens" in humans.

There has been only one study of non-pesticide organic chemicals in the milk of American women. It found 192 organic compounds, many of them well-known industrial poisons like carbon tetrachloride and benzene (both known human carcinogens). From reading the scant literature on this topic, one draws the unmistakable impression that further study would reveal more contamination.

Table 53.1 shows how grossly contaminated the milk of American women is, based on just four pesticides. The first column names the pesticide; column 2 gives typical levels of contamination reported in scientific studies; column 3 gives the FDA's "action level" for each pesticide; this is the level at which the FDA can (if it chooses to) take commercial cows' milk off the shelves because of excessive contamination; column 4 shows the allowable daily intake of each pesticide for an adult (expressed in micrograms of pesticide per kilogram of body weight). [There are 28 grams in one ounce; a kilogram is about 2.2 pounds.] The last column shows the actual daily intake for a nursing

Pesticide	Typical Levels (whole milk)	FDA Action Levels for whole milk (cows')	Allowable Daily Intake (Adult)	Actual Daily Intake (Infant)
	parts per billion		µg/kg	
Dieldrin	1-6	9.0	0.1	0.8
Heptachlor Epoxide	8-30	0.3	0.5	4.0
PCBs	40-100	63.0	1.0	14.0
Total DDT	50-200	38.0	5.0	28.0

Source: Walter J. Rogan and others. "Pollutants in Breast Milk," *New England Journal of Medicine* Vol. 302 (June 26, 1980), Pg. 1451, Table 3.

Table 53.1. *Typical levels of pesticides and PCBs in human milk in the U.S., FDA Action Level, Allowable Daily Intake and Actual Daily Intake of Breast-Fed Infants.*

infant in America. It is clear that the actual daily intake by an infant exceeds an adult's allowable daily intake by anywhere from a factor of 6 to a factor of 14.

No allowable daily intakes have been calculated for infants, but it is known that infants are much more susceptible to toxic chemicals than are adults because an infant's kidneys, liver, enzyme systems, and blood-brain barrier are not fully developed. Furthermore, a newborn has very little body fat available for storage; consequently, the fat soluble chemicals are circulated in the blood throughout the body for a longer period and may interfere more intensely with normal enzyme activity.

For More Information

1. D.B. Jelliffe and E.F.P. Jelliffe, *Human Milk in the Modern World: Psychosocial, Nutritional and Economic Significance.* NY: Oxford University Press, 1978.

2. E.P. Laug, "Occurrence of DDT in Human Milk." *Archives of Industrial Hygiene*, Volume 3, pp 245 - 246, 1951.

3. B.R. Sonawane, "Chemical Contaminants in Human Milk: An Overview." *Environmental Health Perspectives*, Volume 103, Supplement 6, September 1995.

Part Nine

Environmental Risks
to Children

Chapter 54

Children—Unique and Vulnerable: Environmental Risks Facing Children and Recommendations for Response

Children may be more susceptible to exposures to environmental toxins than adults and may be more vulnerable to their effects. Because of this, the health care community and those responsible for children need to be alert to possible environmental factors in identifying and responding to the health problems of children. Their focus should be on the causes of the health problem, emphasizing environmental sources, and not on simply treating the symptoms.

Introduction

Children may be more susceptible to environmental exposures than adults and, because of their developing systems, uniquely vulnerable to their effects.

There is a growing urgency for researchers in the private and public sectors to move to fill gaps in the data and for decision makers to incorporate available information into pollution control and prevention strategies. Damage caused to children can be devastating and permanent, and the latency period for certain effects can be decades.

Because of this potential, the health care community and those responsible for children need to be alert to possible environmental factors in identifying and responding to health problems confronting children. All too often, the immediate focus is on symptoms and their

NIH Publication 65-218. Environmental Health Perspectives Volume 103, Number 6, September 1995.

treatment, rather than causes, and environmental sources of effects are the last considered, if ever.

There are particular environmental exposures, pesticides, and air pollutants for which the combination of increased susceptibility and increased opportunity for exposure combine to increase the hazards and risks for children. One of the most effective strategies immediately available is to prevent pollution and so preclude potentially toxic exposures.

A Changing Environment

With the synthetic organic chemical revolution in the post-World War II period came an enormous influx of new chemical substances together with frequently unchecked releases of pollutants into the air, water, and land. Some of those pollutants, such as DDT, are particularly persistent and pervasive, as Rachel Carson eloquently warned in *Silent Spring*.

Past pollution practices, combined with inefficient use of fossil fuels, served to create an environment in which the air and waterways all too often became living laboratories for toxic damage. Love Canal symbolized what could go wrong when an elementary school was built directly over a hazardous waste disposal site.

Environmental legislation of the 1970s and 1980s responded to the public outcry against the pattern of environmental destruction in America, creating a network of laws and regulations to control it. Congress enacted hallmark statutes, including: the Clean Air and Water Acts; Toxic Substances Control Act; Resource Conservation and Recovery Act; Comprehensive Environmental Response, Compensation, and Liability Act (Superfund law); and Safe Drinking Water Act. States adopted implementing laws and programs, in numerous cases going beyond the federal mandate.

The resulting legislative and regulatory framework delivered substantial benefits to public health and environmental protection. But what is becoming clear is that their predominant emphasis on command-and-control strategies has limits. From the point of view of protecting public health and the environment, pollution prevention is essential. Preventing pollution and consequent exposure to potential environmental risk is all the more necessary to protect children from harm.

This is particularly important in the case of pesticides. The sheer volume of pesticide use necessitates a pollution prevention approach. In 1993, for instance, an estimated 4.23 billion pounds of pesticides were used in the United States, this total is based on the amount of active ingredients only (1). The figure includes conventional pesticides used in agriculture, wood preservatives, disinfectants, and water treatment (such as swimming pool chemicals), as well as use in households and buildings.

NAS Report Examines Diet, Pesticides

One of the primary routes of exposure to potential environmental risk for children is diet, underscoring the importance of scrutinizing pesticides under the two federal statutes governing their use in food— the Federal Insecticide, Fungicide, and Rodenticide Act (FIFRA) and the Federal Food, Drug, and Cosmetic Act.

Concern about the link between pesticide residues in food and children's health prompted Congress in 1988 to ask the National Academy of Sciences (NAS) to examine the issue. NAS established a committee to do so through its National Research Council. The committee examined scientific and policy issues confronted by government agencies, particularly the U.S. Environmental Protection Agency (U.S. EPA), in regulating pesticide residues in foods eaten by children and infants.

The resulting NAS report, *Pesticides in the Diets of Infants and Children*, issued in 1993, includes two major findings of particular importance to the protection of children from pesticide exposures (2). The first is that the federal government is not doing enough to protect children from exposures to pesticides. The second is that risk assessments for pesticides and toxic chemicals do not differentiate between risk to children and risk to adults, but should do so.

Children are not simply little adults, the NAS report emphasized. Children are different from adults in terms of sensitivity because they are growing and their internal organs are developing and maturing. Children are also different in terms of exposures because they have distinctly different behavioral and eating patterns.

Doing a better job of assessing risks for children requires more information about both susceptibility and exposures. Too many critical gaps in existing data persist. Although developing the needed information is a complex matter, scientists in government, academe, and elsewhere have succeeded in filling some of the gaps; and research currently underway needs continued support. At the same time, however, incorporating existing information into the assessment of children's risks must become a priority.

This chapter will examine how children may be more vulnerable to potential toxic effects of chemicals because of the developmental nature of their systems, behavior patterns, and environmental conditions. It will also draw on a series of examples to illustrate risk issues involving children. These include sensitivity, exposure patterns, multiple sources of exposure to the same chemicals, and multiple exposures to chemicals that can act in the same way and ran affect the same child.

Sensitivity and Pesticides

The first case illustrates the importance of considering sensitivity in determining environmental risks to children. Sensitivity, in an environmental context, is the capacity to be harmed. It varies among different populations, ethnic groups, and genetic backgrounds, as well as by age and childhood experience and development. Age-related differences have a significant effect on metabolism (or how humans handle toxic substances), physiology (or how the body works), developmental stages, behavior, and diet.

In 1981, vinclozolin was registered for use as a fungicide on fruits and vegetables, having satisfied registration criteria under FIFRA. Federal regulations allow registration only if there are "no unreasonable adverse health effects" when compared with benefits gained. If that test is met, the risks involved are not considered unreasonable.

However, in 1988, the manufacturer of vinclozolin had important new findings from hormonal studies of rats and reported them to the U.S. EPA, as mandated by law when new significant findings of an adverse effect from a pesticide are found. The company determined that in utero, or during fetal development, vinclozolin was associated with feminization of the male fetus. During in utero development, male fetuses were developing feminine sexual characteristics.

The Health Effects Research Laboratory in the U.S. EPA's Office of Research and Development, which had been working on hormonal effects of pesticides, took a closer look at vinclozolin and determined that effects were found at doses six times lower than those reported when the pesticide was originally registered. Feminization of male fetuses, sterility later in life in the male animals, and other developmental variations were all confirmed. The mechanism of action is vinclozolin, which acts as an anti-androgen, blocking androgen effects (3,4).

As a result, no new uses have been allowed for vinclozolin, and as vinclozolin goes through the reregistration process under the 1988 FIFRA amendments, all uses currently allowed will be reassessed.

The potential implications of the effects of vinclozolin for children are inconclusive, but the data underscore the need for a cautionary regulatory approach and continued vigilance in regulating pesticide residues in food. Growing children are sensitive to imbalances in hormone levels, and the question of potential adverse health effects from exposure to pesticide residues in food needs to be the subject of continued research.

Sensitivity and Wildlife

Evidence of abnormal sexual development possibly due to environmental contaminants also comes from case studies involving wildlife, raising the issue of potential implications for childbearing and children's postnatal development. Much more research needs to be done in this area.

In the highly evolved chain of ecologic connections, air, water, land, vegetation, and animals are linked in a complex web of interactions. For example, pollutants move among air, water, and land and are taken up by plants, which in turn are consumed by animals and humans. What goes into the air from near and far becomes deposited in rivers and lakes, for example, contaminating fish and fowl to varying degrees.

In recent years, scientists have begun observing marked effects on the reproductive systems of wildlife in areas that have been subjected to significant environmental contamination, provoking questions about potential implications for human beings' ability to have healthy children. Many of the instances have involved a group of widely used chemicals called organochlorines.

Perhaps the most noted case involves alligators living in Lake Apopka in central Florida (5). A number of endocrine-related effects were observed, including low hatching rates, males with abnormal reproductive tracts, and females with ovaries bearing abnormal eggs. These effects were inferred to be due to a large quantity of DDE, a potent metabolite of the insecticide DDT, which had been spilled there. DDE's effects apparently led to an imbalance between androgens and estrogens in the developing alligators, which in turn caused abnormal sexual development.

Both DDT/DDE and vinclozolin are endocrine disrupters, substances that mimic or block the action of natural hormones. DDT is an estrogen, and vinclozolin and DDE are antiandrogens. Estrogens are the group of human hormones responsible for many of the more feminine parts of sexual development throughout life, and androgens, mainly testosterone, are responsible for development of many male sexual characteristics. Both males and females naturally have levels of estrogens and androgens; it is the proper balance between the two that results in appropriate sexual development.

Endocrine disrupters such as DDT/DDE may be persistent in the environment. In theory, possible side effects of environmental estrogens and antiandrogens include abnormal pregnancy and sexual development; potential cancer risks, i.e., breast and prostate; and other diseases such as endometriosis. Many endocrine disrupters like DDT/DDE bioaccumulate or concentrate in the food chain. In humans, effects on lactation have been demonstrated. Rogan et al. (6) studied breast milk DDT levels for approximately 800 women in North Carolina. The intent was to look for health effects in children exposed to DDT in breast feeding. Researchers found no evidence of increased illnesses among the children. However, they discovered that women with the highest levels of DDT in their milk breast fed less than 40 percent as long as women with the lowest levels of DDT. Impaired lactation would have profound effects in circumstances where breast milk is the only safe alternative for feeding infants (for example, when there is no safe drinking water for mixing formula).

There have also been concerns about the potential for effects on sexual development and cancer risks that might be hormonally related, such as breast cancer in women and prostate and testicular cancer in men (7).

The U.S. EPA has developed testing protocols for evaluating hormonal effects of pesticides. The revised protocols call for using extended dosing periods, testing for developmental milestones in the animals, and looking for developmental end points after birth or postnatally. The U.S. EPA's Scientific Advisory Panel, comprised of outside experts, endorsed the changes, clearing the way for them to be added to the agency's testing requirements. The new protocols will add a further layer of protection in discerning potential environmental risks to human health, but troubling questions about effects on reproductive systems remain.

Dietary Exposure to Toxicants

On the issue of exposures, children's diets differ significantly from those of adults, the NAS report confirmed (2). They eat more fruit in proportion to their body size; they also have less varied diets. As every parent knows, as children go through the first few years of life, they develop preferences for certain foods and often only will eat those particular foods for months at a time.

But NAS found that knowledge about what children eat is much more limited than it should be. Not only are existing data for children inadequate, current information on the U.S. diet is based on surveys conducted in the late 1970s. Dietary habits have changed substantially since then. Much higher consumption of fresh fruits and vegetables is a key example.

In looking at the diets of infants and children, NAS was critical of the current system for evaluating dietary intake for children because it groups all children between one and six years of age. Data are available for children up to one year of age. However, the differences that exist between the diet of a 1-year-old child and that of a 5-year-old child cannot be taken into account. In assessing exposure and potential risk, NAS recommended more precision about what children eat during the first few years of life by addressing each year of life between one and six separately.

Work is underway with the U.S. Department of Agriculture (USDA) to accomplish that objective. For example, USDA is planning to revise the national food consumption survey, called the Continuing Survey of Food Intake, to characterize more accurately consumption patterns for foods children eat most frequently.

In addition to using the USDA data, the U.S. EPA is planning to use data collected in the National Health and Nutrition Examination Survey to get a better idea of the food children eat. This survey also gathers information about young children, including those from various income and ethnic groups.

The foods children most commonly eat are identified in the NAS report (Table 54.1). In addition to foods that might be expected, such as milk and apples, there are some interesting and unexpected items, like coconut oil, which is in a number of processed foods, including sweet cereals that children often love.

Exposure and Bananas

A specific example of the need to protect children from dietary exposure to risk involves the use of the pesticide aldicarb on bananas, one of the foods that many children prefer. A toddler can easily eat an entire banana. Some can eat several in a sitting, and children typically eat more of them than adults per pound of body weight.

Aldicarb is an insecticide that has been used for a number of years on fruits, nuts, potatoes, and various other vegetables. It is a systemic pesticide, which means it is taken up by the roots of the plant and ends up in the plant itself, and so cannot be removed by simply washing or peeling fruits and vegetables.

Aldicarb is a carbamate pesticide. It acts by inhibiting acetylcholinesterase, an enzyme necessary for the proper transmission of nerve impulses, and can be very toxic to humans, causing a number of effects, including diarrhea, vomiting, and changes in the function of the central nervous system.

Table 54.1. Eighteen foods most commonly eaten by infants.

Milk, nonfat solids	Milk sugar (lactose)
Apple juice	Bananas, fresh
Apples, fresh	Rice, milled
Orange juice	Peas, succulent, garden
Pears, fresh	Beans, succulent, garden
Milk, fat, solids	Oats
Peaches, fresh	Soybean oil
Carrots	Coconut oil
Beef, lean	Wheat flour

The manufacturer of aldicarb notified the U.S. EPA in 1991 of some unexpected aldicarb residues on bananas. Generally, the residues were below the legal limit or tolerance. "Tolerances," the NAS report noted, "constitute the single, most important mechanism by which the U.S. EPA limits levels of pesticide residues in foods. A tolerance is defined as the legal limit of a pesticide residue allowed in or on a raw agricultural commodity and, in appropriate cases, on processed foods. A tolerance must be established for any pesticide used on any food crop"(2). Tolerances are set on the basis of composite samples. Under this approach, bunches of bananas were blended and then analyzed.

The level detected using this sampling method was found to be below the legal limit. However, when bananas were analyzed one at a time, some of these bananas were found to have levels of aldicarb that were up to 10 times greater than the legal limit. When the legal limit was originally established, it was considered safe. This conclusion was based, in part, on the assumption that any exposure to aldicarb would be spread over a day. More recently, it has become apparent that a whole day's exposure could occur in a single serving.

With chemicals like aldicarb, which can produce acute effects, the original legal limits may no longer be considered safe for certain age groups, such as young children.

The U.S. Food and Drug Administration checked aldicarb levels in bananas used for baby food. Those levels were very low, probably because the baby foods are made by blending large numbers of bananas. The problem was high levels of aldicarb in individual bananas that, at random, some children could end up eating. Some of these bananas were not only well above the legal limit but had levels potentially high enough to make a child acutely ill.

The U.S. EPA's dietary risk assessment found that, for the hottest bananas, the allowable daily limit of aldicarb would be exceeded by an adult eating more than one-eighth of a banana and by a child eating more than one bite of a banana. But even for bananas at the legal limit, just one-third of a banana would be an excess for a toddler and one-seventh of a banana would be above the allowable daily intake for an infant.

In 1991, the U.S. EPA and the manufacturer reached an agreement to stop the sale of aldicarb for use on bananas. The registration for bananas has since been canceled and the tolerance revoked. The company also has voluntarily withdrawn its use on white potatoes for the time being because of reasons similar to those that pertain to bananas. Sampling single potatoes revealed a few with residues at or above levels of concern. The company also agreed to reduce the amount of aldicarb used on citrus fruits. The pesticide is currently undergoing special review for groundwater concerns. The situation involving aldicarb residues in bananas is a good example of the need to monitor children's exposures to pesticides in food and to respond accordingly.

A cautionary approach holds true for food imported from abroad. There has been concern for some time about potential risk from pesticides banned or not registered for use in the United States but sometimes detected in imported food. The U.S. Food and Drug Administration (FDA), which oversees the safety of imported food, generally has found a 2- to 3-fold higher violation rate for imported than for domestic foods, usually due to residues of pesticides without tolerances rather than for pesticide residues above prescribed tolerance levels (8).

The food supply in the United States is considered the safest in the world, and adults as well as children should eat a diet high in fruits and vegetables. But efforts to ensure its safety with still higher certainty are key, particularly in view of children's patterns of food consumption and their vulnerability to toxicity.

Variety of Exposure Routes

There are multiple sources and avenues of exposure to pesticides and other toxic substances for children (9). Food and water are obvious sources. There can be direct inhalation and contact with agents inside and outside the home. Some exposures are occupationally related, like parents carrying home chemical residues on their clothing or the transfer to breast milk of chemicals contacted at work. Still other exposures can come from discharges to the air and water, certain waste sites, and, on occasion, industrial accidents.

The task of trying to account for all exposures is complex and difficult. Pesticides, for example, can be ingested during food consumption, inhaled when present in the air, and absorbed through skin contact (Table 54.2). They are commonly found in food and drinking water; in the air; on lawns and gardens; in households; and, for adults, in the workplace.

	Ingestion	Inhalation	Dermal
Food	×		
Water	×	×	×
Air	×		
Lawn/garden	×		×
Household	×	×	×
Occupational	×	×	×

Table 54.2. *Multiple sources and routes of exposure to pesticides for children.*

Infants, for example, individually can face a higher level of exposure than adults to the same level of toxic contaminants in drinking water (12). This would include pesticides. Although infants typically weigh only one-tenth as much as adults, they drink about one-third as much water each day. In addition, water constitutes a higher percentage of their body weight. They also have a higher daily rate of water replacement. These factors combine to increase the exposure of infants to toxic contaminants in water, compared with that of adults, underscoring the need for preventive action to protect them.

In communities with contaminated air, improving overall air quality is vitally important for disease prevention. In terms of protecting children's health, specifically, pediatric asthma is a major concern. Poor air quality conditions exacerbate asthma for children and possibly lead to an increased incidence of attacks, a number of studies have shown (12,13).

But indoor air environments cannot be ignored. There are a number of important sources of pollutants in indoor environments, including tobacco smoke, stove and fireplace fumes, household cleaners, paints and glues, and synthetic fabrics, as well as pesticides.

A U.S. EPA study completed in 1990, titled *The Non-Occupational Pesticide Exposure Study*, found that 85 percent of the total daily exposure to airborne pesticides comes from breathing air inside the home (11). Because of this finding, the U.S. EPA developed a new residential exposure research strategy. Developing additional information about how these exposures occur will be increasingly necessary.

Some of the ways in which children can be exposed involve hand-to-mouth behavior, like sucking on thumbs and fingers. Other behaviors include object-to-mouth, elbow-to-lawn, hand-to-surface, and elbow-to-floor. There are many permutations of these. As a result, residues that persist on such things as carpets, floors, furniture, grass, soil, and playground equipment may be sources of exposure for children.

The U.S. EPA programs that evaluate the risks of toxic substances need to pay more attention to the question of whether and how products in homes and the workplace lead to indoor air pollution problems. They also need to take a more preventive strategy. This means preventing chemicals in these products from being present in indoor environments in the first place and so precluding exposure to children and others.

Health Effects and Lead

The medical community played an important role in uncovering the link between children's exposure to lead and the effects on their health. In decades past, paint containing lead was widely used in the interior of American homes. As homes began to deteriorate and suffered from the lack of upkeep, children frequently ingested the paint chips; this was particularly true in lower economic areas. Children experienced various symptoms, ranging from constipation and retardation to encephalopathy, with coma, convulsions, and even death. Still the link with lead was unclear.

In the 1980s, however studies tracking children from birth resulted in credence being given to the idea that exposure to lead caused behavioral disorders and a lowering of intelligence. Further, the effects were detected at much lower levels than expected and lasted longer than expected; these exposures were at levels once thought to be safe.

Fortunately, lead levels are coming down, due to government action to reduce lead exposure not only from house paint, but also from gasoline, drinking water, and household products. There is still much to be done, however, particularly to protect children living in lower income areas.

Role of Clinicians

Identifying children's exposures to the multitude of potential hazards is difficult. Following are cases that illustrate not only the problems involved but also the crucial role clinicians can play in helping to identify environmental sources of toxicity and responding to them.

The first case involves an 8-month-old infant girl who was diagnosed with chronic diazinon poisoning (14). A routine physical examination at 12 weeks of age found excessive muscle tone in her legs. A month later, when symptoms did not improve, a specialist examined the infant and found increased tone in both her arms and her legs. The specialist suspected a mild case of cerebral palsy and began treatment and therapy.

Fortunately, the clinician discovered several months later that the home had been sprayed with diazinon prior to the first examination. He recommended testing and diazinon residues were found in the home. The child also had an elevated urinary alkyl phosphate level, comparable to the levels found in farm workers who work with the pesticide. Alkyl phosphate is a metabolite of diazinon. Happily, six weeks after leaving the home environment, the child's signs resolved.

The unusual features in this case are that the clinician took the time to take the history, which revealed this exposure and understood what was needed to do the laboratory work, to identify diazinon in the home, and to find metabolites in the child's urine. Under other circumstances, this child might have gone on to have chronic neurologic damage from the exposure and no one would have known why.

The second example concerns chronic mercury toxicity in a child, as reported in Morbidity and *Mortality Weekly Reports* in 1991 (15,16). The case involves a 4-year-old child from Michigan with sweating, itching, headaches, difficulty walking, gingivitis, hypertension, and red discoloration of the palms and the soles of the feet. The physician involved suspected mercury poisoning. Fortunately, this doctor remembered the days when mercury compounds were used for teething powders.

He also knew the significance of a particular array of symptoms that are characteristic of acrodynia, which is pathognomonic for, that is, always linked with mercury exposure.

What the physician learned from the patient's history was that much of the inside of the home had recently been painted with latex paint, and the family had closed the windows and used air conditioning. Since that was the only change in the environment, he investigated further and found not only elevated urinary mercury levels in the child's urine but also mercury vapors in the house. He learned that mercury had been used as a fungicide in the paint.

Since then, the mercury compound involved has been banned for use in house paints, but this case raises the question of whether there have been a number of instances of exposure for children in the past that went unrecognized.

Multiple Exposures

Children may have multiple chemical exposures, which are difficult to identify and evaluate. Suppose, for example, that a child's home is treated with one pesticide. Others are used to treat the child's school for pests. Still other pesticides are in the food the child eats. All may have the same mechanism of action.

Several classes of pesticides contain specific chemicals that are likely to act by the same method of action. Examples include the organophosphates and carbamates, both of which inhibit acetylcholinesterase.

It is not known how to combine the effects from these exposures and so estimate potential risk. Not known, for example, is whether these exposures are simply additive, if these pesticides sometimes inhibit each other, or if they sometimes are additive or synergistic, multiplying each other's potential effects on children.

The NAS recommended research to evaluate the issue of multiple exposures to pesticides that act by the same mechanism. Such information could lead logically to developing procedures to take multiple exposures into account in the regulatory process. Work on this issue needs to be accelerated.

There are still many unknowns about the effects of pesticides on people and on infants and children in particular. Filling the information gaps on effects and exposures, primarily nondietary exposures, is essential, but achieving that goal will take time, focused effort, and unwavering support for research dedicated to this end.

Clinicians can play an important role in accomplishing this goal through special awareness of the potential effects of pesticide poisoning. Although environmental toxicity typically is not the first item on a doctor's mind in making a diagnosis, increased alertness to environmental toxicity can be a direct route to identifying causes of disease. Parents can contribute as well by identifying possible environmental links and advising the physician involved in treating the child's health problem about them.

One of the major strategies immediately available for protecting children from exposures to environmental risk is pollution prevention. It is time for parents and schools to take a careful look at how pesticides and other toxic chemicals are used around children. Pesticide users must learn how to use the safest possible methods of pest control to prevent exposure to children. First and foremost, pesticides should not be used on a "preventive" basis but rather to treat specific pest problems. When pest control is needed, it is important to use Integrated Pest Management (IPM) techniques to avoid the use of pesticides. Around the home and around schools, this means keeping pests out in the first instance and denying them access to food and shelter. If a pesticide is needed, use the safest product available and follow label instructions carefully. Be sure that any pest control contractors are licensed. And stay out of the house or school during treatment, ventilating it well before reoccupying it. Likewise, it is important to reduce the risks of agricultural pesticides. The U.S. EPA is working with farmers and the USDA to reduce unnecessary use, encourage IPM practices, and help the transition to safer alternatives. We are working to strengthen regulation of pesticides to protect children. What these changes will mean is fewer pesticide residues in children's environments, in drinking water, and on food.

— by Lynn R. Goldman, U.S. Environmental Protection Agency.

References

1. U.S. EPA. Quantities of Pesticides Used in the United States Information Sheet. Washington: U.S. Environmental Protection Agency, 1994.

2. National Academy of Sciences. Pesticides in the Diets of Infants and Children. Washington: National Academy Press, 1993.

3. Kelce WR, Monosson E, Gamcsik MP, Laws SC, Gray LE Jr. Environmental hormone disruptors: evidence that vinclozolin developmental toxicity is mediated by antiandrogenic metabolites. Toxicol Appl Pharmacol 126:276-285 (1994).

4. Gray LE, Jr, Ostby JS, Kelce WR. Developmental effects of an environmental antiandrogen: the fungicide vinclozolin alters sex differentiation of the male rat. Toxicol Appl Pharmacol 129:46 52 (1994).

5. Hileman B. Environmental estrogens linked to reproductive abnormalities, cancer. Chem Eng News, January 31, 1994.

6. Rogan WJ, Gladen BC, McKinney JD, Carreras N, Hardy P Thullen J, Tingelsad J, Tully M. Polychlorinated biphenyls (PCBs) and dichlorodiphenyl dichloroethene (DDE) in human milk: effects on growth, morbidity, and duration of lactation. Am T Public Health 77(10):1294-1297 (1987).

7. McLachlan JA. Functional toxicology: a new approach to detect biologically active xenobiotics. Environ Health Perspect 101(5):386-387 (1993).

8. U.S. Food and Drug Administration. Pesticide program- residue monitoring 1993. J AOAC Int 77(5):161A-85A (1994).

9. Rogan WJ. The sources and routes of childhood chemical exposures. J Pediatr 97(5):861-865 (1980).

10. David DL, Miller Poore L, Levin R. Chemical contamination of food and water. In: Textbook of Clinical Occupational and Environmental Medicine (Rosenstock L, Cullen MR, eds). Philadelphia: W.B. Saunders Company, 1994;47-53.

11. Immerman FW, Schaum JL. Nonoccupational Pesticides Exposure Study. Document no 600/S3-90/003. Washington: U. S. Environmental Protection Agency, 1990.

12. Morgan WJ, Martinez FD. Risk factors for developing wheezing and asthma in childhood. Pediatr Clin North Am 39(6):1185-1203 (1992).

13. Bloomberg GR, Strunk RC. Crisis in asthma care. Pediatr Clin North Am 39(6):1225-1241 (1992).

14. Wagner SL, Orwick DL. Chronic organophosphate exposure associated with transient hypertonia in an infant. Pediatrics 94(1):94-97 (1994).

15. Acute and chronic poisoning from residential exposures to elemental mercury, Michigan, 1989-1990. MMWR 40(23):393-395 (1991).

16. Blondell JM, Knott SM. Risk analysis for phenylmercuric acetate in indoor latex house paint. In: Pesticides in Urban Environments: Fate and Significance (Racke K, Leslie A, eds). Washington: American Chemical Society, 1993.

Chapter 55

Growing Pains: Children in the Real Environment

While most people would do anything to protect their children from environmental hazards, many parents would be shocked to learn that children's exposure to toxicants can be much higher than their own. Far from being "little adults," children are very different both behaviorally and physiologically. For instance, children's habit of putting things in their mouths can increase their relative exposure to environmental toxicants such as lead. Moreover, children are particularly vulnerable to toxicants and other environmental hazards because many organ systems, including the gastrointestinal, central nervous, immune, and reproductive systems, are still developing after birth. In general, the younger the child, the greater any potential health effects.

Despite differences in behavior and physiology between children and adults, few studies have focused on the effects of these differences on risks to children's health of environmental exposures. "Children are not routinely included in risk assessment processes, and most environmental regulations are based on exposure data of adult males," write Joy Carlson and Katie Sokoloff of the Children's Environmental Health Network in the 1995 *Environmental Health Perspectives Supplement* on child health.

The lack of studies notwithstanding, there are indicators that children's environmental health may be declining. Asthma in children has increased by more than a third over the past 15 years, afflicting

NIH Publication 96-218. *Environmental Health Perspectives* Volume 104, Number 2, February 1996.

an estimated 4.2 million children under the age of 18 nationwide, according to the American Lung Association (ALA). "Asthma is now the leading cause of admissions to hospitals in children. It's reached epidemic proportions," says Philip Landrigan, professor of community medicine at the Mount Sinai Medical Center in New York, who authored the 1994 book *Raising Children Toxic Free* with Herbert Needleman, professor of child psychiatry and pediatrics at the University of Pittsburgh School of Medicine. Similarly, the rates of the two most common childhood cancers have increased significantly over the past 15 years: acute lymphocytic leukemia is up more than 10 percent and brain rumors are up more than 30 percent. While these increases may in part reflect better diagnoses, environmental hazards such as air pollution, pesticides, and industrial chemicals are also likely to play a role.

Lead

Lead is considered by many to be the, greatest environmental health threat to children in the United States, especially along the eastern seaboard and in the Midwest. While adults absorb about 10 percent of the lead they ingest, children's less mature digestive systems can absorb as much as 50 percent because lead resembles calcium and children's gastrointestinal tracts take up calcium at greater rates than adults'. Young children's nervous systems are particularly susceptible to detrimental effects of lead because the "blood-brain barrier" (which protects the brain from many substances) is not completely functional until three years of age, a period when neurons are still migrating and synapses are still forming.

While high levels of lead can cause mental retardation and even death, most of the lead poisoning in U.S. children is at levels so low that it goes undetected because there are no overt symptoms. "The effects typically don't manifest until school age. [Lead-poisoned] children have attention deficits, decreased hearing, and increased impulsivity, all of which can lead to difficulty in learning," says Janet Phoenix, manager of public health programs at the National Lead Information Center in Washington, D.C.

These neurological effects are seen at blood lead levels near 10 micrograms per deciliter (μg/dl), which the Centers for Disease Control classifies as a "level of concern." Moreover, decreases in IQ and growth can occur even below 10 μg/dl, according to the 1992 report *Lead Toxicity* by the Agency for Toxic Substances and Disease Registry

(ATSDR) in Atlanta. In fact, no minimum level for lead toxicity has been identified, according to the 1993 American Academy of Pediatrics report *Lead Poisoning: From Screening to Primary Prevention.*

Three to four million U.S. children (17 percent of all children) had blood lead levels above 15 μg/dl in 1989, according to the ATSDR report. "Most parents are not aware that lead is still a problem," says Maurci Jackson of United Parents Against Lead. "Our children are used as the lead detectors. We've got to reverse that and put the emphasis on prevention just as we do with immunizations. Lead testing needs to be standard for all children across the country."

The main source of lead poisoning in children is old lead-based paint. Prior to 1955, much of the white interior paint in the country was half lead and half linseed oil, a durable but toxic combination. While lead-based paint was banned in the United States in 1971, the EPA estimates that more than three quarters of the homes in the United States still contain some. Children can be exposed to lead by eating chips that fall off the walls as the paint ages, by chewing on painted cribs, or by breathing dust when paint is sanded off walls during renovation.

Other sources of this toxicant include drinking water from lead-soldered plumbing and soil that contains lead residues from motor vehicle exhaust. Cultural practices can also expose children to lead. For example, the traditional pottery made by Hispanic people in the southwest United States, as well as much imported pottery, is fired at temperatures too low to fix the lead in the pigments, and kohl, a southeast Asian folk remedy that is applied around the eye, can be 80 percent lead.

Air Pollution

While lead is the major environmental hazard to children in much of the United States, air pollution may pose an even greater threat to children in urban areas. Children are more vulnerable to air pollution in part because lungs continue to develop throughout childhood, adding new alveoli until about age 20. Damage from air pollution can impede lung development and may lead to chronic lung disease later in life, according to the ALA's 1995 report *Danger Zone: Ozone Air Pollution and Our Children.*

Children's exposures to air pollution are likely to be much greater than adults' for several reasons. Due to their higher metabolic rates, children need more oxygen and therefore breathe more air—twice as much air per pound of body weight compared to adults. In addition, children often play outside on warm, sunny afternoons, which is when ozone levels peak. Children also breathe air closer to the ground, where respirable particles settle, and can be so much more active that they breathe air pollutants deeper into their lungs than adults.

The ozone and particulate air pollution that children breathe comes primarily from motor vehicles. Ozone can damage the cells that line the respiratory tract, making airways narrower and causing wheezing, chest pain, bronchitis, and asthma. These effects are greater in children because their airways are narrower than those of adults. Ozone can also decrease resistance to respiratory infection, make airways more sensitive to airborne allergens, and act synergistically with airborne acidity to damage deep lung tissues, according to the 1993 American Academy of Pediatrics' report *Ambient Air Pollution: Respiratory Hazards to Children*. While the Federal standard for ozone is 120 parts per billion averaged over an hour, wheezing and other symptoms can occur at exposures to lower levels over longer periods of time, according to the ALA.

Besides diesel vehicle and car exhaust, sources of particulate air pollution include wood fires and factory and utility smokestacks. Particulate air pollution comprises solid and liquid particles less than 10 microns in diameter. Particles this small can be inhaled deep into the lungs, causing wheezing and coughing, and triggering asthma attacks, and are also associated with pleurisy and pneumonia. Symptoms can occur below the Federal standard of 150 micrograms per cubic meter, according to Landrigan.

While there have been no direct studies of the effects of air pollution on children, autopsies of 100 Los Angeles children who died for unrelated reasons in 1990 revealed that more than 80 percent had subclinical lung damage, says spokesman Jerry Martin of the California Air Resources Board. "We're pretty certain that the only thing they had in common was living in polluted air," he says. This pilot study led to an ongoing, long-term study to determine the effects on developing lung tissues of growing up in polluted air.

Pesticides on Food

Besides having greater exposures to lead and air pollution compared to adults living in the same environment, children can also be exposed to greater amounts of pesticides because they generally eat much more of certain foods than adults do.

For example, children eat up to seven times more apples, bananas, grapes, pears, and carrots in proportion to their body weight. Standards for food pesticide levels are inadequate for protecting children because they are based on adult exposures, says Landrigan, who chaired the National Academy of Sciences committee that authored the 1993 study *Pesticides in the Diets of Infants and Children.* The report called for new pesticide residue standards that reflect the critical differences in children's diet and physiology. "We agree with the general thrust of the [NAS] recommendations but the methods are not necessarily available," says John McCarthy, vice president for scientific and regulatory affairs of the Washington, D.C.-based American Crop Protection Association.

Children of farm-workers are probably exposed to the highest levels of pesticides used on food but there are no good studies showing this, says Valerie Wilk, a health specialist with the Farm-worker Justice Fund in Washington, D.C. "Temporary housing is right on the fields and the concentration of pesticides inside them is high. And most often the whole family is out in the fields and the kids are crawling around in pesticide-contaminated soil," she says. A recent pilot study by the California Department of Health suggested that agricultural pesticide levels are indeed elevated in houses within a quarter mile of fields, according to Lawrie Mott of the Natural Resources Defense Council in San Francisco. McCarthy agrees that pesticide exposures of farm-workers are a problem. "We are champions of the 1992 EPA worker protection standards," he says. "For example, we are helping to train and educate farm-workers—those who plant and harvest the crops—and pesticide applicators."

Pesticides Used in the Home

For most children, however, pesticides used in the home and yard may pose a greater threat than pesticide residues on food. Compared to adults, children can be exposed to higher levels of pesticides in flea bombs, pest strips, herbicides, and other pesticides used at home because they are more likely to play on floors and lawns. For example, after flea bombs are used, concentrations of the insecticide Dursban (chlorpyrifos) are much higher one foot above the floor, where babies play, than six feet above the floor, where adults breathe. The EPA estimates that 84 percent of U.S. households use pesticides. Unfortunately, there are no regulations for home pesticide use, says Landrigan. For example, the highly toxic organophosphate pesticide diazinon (Spectocide) is allowed for use in homes and by commercial lawn care companies but is banned for use on golf courses, corn, and alfalfa fields, he says.

While several studies have suggested that home exposure to pesticides can cause brain cancer and leukemia in children, the results are not conclusive. "There are no data on children [and pesticides] period," says Sandra Schubert, program director of the National Coalition Against the Misuse of Pesticides in Washington, D.C.. "Until recently there has been no concerted effort to look at children's issues. Half of the problem is lack of education—people assume that if the EPA approved a product, then it's safe." Wendy Gordon, executive director of Mothers and Others for a Livable Planet, an advocacy group for children's health issues, agrees: "At the Federal level, the laws are very protective. But when the laws are translated into regulations, they are designed to protect industry. Chemicals are innocent until proven guilty."

Endocrine Disrupters

There is rising concern that DDT and its metabolites, some PCBs, and a host of other compounds can disrupt the endocrine system and thus have disastrous effects on sexual development and reproduction. The DDT metabolite DDE, for instance, mimics the effects of estrogen by binding to the hormone's receptors. In wildlife from salmon to alligators and eagles to whales, endocrine disrupters are associated with reproductive effects such as decreased fertility, feminization of males, and masculinization of females. "The evidence is pretty good for wildlife but is less dear for people—it's all epidemiological," says Michael Fry of the Department of Avian Sciences at the University of California at Davis, who is a member of a National Academy of Sciences and reviewing data on the effects of endocrine disrupters on wildlife and people. "People are exposed to such a wide range of toxins that it's hard to show a cause," says Schubert. "But endocrine disrupters are particularly scary because people have found parallels between wildlife and the human population."

While DDT and PCBs have been banned in the United States for about 20 years, they are still used extensively in developing countries and are widespread in the environment. In addition, the DDT analogues dicofol, kelthane, and methoxychlor, as well as many other endocrine-disrupting compounds, are currently used in the United States. In light of the effects of endocrine disrupters on wildlife, Theo

Colborn of the World Wildlife Fund in Washington, D.C. calls for re-examining the endocrinological effects of new and currently used pesticides. Colborn says that most tests assess only acute toxicity, carcinogenicity, or mutagenicity, and that we need to do, for example, *in vitro* assays for hormone receptor binding. "We respectfully disagree," says the American Crop Protection Association's McCarthy. "The current routine testing required for pesticides is good enough." Others suggest getting rid of endocrine-disrupting compounds entirely. "We think we know enough about many of these compounds to ban them," says Monica Moore, program director of the Pesticide Action Network's North American Regional Center in San Francisco.

Hazardous Waste

There are an estimated 30,000 to 40,000 hazardous waste sites in the United States, according to Jeffrey Lybarger, director of health studies at the ATSDR. Nearly 1,300 of these are Superfund sites, 42 percent of which are landfills or waste storage/treatment facilities, 31 percent are abandoned manufacturing facilities, 8 percent are waste recycling facilities, 5 percent are mining sites, and 4 percent are government properties, according to a 1995 *Chemosphere* article by Assistant Surgeon General Barry Johnson. To date, more than 2,000 toxicants have been identified at Superfund sites, and 275 of these are ATSDR/EPA priority substances—those that pose the greatest health risks. Lead is ranked first on the list, PCBs are seventh, and DDT is twelfth.

Hazardous waste sites are largely uncharacterized. "We don't know the extent of the contamination so we can't assess the health risk," says Lybarger. But, he says, children's behavior makes them more at risk for increased exposure to hazardous waste because they play outside more, play in dirt, and are curious. "They may play in an abandoned drum," he says. "They may not have the wisdom to leave it alone."

The many epidemiological studies of the adverse health effects of hazardous waste sites have been inconclusive. But while the overall impact of hazardous waste is unknown, investigations at specific sites have documented symptoms ranging from headaches and neurobehavioral problems to cardiac anomalies and cancer, according to a 1993 NRC review *Environmental Epidemiology: Public Health and Hazardous Wastes*. The EPA ranks Superfund sites eighth on their list of the top 29 environmental causes of cancer. "Although the hazard posed by an individual site to public health and ecosystems remains some-what controversial, the evidence is mounting that many sites do present a hazard to human health because of releases of contaminants into groundwater and other environmental media," writes Assistant Surgeon General Johnson.

Pesticide exposures related to childhood brain cancer		
Exposure	**Time Period**	**Odds Ratio**
Pesticides used for nuisance pests	Child	3.4
Bomb used for nuisance pests	Pregnancy	6.2
No-Pest-Strip used for nuisance pests	Pregnancy	5.2
No-Pest-Strip used for nuisance pests	Child	3.7
Termite pesticides	Any period	3.0
Kwell shampoo used for head lice	Child	4.6
Flea collar used on pets	Infant	5.5
Flea collar used on pets	Child	2.4
Insecticides used in the garden	Child	2.6
Carbaryl used in the garden	Any period	2.4
Diazinon used in the garden	Any period	4.6
Herbicides used in the yard	Infant	3.4
Herbicides used in the yard	Child	2.4

Source: Davis JR. Childhood brain cancer linked to consumer pesticide use. *Pesticides and You* Spring, 18–20 (1993). Adapted from Davis JR, et al. Family pesticide use and childhood brain cancer. *Arch Environ Contam Toxicol* 24:87–92 (1993).

Table 55.1.

Radiation

Radiation can have devastating effects on children. While very high doses can cause blindness, intractable bloody diarrhea, and death, lower doses have more subtle effects such as genetic mutations, he-matopoietic disorders, and cancer. A 1990 NAS report concluded that there are no safe levels of radiation. The younger the child and the greater the radiation dose, the greater the risk of cancer. Studies of atomic bomb survivors show that children who were under the age of 20 when exposed to the radiation were at greater risk of developing cancer. Similarly, atomic bomb survivors who had received heavier doses were more likely to develop leukemia. Repeated exposure to x-rays can cause a wide range of childhood cancers including brain can-cer, leukemia, lung cancer, and thyroid cancer.

Historically, Department of Energy nuclear weapons manufactur-ing facilities released radioactive compounds into the environment, which may have affected children living nearby. For example, from the mid-1940s to the mid-1950s, the Hanford nuclear weapons manufacturing facility in eastern Washington released radioactive iodine into the air; the facility was closed in the late 1980s. "A lot of radiation was released (700,000 curies total) and native Americans were potentially affected by the radiation," says Michael Sage, deputy chief of radiation studies at the National Center for Environmental Health in Atlanta. The CDC is three years into a study of whether people in the Yakima and Umatilla Nations who lived near the site during the time of the releases have higher incidences of thyroid diseases such as hypothyroidism, hyperthyroidism, and cancer.

Commercial nuclear power plants are safer than DOE facilities on a day-to-day basis in part because the reactors are newer and do not produce nuclear material. "The big issue is potential accidents like Three Mile Island," says Sage. Landrigan adds that nuclear waste is the greatest long-term risk of nuclear power generation, pointing out that we have yet to find a safe disposal method.

Today some argue that the most significant source of radiation exposure in children is radon, a gas produced from uranium-rich soils. Radon seeps into houses through cracks in basements and gaps around pipes. Radon breaks down into radioactive particles that can be retained in the lungs. While there have been no studies in children, studies have shown that radon can cause lung cancer in miners. Residential exposure to radon may account for 13,000 lung cancer deaths per year, according to the 1989 American Academy of Pediatrics' report *Radon Exposure: a Hazard to Children*. Children are at greater risk for radon exposure because they breathe more per body weight and are closer to the floor, where radon breakdown products accumulate. Compared to an adult, a six-month old baby will receive about twice the radon exposure per body weight.

EMFs

There is no consensus on the effects of electric and magnetic fields (EMFs) on children's health. Four out of 14 studies suggest that there is a link between proximity to power lines and childhood cancers such as leukemia, according to the 1995 NIEHS/DOE booklet *Questions and Answers About EMF: Electric and Magnetic Fields Associated with the Use of Electric Power*. One of the studies suggests that living within 130 feet of high-current power lines may increase children's risk of leukemia several fold. "Some studies have shown risks, some haven't.

The studies that have [shown risk] are convincing enough that we can't say there's no risk— but it's probably not that great," says Anne Mellinger, medical epidemiologist at the National Center for Environmental Health's Radiation Studies Branch.

Poor and Minority Children

While all children are vulnerable to environmental hazards, poor and minority children are particularly at risk because they tend to live in less healthy environments. For example, poor and minority children are more likely to be exposed to pesticides used on crops because more than 70 percent of seasonal farm-workers are Hispanic, according to the EHP Supplement on child health. And the areas with three of the five largest hazardous waste sites nationwide have twice as many people of color as areas without such sites, says Jerry Poje, director of minority health programs at the NIEHS.

Although children's average blood lead levels are down nationwide, there has been no such decrease in minority populations, says Poje. Of the several million U.S. children with lead poisoning, 55 percent are poor and black while 26 percent are poor and white, according to the 1989 ATSDR report on lead toxicity. Poor and minority children are more likely to be exposed to higher levels of lead because low-income housing tends to be poorly maintained and more likely to have old, peeling paint. To make matters worse, poor children can absorb lead more readily because their diets can be deficient in protein, calcium, iron, and zinc.

Poor and minority children are also at greater risk for exposure to air pollution in part because ozone and particulates from motor vehicles are concentrated in inner cities. The ALA estimates that 69 percent of Hispanics, 67 percent of Asian-Americans, 61 percent of blacks, and 51 percent of whites live in areas where ozone levels exceed the EPA standard.

While there are many reasons to be concerned about children's environmental health, "environmental diseases are in part the result of personal and collective choices in the way we live, in the way we consume our resources, and dispose of our waste products," write Landrigan and Needleman. "There is cause for optimism in this observation. If a disease is made by human beings, we should be able to prevent it." As a nation, preventing disease in our children is the only way to protect our future.

Making Children a Policy Priority

Recognizing the special vulnerabilities of children to environmental hazards, the EPA has instituted a new policy that requires evaluations of environmental health risks to infants and children in all of the agency's risk assessments, risk characterizations, and environmental public health standards. In announcing the new policy, EPA Administrator Carol Browner said that the policy "will encourage new, much needed research to provide the child-specific data we will need to thoroughly evaluate health risks children and infants face from pollution in our air, land, and water."

Although the EPA has considered children's health risks in many of the agency's programs, the new policy will require risk assessments during the decision-making process for setting environmental standards. The agency will develop a separate assessment of risks to infants and children or state clearly why this is not done (for example, in instances where children are not exposed). As part of these assessments, the EPA will consider age-related variations in susceptibility, including factors such as differences in pharmacokinetics, pharmacodynamics, body composition, maturity of biochemical and physiological functions, and differences in types and levels of exposure.

The policy, which became effective on 1 November 1995, was sponsored by the 44 EPA Science Policy Council which evaluates agency science policy issues.

—by Robin Meadows

Part Ten

Global Concerns

Chapter 56

Anticipated Public Health Consequences of Global Climate Change

Introduction

Human activities are placing enormous pressures on the biosphere. The introduction of new chemicals and the increasing ambient levels of existing chemicals have resulted in atmospheric degradation. This chapter reviews some of the adverse effects of stratospheric ozone depletion and global warming. Because the atmospheric effects of ozone depletion are fairly well characterized, quantitative risk estimates have been developed. However, because the atmospheric effects of global warming are less understood, public health problems that could be intensified by climate change are assessed qualitatively. The interactive effects of these two phenomena are also discussed.

Human activities are resulting in phenomena that are changing our world in unprecedented ways. Use of non-conservative land practices in the development of food sources to feed a growing global population has resulted in vast areas of deforestation and desertification. Use of the manufactured chemicals, chlorofluorocarbons (CFCs), has resulted in degradation of the stratospheric ozone layer, and there is every indication that this will continue for many years to come, eventually resulting in measurable increases in ultraviolet radiation on the earth's surface. Increasing energy usage and the production of meat and grain to support economic development have resulted in increases in the ambient concentrations of CO_2, methane, nitrous

NIH Publication 96-218. *Environmental Health Perspectives* Volume 96, 1991.

oxide, and CFCs. Such increases will contribute to an increase in mean temperature at the earth's surface and may have serious consequences for climatic conditions across the globe. All of these activities contribute to a changing globe and most if not all will contribute to some extent to changes in the global climate and, by extension, contribute to changes in human health. This chapter, however, focuses principally on the anticipated consequences of stratospheric ozone depletions and global warming resulting from the greenhouse effect.

Stratospheric Ozone Depletion

Background

Ozone (O_3) has conceptually been thought of as existing in two layers in the earth's atmosphere: a stratospheric layer and a tropospheric layer. The tropospheric layer hugs the surface of the earth and is part of the air we breathe. In it, ozone is a noxious pollutant, exposure to which has been associated with lung damage and respiratory problems. In the stratospheric layer, however, ozone acts like a protective shield, preventing much of the sun's ultraviolet radiation (UVR) from reaching the earth. This protection is selective, with shorter wavelengths being absorbed preferentially. Thus, energy in the UV-C wavelengths (200 to 290 nm) is completely absorbed by the ozone layer, while the UV-B (290 to 320 nm) is only partially absorbed, and the UV-A (320 to 400 nm) is not absorbed at all. In addition, UVR varies by time and location due to the length of its path through the ozone layer. Radiation entering over the equator has the shortest path length and thus encounters less ozone, so more reaches the surface than radiation hitting the surface at the poles. Figure 56.1 shows model-based estimates of the variation by time of day in UVR by wave band for clear days in Washington, D.C.. Similar variation is seen by time of day, latitude, and altitude.

Currently, production and release of CFCs have begun to result in a decrease in the concentration of ozone in the stratosphere. With depletion of the stratospheric ozone layer, it has been predicted that more UV-B, particularly in the shorter wavelengths, will reach the earth. The amount of UV-A will remain unchanged, and UV-C is still expected to be completely absorbed. Both UV-B and UV-A are biologically active; however, UV-B, especially the shorter wavelengths, is generally more effective than UV-A for any given effect. The U.S. Environmental Protection Agency (EPA) has been charged with assessing

June 21. No Cloud Cover. Half Hour Intervals

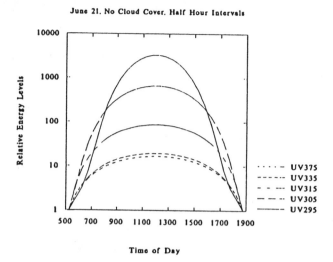

Figure 56.1. *Relative changes in radiation for five wavelengths. Estimates taken from the NASA satellite-based model of UV flux developed by Serafino and Frederick (1) and adapted by Pitcher and Longstreth (2).*

the potential risks associated with stratospheric ozone depletion; as part of that assessment (3), the potential impacts on human health of increased UV-B were evaluated. Much of the material presented below has been drawn from that evaluation.

Health Effects of Ozone Depletion

The principal targets of UVR in humans are the skin and the eye; important effects include skin cancer, cataracts, and effects on the immune system. UVR is biologically active chiefly because there are molecules in the skin and the eye that can absorb its energy. Perhaps one of the most important of such molecules, DNA, undergoes a variety of changes upon absorption, including the formation of a number of pyrimidine photo products, e.g., cyclobutadiene dimmers. Such photo products, if not repaired or if misrepaired, are thought to lead to changes in cell function, which may culminate in transformation and neoplasia.

All wavelengths are not equally effective at inducing such effects. Rather, there is a spectrum of energy that for most of the direct effects of UVR cover principally the UV-B region and may in some instances extend into the UV-A region. Each effect has its specific spectrum of effective energy; this has been termed its action spectrum. The exact spectra for effects observed in humans are not known and may never be known. However, spectra have been determined for DNA damage and for carcinogenesis in the mouse; these are presented in Figure 56.2.

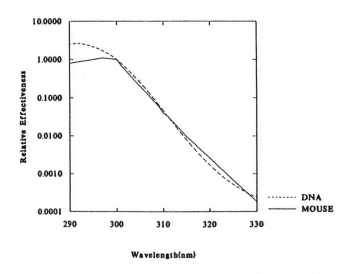

Figure 56.2. *Mouse carcinogenesis and DNA action spectra.*

Skin Cancer. Exposure to sunlight (and by inference, UV has been associated with three forms of skin cancer: basal cell and squamous cell carcinoma (the so-called non-melanoma cancers) and cutaneous melanoma (CM). Basal cell and squamous cell carcinoma (BCC and SCC, respectively) are both malignancies of the epidermal keratinocyte, the major cell of the epidermis. Melanoma occurs via the neoplastic transformation of the pigment-producing cell in the skin, the melanocyte. The linkage between sunlight and non-melanoma skin cancer (NMSC) is generally thought to be more solid than that for CM. NMSC occurs with greater frequency on the most highly exposed sites, e.g., the hands and face; individuals with fair skin and with the most outdoor exposure, e.g., farmers and fisher men, are at greatest risk. There is also a latitude gradient with individuals living near the equator being at greater risk than those living farther from it. BCC and SCC are much more common but, also relatively benign tumors. These two factors have led to a paucity of statistics on these tumors. They are so benign that they are often removed by dermatologists or even general practitioners and not sent for pathologic confirmation, and they are so common that tumor registries would be overwhelmed if reporting became mandatory (which would also require pathologic confirmation).

The United States has not had a survey to determine incidence on NMSC since 1978 (4); the data gathered then indicated that between 400,000 and 500,000 individuals developed NMSC annually. This represented a 15 to 20 percent increase in incidence when compared to a similar survey performed in 1970-1971 (4). Using these data, the U.S. EPA (3) estimated that for every 1 percent decrease in ozone, there would be between a 2 and 3 percent increase in NMSC. Assuming no controls and growth rates of 1.2 to 5.0 percent in CFC production, it was estimated that there would be between about 11 and 260 million additional cases of NMSC in individuals alive in 1985 or born through 2074.

However, those estimates my have started with too low a base case. A much more recent study, but of a selected population (those enrolled in a Kaiser-Permanente health plan in Portland, Oregon and Vancouver, Washington) presents a much greater increase (5). This study examined pathology records on SCC and CM for the study population spanning the years 1960 to 1986. During that time period, the age-adjusted incidence rates for SCC increased from 9.7 to 29.8 per 100,000 for females and from 41.6 to 106.1 per 100,000 for males. More disquieting, however, was the fact that a comparison of the data from this current study to data from the Seattle population included in the Scotto et al(4) study indicated about a 2-fold discrepancy between the estimates, with the latter study being the lower of the two. There might be several explanations for this discrepancy; two plausible ones are,

- the techniques of routine biopsy and pathologic examination of all lesions result in an output that more accurately reflects the true incidence of these lesions than the methodology used in the Scotto et al. (4) study, or

- the Kaiser Permanente population, by virtue of being middle class and employed, may be at greater risk, possibly due to more risk associated behavior, e.g., sunny recreational activities.

Either way, the population, or perhaps a specific portion of it, is at greater risk than would be predicted on the basis of earlier studies.

The evidence linking CM to sunlight (and presumably UVR) has traditionally been thought to be less compelling than that cited for NMSC. However, recent evidence, particularly viewed in the context of what was already known, suggests that there are strong reasons to believe that excessive exposure to UV is associated with an increased risk of melanoma. In the past few years, analysis of a number of major case-control studies [reviewed in Longstreth (6)] has revealed, almost without exception, an association between melanoma risk and measures that assess increasing intensity of sun exposure. In addition, like NMSC, melanoma affects fair-skinned individuals more than dark-skinned ones and has a latitude gradient, with individuals living nearer the equator being at greater risk than those living farther from it. Unlike NMSC, however, individuals at greatest risk are not those who have the highest sun exposure but rather are indoor workers. The preferred sites also differ with face and hands being major sites for NMSC and the trunk in males and legs and back in females being the major sites for CM.

Eye Disease. When an individual is outdoors, the eye, like the skin of face and hands, is continually exposed to UVR unless protected by glasses or clothing. UVR-induced damage has been documented for the cornea, lens, and retina (7). The most common form of damage to the cornea is "snow-blindness," or photokeratitis, the ocular equivalent of a sunburn. Unlike the skin, however, which develops a partial tolerance to the effects of sun through thickening or darkening, the cornea develops no resistance with repeated exposure. This is a common problem among skiers, and it is likely that with ozone depletion enough additional UVR will reach the surface that the risk of this condition will measurably increase.

The most common form of lenticular damage associated with UVR exposure is cataract. There are several forms of cataract; the three most common, cortical, nuclear, and posterior subcapsular cataract, have recently been evaluated in epidemiologic studies for their etiologic relationship to UVR exposure. In these studies, cortical (8) and posterior subcapsular cataract (9) both showed an association with increasing cumulative UV-B dose or with average annual UV-B dose. Cataract is an increasing problem as the world's population ages (10); with increased UV-B due to ozone depletion, even larger impacts are likely.

Immunosuppression. It has been known for some time that UVR has a suppressive effect on the skin immune system. This was originally discovered in experiments done in a non-melanoma skin cancer model in mice (11); it has since been extended to antigens administered in protocols to examine both contact (12) and delayed hypersensitivity

(13) and, very recently, to a variety of infectious diseases when studied in animal systems [reviewed in van der Leun et al. (15)]. The immunosuppression that is induced may be either local, i.e., limited to the skin, or systemic; generally, systemic immunosuppression requires a larger total dose to achieve than that required to induce the local effect (15). The exact mechanism underlying this immunosuppression is unknown; however, one of the first events observed is loss of activity in a class of antigen-presenting cells in the skin—the Langerhans cells. Shortly after the loss of antigen-presenting activity by Langerhans cells, the subset of lymphocytes responsible for suppression of cell-mediated immunity (T-suppressor cells) appears in the skin. Action spectra for the immunosuppressive effects of UVR demonstrate the greatest activity in the UV-B region (3). Of concern *vis-a-vis* ozone depletion, therefore, is the potential impact that additional UV may have on infectious diseases in human populations. The impact could be not only one of perhaps increasing the incidence or severity of various diseases, but it is also possible that vaccination programs designed to protect populations could be ineffective if administered to heavily sun-exposed populations.

Effects Due to Air Pollution. Stratospheric ozone will allow UVR to penetrate deeper into the earth's atmosphere, and there is evidence that tropospheric air quality could be adversely impacted (16). To the extent that air pollution increases, individuals with respiratory problems who are sensitive to a variety of pollutants will suffer, potentially resulting in an increase in the number of hospital visits by such people. In addition, there is some evidence that urban smog contributes to respiratory carcinogenesis so that any increase in pollution may eventually result in additional lung cancer incidence (17).

Global Warming

Background

The seasonality of disease—flu during the winter, measles in the fall, and sunburn in the summer—is something with which we are all familiar. There is a whole field, biometeorology, devoted to the study of the impact of weather or climate on biologic systems and a rather voluminous literature on the subject (particularly as it relates to human disease) going back to the time of Hippocrates (18). With human activities generating ever increasing concentrations of CO_2 and other radiatively important trace gases, changes in global temperature are likely and with them changes in climatic conditions. How this may affect human health is still somewhat of a speculative question because there are such complexities involved in even assessing the role normal weather plays in human disease, and there are also vast uncertainties in the precise changes in weather anticipated with global warming. The EPA was charged, however, with developing a Report to Congress on the Potential Consequences of Global Climate Change for the U.S., including an evaluation of potential impacts on human health (19). Much of the material presented below has been drawn from that evaluation. As with all such assessments, often the analytical exercise of evaluating what may happen can provide important clues to what scientists and policy makers should be following to determine if a risk is real or imagined.

Health Effects of Global Warming

The health effects of global warming are much less easy to identify than those likely to be associated with stratospheric ozone depletion. With ozone depletion there is an easily identified culprit: an increase in UV-B, with fairly well-defined effects. As shown in Figure 56.3, with global climatic change, the impacts will be secondary and even tertiary, i.e., few of the predicted effects are directly related to the direct impact of heat on a cell or an organ such as would be observed with a burn; they are likely to be the result of what the impacts of heat would be on ecosystems such as forests and farmland.

Heat Stress. Perhaps the easiest adverse effect to predict from global warming is the impact of increased temperatures. Heat places stress on the thermoregulatory system, which is intimately tied to the circulatory system. In individuals whose circulatory systems are already compromised by heart, respiratory, or vascular problems, additional stress brought about by increased temperature can be disastrous, resulting in significant increases in morbidity and mortality. In a study performed for the EPA, Kalkstein (20) evaluated the potential impact of global warming on temperature-related mortality in 15 cities across the United States. The outcome was highly dependent on the degree of acclimatization predicted. With complete acclimatization, little or no effect was predicted. However, with moderate acclimatization, a net increase in mortality for the 15 cities was predicted, even when taking into account that the number of cold-related deaths would probably drop.

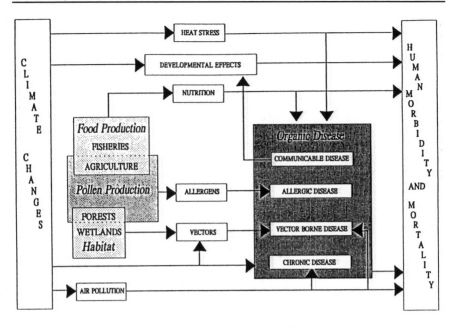

Figure 56.3. Public health impacts of global climatic change.

The Kalkstein study (20) found that generally, cities in the South did not show summertime heat-related increases in mortality presumably because their populations became acclimatized in some fashion to hot weather. If, with global warming, populations in Northern cities became like those in the South, then full acclimatization will have occurred and little or no impact of global warming is predicted. If populations in Northern cities continue to behave in their current fashion, i.e., do not acclimatize, then a significant increase in heat-related mortality is predicted.

Vector-borne Disease. Potential changes in weather that may occur due to global warming include changes in temperature and rainfall. The most likely scenarios include regions becoming either warmer and wetter or warmer and drier than before, but it is also conceivable that some places will become colder and wetter or dryer at least at particular times of the year. Vector-borne diseases are spread to man from insect and arachnid vectors such as mosquitoes and ticks. The natural history of most vector-borne diseases is almost always tied to such weather parameters as humidity and temperature either directly or via the impact that these parameters have on forests and wetlands that are critical habitats for such organisms. Thus, it seems

587

entirely plausible that changes in climate may result in changes in the distribution and quantity of vectors and thus may affect such diseases (21). It should be noted, however, that modeling the impact of weather on such diseases is a very complex process because these diseases are dependent on having just the right weather, habitat, and intermediate hosts at exactly the required time in their life cycles. Since all of these factors will vary depending on how the weather changes, determining the precise impact of global warming on these diseases requires knowing with a fair degree of precision the regional impacts of a phenomenon that is even now only poorly characterized at a global level.

For the Report to Congress on the Potential Impacts of Global Climate Change (19), one study was commissioned that attempted to evaluate the likelihood that global warming would make the United States a more hospitable place for either malaria or Rocky Mountain spotted fever (RMSF)(22). The conclusions of that study, which used models for the relationship of malaria or the dog tick (vector for RMSF) to various weather/climate parameters, were that the southern portion of the United States would become no more hospitable than it already is for malaria, and that it seems likely that the habitat for the dog tick would spread north into Canada. It should be noted, however, that in both of these modeling exercises, the parameterizations for habitat and intermediate host availability were not changed when the other parameters were modified to account for global warming. Thus, the conclusions from this exercise have to be accepted with caution.

Respiratory Disease. Individuals with pre-existing respiratory disease are likely to be adversely impacted by increased heat stress as mortality due to respiratory disease increases with elevated temperatures (23), presumably due to combined insults of disease and temperature on the circulatory system. Increases in temperature are also likely to have an impact on the degree of air pollution experienced in U.S. cities with high levels of pollutants such as ozone being achieved earlier in the day and maintained longer (19). Asthmatics and individuals with other respiratory problems will have greater difficulty as such occurrences become more frequent, and it is conceivable that such episodes could also elevate the frequency of respiratory cancer (17).

Allergic Disease. Global warming is likely to have impacts on forests, farmland, and wetlands. To the extent that these latter impacts result in changes in the degree or quality of vegetation, there are likely to be quantitative and/or qualitative changes in the airborne concentration of allergens, e.g., molds and pollens. This in turn could lead to changes in the prevalence or intensity of asthma and hay fever episodes in affected individuals.

Developmental Effects. Impacts of elevated body temperature on fertility (24) and on neonatal development (25) are well recognized; however, there is very little information in the literature indicating that such an effect could be associated with elevated environmental temperatures. Recently, reports have appeared in the literature indicating a seasonal (summertime) increase in perinatal mortality (26) and/or preterm birth (27) in two large-center studies. Further investigation of these observations is needed to evaluate whether the observed summertime peak in perinatal mortality or preterm birth is a general one and whether an association can also be demonstrated with elevated temperatures. The United States has a poor record in this area already, and if temperature does play a role in these phenomena, then current efforts to reduce infant mortality need to take such a relationship into consideration.

Impacts Due to Malnutrition and Lack of Water. Increases in global temperature are likely to cause droughts and associated disruptions in agriculture and water supplies. The United States and other highly developed nations probably have the resources and the infrastructure to adjust, with regional impacts being ameliorated by national distribution systems. In the less well-developed nations, it is likely that these effects will result in famines, thereby contributing to malnutrition and increased susceptibility to a variety of infectious diseases. The World Bank has estimated that there are at least 100 million individuals in Africa who do not have enough food (28); the additional problems due to global warming can only serve to make such a bad situation worse.

Impacts Due to Crowding. As global temperatures rise, so will the sea level, eventually placing many thousands of hectares of land under water. Much of the world's populations live on coastlines that will be threatened, and as the coastlines disappear, their residents will be crowded into less land area. Such crowding is likely to exacerbate many of the problems already encountered in the mega-cities housing much of the population in developing nations.

Interactions

Although the potential impacts of stratospheric ozone depletion and global warming have been evaluated as if these were separate or discrete phenomena, there is no question that the impacts associated with them will co-occur. Thus, it is critical to evaluate what if any systems might be jointly impacted. Two such health effect areas come to mind. The first are respiratory effects in that both global warming and stratospheric ozone depletion will result in increases in air pollution. Not only that, but industrialization, as it progresses in the developing nations, will also contribute to air pollution problems. Thus, it seems likely in the coming decades that one of the largest public health issues will be respiratory diseases brought about by increased air pollution. This issue has both local and global implications. Local controls will help reduce the industrial emissions, but global controls will be required to reduce the contribution to these problems made by global warming, stratospheric ozone depletion, and acid aerosols.

The second effect that has the potential to be affected both by ozone depletion and global warming is infectious/communicable diseases. As UV-B increases with ozone depletion, it may potentially affect immunity to such diseases at the same time that changes in climate due to global warming may result in the expression of diseases in areas that have never dealt with them before. This could cause a situation where a population has a depressed immunity to a disease and is exposed to it in an area where public health facilities are ill prepared to deal with it.

Conclusions

There is still much that is unknown about the potential health effects of global climate change. The various phenomena that can be said to contribute to the rubric include stratospheric ozone depletion, global warming, acid aerosol formation, desertification, and deforestation. At the current time, these phenomena are being investigated separately, yet the case can and should be made that these things are happening concurrently and there are many instances where interactions are possible as well as likely. Thus, a more global view is required, particularly with regard to the science, but also with regard to policy. These phenomena are not occurring independently, and to analyze them and try to develop responses to them as though they were, seems an exercise designed to fall short of the optimum solution. Although it is sometimes helpful to divide a problem into components in order to analyze what contributions are made by the various pieces, at some point the analyst has to reassemble the parts and look for the sum of the effects. This has not yet been done in the public health arena regarding global climate change, and there is very little evidence that it is being done in other important areas such as agriculture and natural resources.

Acknowledgement

This work was partially supported by EPA contracts 68-02-4601, 68-D90068, and 68-01-7289 to ICF, Inc. and Clement Associates. The information presented is totally the responsibility of the author and should not be construed as EPA position or policy. The author thanks John Hoffman, Dennis Tirpak, and Joel Smith for their support, Hugh Pitcher for the development of some of the graphics, and Hugh Pitcher and C. Suzanne Lea for many helpful discussions.

This work was performed by Pacific Northwest Laboratory, which is operated for the U.S. Department of Energy by Battelle Memorial Institute under contract DE-AC06-76RL0 1830.

References

1. Serafino, G., and Frederick, J. Global modeling of the ultraviolet solar flux incident on the biosphere. In: Assessing the Risks of Trace Gases That Can Modify the Stratosphere. EPA 400/1-87/001H. Government Printing Office, Washington, D.C., 1987, Appendix H.
2. Pitcher, H.M., and Longstreth, J.D. Melanoma mortality and exposure to ultraviolet radiation: an empirical relationship. Environ. Int. 17: 7-21(1991).
3. U.S. Environmental Protection Agency. Assessing the Risks of Trace Gases That Can Modify the Stratosphere. EPA 400/1-87/OOlA-H. Government Printing Office, Washington, D.C., 1987.
4. Scotto, J., Fears, T.R., and Fraumeni, J.E, Jr. Incidence of Non-melanoma Skin Cancer in the United States. (NIH) 82-2433. National Cancer Institute, U.S. Department of Health and Human Services, Washington, D.C., 1981.
5. Glass, A.G., and Hoover, R.N. The emerging epidemic of melanoma and squamous cell skin cancer. J. Am. Med. Assoc. 262: 2097-2100 (1989).
6. Longstreth, J.D., Ed. Ultraviolet Radiation and Melanoma with a Special Focus on Assessing the Risks of Stratospheric Ozone Depletion. EPA 400/1-87/001D. Government Printing Office, Washington, D.C., 1987.
7. Pitts, D.G. Optical radiation and cataracts. In: Visual Health and Optical Radiation (M. Waxler and V. Hitchens, Eds.), CRC Press Inc., Boca Raton, FL 1987.

8. Taylor, H.R., West, S.K., Rosenthal, E.S., Beatriz, M., Newland, H.S., Abbey, H., and Emmett, E.A. The effect of ultraviolet radiation on cataract formation. N. Engl. J. Med. 319: 1411-1415 (1988).

9. Bochow, T.W., West, S.K., Azar, A., Munoz, B., Sommes, A., and Taylor, H.R. Ultraviolet light exposure and the risk of posterior subcapsular cataract. Arch. Opathalmol. 107: 369-372 (1989).

10. Maitchouk, I.F. Trachoma and cataract: two WHO targets. Int. Nurs. Rev. 32: 23-25 (1985).

11. Kripke, M.L., and Fisher, M.S. Immunologic parameters of ultraviolet carcinogenesis. Natl. Cancer Inst. 57: 211-215f (1976).

12. Elmets, C.A., Bergstresser, P.R., Tigelaar, R.E., Wood, P.J., and Streilein, J.W. Analysis of the mechanism of unresponsiveness produced by haptens painted on the skin exposed to low dose ultraviolet radiation. J. Exp. Med. 158: 781-794 (1983).

13. De Fabo, E.C., and Noonan, E.P. Mechanism of immune suppression by ultraviolet irradiation in vivo. I. Evidence for the existence of a unique photoreceptor in skin and its role in photoimmunology. Photochem. Photobiol. 32: 183-188 (1983).

14. Van der Leun, C., Takizawa, Y., and Longstreth, J.D. Human health. In: Environmental Effects Panel Report, November 1989 [Pursuant to Article 6 of the Montreal Protocol], United Nations Environment Programme, Nairobi, Kenya, 1989, pp. 1-24.

15. Kripke, M.L. Photoimmunology: the first decade. Curr. Probl. Dermatol. 15: 164-175(1986).

16. Gery, M.W. Tropospheric air quality. In: Environmental Effects Panel Report, November 1989 [Pursuant to Article 6 of the Montreal Protocol], United Nations Environment Programme, Nairobi, Kenya, 1989, pp. 49-54.

17. Grant, L.D. Health Effects Issues Associated with Regional and Global Air Pollution Problems. Draft Document prepared for World Conference on the Changing Atmosphere, Toronto, 1988.

18.Kutschenreuter, P.H. A study of the effect of weather on mortality. Ann N Y. Acad. Sci. 22: 126-138 (1959).

19.Smith, J., and Tirpak, D., Eds. The Potential Effects of Global Climate Change on the United States. Report to Congress. Office of Policy, Planning, and Evaluation, Office of Research and Development, U.S. Environmental Protection Agency, Washington, D.C., 1989, pp. 1-1 - 1-35.

20. Kalkstein, L.S. The impact of CO_2 and trace gas-induced climate change upon human mortality. In: The Potential Effects of Global Climate Change on the United States. EPA 230-05-89-057. Office of Policy, Planning and Evaluation, U.S. Environmental Protection Agency, Washington, D.C. 1989, pp. 1-1 - 1-35.

21. Longstreth, J.D., and Wiseman, J. The potential impact of climatic change on patterns of infectious disease in the United States. In: The Potential Effects of Global Climate Change on the United States. EPA-230-05-89-057 Office of Policy, Planning and Evaluation, U.S. Environmental Protection Agency, Washington. D.C., 1989, pp. 3-1 - 3-41.

22. Haile, D.G. Computer simulation of the effects of changes in weather patterns on vector-borne disease transmission. In: The Potential Effects d Global Climate Change on the United States. EPA 230-05-89-057. Office Of Policy, Planning and Evaluation, U.S. Environmental Protection Agency, Washington, D.C., 1989, pp. 2-1 - 2-11.

23. White, M.R., and Hertz-Picciotto, I. Human health: analysis of climate related to health. In: Characterization of Information Requirements for Studies of CO_2 Effects: Water Resources Agriculture, Fisheries. Forests, and Human Health, DOE/ER/0236 (M.R. White, Ed.), Department of Energy, Washington, D.C., 1984.

24. Mieusset, R., Bujan, L., Mondinat, C., Mansat, A., Pontonnier, F., and Grandjean H. Association of scrotal hyperthermia with impaired spermatogenesis in infertile men. Fertil. Steril. 6: 1006-1011 (1987).

25. Edwards, M.J. Hyperthermia as a teratogen: a review of experimental studies and their clinical significance. Teratog. Carcinog. Mutagen. 6: 563-582(1986).

26. Keller, C.A., and Nugent, R.P. Seasonal patterns in perinatal mortality ad preterm delivery. Am. J. Epidemiol. 118: 689-698 (1983).

27. Cooperstock, M., and Wolfe, R.A. Seasonality of preterm birth in the collaborative perinatal project: demographic factors. Am. J. Epidemiol. 124: 234-241 (1986).

28. Leaf, A. Potential health effects of global climatic and environmental changes. N. Engl. J. Med. 321: 1577-1587 (1989).

—by Janice Longstreth,
Battelle Washington Operations,Washington, D.C.

Index

Index

Page numbers in *italics* refer to tables and illustrations; the letter "n" following a page number refers to a note.

A

AAEM *see* American Academy of Environmental Medicine
acid rain 35
Ackerman, Stephen J. 505
acrodynia (pink disease) 177
Addiss, D. G. 147, 148
aero allergens 93
aerosols 258
  described 107
  nasal irritation 114
  non-respirable 109
aflatoxins 493
age factor
  allergies 57
  hearing impairment 34
  immune function 39, 40
  indoor air pollution 230
  indoor air quality 187
  noise and sleep 440
Agency for Toxic Substances and Disease Registry (ATSDR) 55, 416, 566–67, 571

Agent Orange 42, 345–47, 351
agrichemicals 333
  see also pesticides
agricultural dust 335–42
agriculture
  biotechnology 500–501
  environmental hazards 333–44
  pesticides 329–32
  water pollution 129–30, 133, 135, 141, 143
AIDS (Acquired Immune Deficiency Syndrome) 17, 38
air cleaners 195–96, 198–99, 292, 302
air conditioners 274, 277, 278
  see also heating, ventilation, and air conditioning (HVAC)
air filters 196, 301, 306–7
air handling systems 189, 209, 302
  see also ventilation
air pollution 34–35, 75–80, 585
  children 567–68
  ear nose and throat 105–15
  households *190–91*
  offices 288–89
  pesiticides 384–86
air quality
  improvements 100
  office buildings 287–93
  standards 76–78, 81–82
Alar 466

597

N